KEY TOPICS IN

ORAL AND MAXILLOFACIAL
SURGERY

The KEY TOPICS Series

Advisors:

T.M. Craft *Department of Anaesthesia and Intensive Care, Royal United Hospital, Bath, UK*
C.S. Garrard *Intensive Therapy Unit, John Radcliffe Hospital, Oxford, UK*
P.M. Upton *Department of Anaesthetics, Treliske Hospital, Truro, UK*

Anaesthesia, Second Edition

Obstetrics and Gynaecology

Accident and Emergency Medicine

Paediatrics

Orthopaedic Surgery

Otolaryngology and Head and Neck Surgery

Ophthalmology

Psychiatry

General Surgery

Renal Medicine

Chronic Pain

Trauma

Oral and Maxillofacial Surgery

Forthcoming titles include:

Oncology

Obstetrics and Gynaecology, Second Edition

Cardiovascular Medicine

Neonatology

Critical Care

Orthopaedic Trauma Surgery

Respiratory Medicine

Thoracic Surgery

KEY TOPICS IN

ORAL AND MAXILLOFACIAL SURGERY

K. RIDEN
FRCS, FDSRCS
Southmead Department of Maxillofacial Surgery, Southmead Hospital, Bristol, UK

Present address
Department of Oral and Maxillofacial Surgery, Derriford Hospital, Plymouth, UK

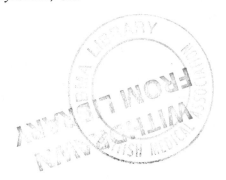

βIOS
SCIENTIFIC
PUBLISHERS

© BIOS Scientific Publishers Limited, 1998

First published 1998

A CIP catalogue record for this book is available from the British Library.

ISBN 1 85996 030 8

BIOS Scientific Publishers Ltd
9 Newtec Place, Magdalen Road, Oxford OX4 1RE, UK
Tel. +44 (0)1865 726286. Fax. +44 (0)1865 246823
World Wide Web home page: http://www.Bookshop.co.uk/BIOS/

DISTRIBUTORS

Australia and New Zealand
   Blackwell Science Asia
   54 University Street
   Carlton, South Victoria 3053

India
   Viva Books Private Limited
   4325/3 Ansari Road, Daryaganj
   New Delhi 110002

Singapore and South East Asia
   Toppan Company (S) PTE Ltd
   38 Liu Fang Road, Jurong
   Singapore 2262

USA and Canada
   BIOS Scientific Publishers
   PO Box 605, Herndon
   VA 20172-0605

Production Editor Andrea Bosher.
Typeset by Chandos Electronic Publishing, Stanton Harcourt, UK.
Printed by Redwood Books, Trowbridge, UK.

CONTENTS

ABBREVIATIONS

ACE	acetylcholinesterase
AF	atrial fibrillation
ANS	anterior nasal spine
ARDS	adult respiratory distress syndrome
AV	anterio-venous
BAHA	bone anchored hearing aid
CABG	coronary artery bypass graft
CMCC	mucocutaneous candidal syndrome
CNS	central nervous system
CSF	cerebrospinal fluid
CT	computerized tomography
CVA	cerebrovascular accident
DIC	disseminated intravascular coagulation
DM	diabetes mellitus
DSA	digital substraction angiography
DVT	deep vein thrombosis
EBV	Epstein–Barr virus
ECG	electrocardiograph
EEG	electroencephalograph
EGF	epidermal growth factor
EMLA	effective mixture of local anaesthetic
ENT	ear, nose and throat
FCPD	fibrocalculus pancreatic diabetes
FESS	functional endoscopic sinus surgery
FNAC	fine needle aspiration cytology
FP	Frankfurt plane
GA	general anaesthetic
GABA	γ-aminobutyric acid
GCS	Glasgow Coma Scale
GI	gastrointestinal
HBO	hyperbaric oxygen
IAM	internal auditory meatus
IDDM	insulin-dependent diabetes mellitus
IGT	impaired glucose tolerance
IMF	intermaxillary fixation
INR	international normalized ratio
ITU	intensive care unit
LA	local anaesthetic
LMN	lower motor neurone
MHC	major histocompatibility complex

MI	myocardial infarction
MnP	mandibular plane
MODY	maturity onset diabetes of youth
MP	maxillary plane
MRDM	malnutrition-related diabetes mellitus
MRI	magnetic resonance imaging
NAI	non-accidental injury
NG	nasogastral
NIDDM	non-insulin-dependent diabetes mellitus
NSAID	non-steroidal anti-inflammatory drug
OAF	osteoclast-activating factor
OPG	orthopantomographs
OSA	obstructive sleep apnoea
PAF	periodic acid Schiff
PCA	patient controlled analgesia
PCS	patient controlled sedation
PDPD	protein deficient pancreatic diabetes
PE	pulmonary embolism
PEG	percutaneous endoscopic gastrostomy
PNS	posterior nasal spine
PSIS	posterior superior iliac crest
PTA	pure tone audiometry
PTH	parathyroid hormone
RA	relative analgesia
ROU	recurrent oral ulceration
SMAS	superficial musculoaponeurotic system
TB	tuberculosis
TENS	transcutaneous nerve stimulation
TMJ	temporomandibular joint
TNM	tumour nodes metastases
UICC	International Union Against Cancer
UMN	upper motor neurone
UVPPP	uvulopalatopharygoplasty
VSS	vertical subsigmoid
ZC	zygomatic complex

PREFACE

Oral and maxillofacial surgery has an extensive body of literature on which its exponents may call and make their own contributions. In spite of this there is no single book aimed at the trainee and those new to the speciality. The twin demand for a clinically useful manual and a source for examination candidates is, like most other specialities, almost impossible to resolve adequately.

The twin undergraduate degrees required, at least currently, by junior maxillofacial surgeons gives a very solid basis in basic medical and dental sciences and the need to sit two final fellowship exams requires broad general professional training. Even though the pattern of exam success expected of surgical trainees is changing, the need for a text for candidates is not. The exit examination is a new hurdle for higher surgical trainees and the specific needs of its candidates changes as the exam evolves. There is enough in this book to satisfy fully the needs of undergraduates, to sate almost entirely the appetite of junior hospital staff and provide a reference text for general medical and dental practitioners.

The reading advice identifies areas of interest and essential reading for exam candidates without being to didactic or directed in identifying specific books or journals. Most people rapidly evolve their own favourite sources in any case but each chapter of this text provides a sensible framework which can be 'fleshed out' with further reading as suggested according to personal needs and interests.

As with most books the thanks and acknowledgements owed are many but any errors are entirely mine. Some of the initial material for the chapters on burns, tumour classification and salivary gland disease were provided by Paul Wilson. Many colleagues both junior and senior had a hand in reading the drafts and passing helpful comments on the emerging texts at various stage of writing. Feedback during SHO teaching is always freely offered and uncompromising in the frankness of its criticisms. The 'beta testing' of some of the chapters has therefore been extensive and the user friendliness testing has exposed the breaking strain of some of my English prose!

Particular thanks are due to my consultant colleagues for their efforts in reading and offering corrections to the final chapter drafts. My thanks to Sandy Davis, Geoff Jones, Gordon Irvine, Phil Guest, Surgeon Captain George Rudge, and Professor Peter Ward Booth for his work on some of the early drafts. Jonathen Sandy's reading of the orthognathic chapters is acknowledged. I owe a debt of gratitude to various able members of my family for their contribution to the tasks of typing and retyping drafts and for invaluable assistance with compilation of the index. In particular Mrs Lesley Riden and Mrs Mavis Riden made invaluable contributions and their typing marathons are gratefully acknowledged. Many other aspects of life have been sacrificed in order to get this volume to production and my family can attest to my preoccupation with it at various times. My thanks to them also.

The one hundred key topics chosen represent my view of the essence of this speciality and go some way to defining its scope. There will inevitably be differences of opinion as to my sins of omission and commission but for the people for whom this book was written there is no equivalent text. It is to them I offer it to be used and abused at will with the hope that it answers their needs for appropriate and accessible information about this speciality.

Keith Riden

ALVEOLAR BONE GRAFTING

Cancellous bone grafting of an alveolar cleft is a well-established procedure for patients during the mixed dentition phase. It forms an integral part of the sequence of operations performed for cleft lip and palate patients.

Bone grafting of the alveolar cleft allows union of the alveolar segments to occur and provides a more physiological pattern of bone environment to encourage eruption of the canines. Because the operation is performed in the early mixed dentition phase, removal of badly deformed teeth and supernumeries is possible at the same operation.

Anaesthetic

General anaesthesia is preferred as patients are young and bone harvest is unpleasant under local anaesthesia.

Bone harvest

1. Cancellous only harvest is required. The presence of cortical bone or cartilage fragments is likely to impede the alveolar union and cancellous bone forms the best medium to permit canine eruption.

2. Bone source. Bone is removed from the anterior superior iliac crest by open operation or from the upper tibia by trephine. The iliac wound must be closed in layers over a vacuum drain and an epidural catheter inserted into the wound permits local anaesthetic infusion to be given post operatively. Early mobility is possible in children but active sport must be advised against usually for 3 months after tibial bone harvest.

Intraoral procedure

1. Buccal mucosal approach. A mucoperiosteal flap is developed and relieved at the first molar region. The palatal gingiva is raised as necessary depending on the extent of clefting on the palatal side of the alveolus.

2. Removal of teeth. It may be advisable to remove badly positioned or malformed teeth or supernumeries.

3. Curettage of cleft scar tissue must be performed thoroughly and completely.

4. Repair of nasal mucosal floor may be required. This stage of the procedure is performed via the oral wound and non-resorbable sutures are used. Nasal packing is not commonly required even if nasal mucosal repair has been performed.

5. *Cancellous bone* is grafted into the cleft and compressed firmly into the defect. Good bone-to-bone contact is essential. A variety of techniques are available to achieve this. Large cancellous fragments may be secured by friction and hammered graft insertion is preferred in some centres.

6. *Bone graft* augmentation of the lateral nasal maxilla, alar 'sill' and alar base is possible via the same intra-oral incision.

7. *Mucosal advance.* Periosteal release will permit the muco-periosteal flap to be advanced to cover the grafted area of alveolus. The exposed molar region bone will rapidly become covered in mucosa without the need for grafting.

8. *Closure.* Watertight closure of the oral mucosa over the bone graft is essential. Non-resorbable monofilament sutures are preferred.

Aftercare

1. *Early mobilization* is possible with good analgesia and the local analgesia infusion to the donor site aids this process

2. *High dose IV antibiotics* are given prophylactically in the peri-operative period but the need for oral antibiotics after hospital discharge is not proven.

3. *Fluids.* Clear fluids only are given for the first 24 hours after surgery. In some units the patient is maintained on a 'nil by mouth' regimen for the first 24 hours before clear fluids are allowed. A nasogastric tube may be preferred if such delayed establishment of oral fluid intake is planned. Oral fluids are re-introduced thereafter with a liquid or semisolid diet permitted after 48 hours.

4. *Discharge.* The patient should be ready to return home on the 3rd post operative day.

Follow up

1. *Surgical follow up* is arranged at 1 week, 2 weeks, 4 weeks and 3 months. Thereafter orthodontic review continues.

2. *If excess bone is shed* via the wound it is possible to re-graft but results are poorer than if the first operation is successful.

3. *Successful grafting* produces an intact alveolus with a normally maturing dentition. It allows easier orthodontic treatment and if subsequent osteotomies are required a grafted alveolus provides a good basis for orthognathic surgery without recourse to segmental surgery.

Late presentation

In patients who present late with an ungrafted alveolar cleft and midface retrusion and who express a desire for restoration of normal facial aesthetics there are several surgical options. Surgery may be performed in stages with alveolar bone grafting preceding orthognathic surgery by a period of 6–9 months. Bone grafting and maxillary osteotomy can be performed at a single operation and some patients may require segmental maxillary osteotomies. Segmental surgery is not usually the preferred option as results from a Le Fort I advancement are often better. This operation is considerably easier in a previously bone grafted patient.

Related topics of interest

Bone grafts (p. 25)
Cleft lip and palate (p. 69)

Revision points

Embryology of the palate and alveolus
Presurgical orthodontics
Healing of bone and physiology of bone remodelling

ANALGESIA

The use of analgesics is central to good surgical management and, in addition, there are a wide variety of non-pharmacological techniques available for moderation of pain responses and pain-related behaviour in surgical patients.

Pain physiology

Pain sensation arises from receptors in peripheral tissues and is conducted centrally by small diameter axons of the A delta and C subtypes. In the spinal cord, the substantia gelatinosa is the main relay site for onward transmission. The modulation of incoming nociceptive afferent fibre action potentials by larger A class axons is the basis of the gate theory of pain transmission. The lateral spinal thalamic tracts in the spinal cord contain the second order neurones and conduct pain sensation to the brain stem via the medial lemniscus. In the pons and mid brain, the peri aquaductal grey matter and nucleus of raphe magnus are the sites of maximum opiate receptor concentration, and the locus cerueleus is a secondary centre. The ventrolateral thalamic nuclei contain relay sites for onward transmission of nociceptive input to the cerebral cortex and conscious appreciation of pain sensation.

Production of endogenous opioids occurs throughout the brain stem and spinal cord. These endorphins, dynorphins and encephalins inhibit action potential propagation in the relay neurones in the spinothalamic tracts and thereby reduce transmission of incoming primary afferent pain sensation. Substance P, glutamate and γ-aminobutyric acid (GABA) are agonists at these relay neurones whereas encephalins and endorphins are antagonists. In the mid brain, the neurotransmitters serotonin and noradrenalin are also thought to be antagonists to pain transmission. Gut neuropeptides have a putative but as yet incompletely understood role in pain modulation and transmission.

There are three families of endogenous opioids, the endorphins, encaphalins of met and leu varieties and the dynorphins. They have different distributions in the central nervous system (CNS) and operate at a variety of receptor sites of which there are three main subtypes mu, delta and kappa. Mu receptors are concentrated maximally in the nociceptive areas of the brain stem and are stoichiometrically the most closely matched to prescribed morphine-like drugs. The delta and kappa receptors have a higher affinity for encephalins and dynorphins respectively. *Drug action* at all of these sites is antagonized specifically by naloxone, with increasing doses being required to inhibit action at mu, delta and kappa receptors respectively. Some drugs such as the partial agonist pentazocine produce both stimulant and sympathomimetic effects by actions at sigma receptors; actions which are not blocked by naloxone.

Narcotic analgesics

These drugs are naturally occurring plant-derived alkaloid compounds which mimic endogenous opioids causing prolonged activation at the opiate receptors. Central analgesia, respiratory depression, euphoria and sedation all occur and vasomotor centre depression causes postural hypotension. Cough suppression, nausea and vomiting, due to stimulation of the chemotactic trigger zone, and constipation are frequently observed. Biliary tract spasm and sphincter spasm are also common. Histamine release may be stimulated, causing peripheral vasodilatation and itching. There are complex effects on gut nerve plexuses resulting in constipation. Continuous treatment with narcotic analgesics therefore needs adjunctive anti-emetics and laxative treatment.

1. Tolerance and dependence are observed in narcotic addicts. In terminally ill patients with continuous or prolonged administration, drug dosage may have to be increased to maintain analgesic effects. A steady increase in opioid dose is possible and where this is necessary due to increasing pain, tolerance and dependence do not seem to occur.

2. Clinically useful drugs. Morphine typifies the strong opiate class of drugs. Pethidine is similar in action to morphine. Equi-analagesic doses depress respiration about equally but exhibit less cough-suppressive and more constipating action. Pethidine has more weak atropine-like activity and causes less miosis than morphine. The weaker narcotic analgesics are useful in moderate pain. They may cause dependence and are still subject to abuse. Codeine has about one-twelfth the analgesic potency of morphine. It is preferred after head injury as it causes minimal miosis and does not mask the ocular signs of intracranial pressure increase.

Dihydrocodeine and dextropropoxyphene are similar in potency and side effects to codeine and are widely used in combination with aspirin or paracetamol.

Omnopon or papaveratum is useful and has recently been introduced in a noscopine-free preparation available for use in women of child-bearing age.

3. Prescribing and administration. Morphine is available in parenteral and oral preparations. Elixirs are useful in terminal care, and morphine sulphate continuus tablets are a slow release preparation and are increasingly widely used in analgesia for cancer patients. Combination with cyclizine as an anti-emetic is often necessary.

Rectal administration is possible for some non-steroidal anti-inflammatory drugs (NSAIDs) and paracetamol, and buprenorphine is available sublingually to avoid first pass hepatic metabolic destruction of the active agent.

Patient-controlled analgesia (PCA) by IV infusion pump is increasingly used in pain control after major head and neck operations.

Non-steroidal anti-inflammatory analgesics

The NSAIDs are a large group of drugs with varying degrees of analgesic, anti-inflammatory and anti-pyretic actions. The NSAIDs are a diverse group biochemically but all have the ability to inhibit cyclo-oxygenase enzymes resulting in inhibition of prostaglandin and leukotriene synthesis. This is the mechanism responsible for their therapeutic effects and also for the gastric mucosal damage due to hydrogen ion trapping and mucolysis resulting in pre-pyloric ulceration and bleeding in the susceptible.

1. The physiology of phosphilipids and arachidonic acid. Phosphilipids form the precursor metabolites from which all prostaglandins are produced. Inflammatory stimuli induce conversion by cyclo-oxygenase of phospholipase A2 to cyclic endoperoxide; a step which is modified by steroids which increase lipocortin levels. Serial enzyme conversions from cyclic endoperoxide result in the formation of leukotrienes, prostaglandins, thromboxanes and prostacyclins. The cyclo-oxygenase step is antagonized by non-steroidal drugs.

2. Pharmacology of NSAIDs. The peripheral actions of NSAIDs include reduction of the effect of acute inflammatory mediators such as histamine and the kinin enzymes, thereby ameliorating the effects of painful inflammatory foci. Inhibition of activation of nociceptors and opposition to their pain-inducing effects account for the analgesic properties of these drugs. Central actions include mild respiratory stimulation and ototoxicity resulting in tinnitus. The nephropathy due to renal tubular epithelium damage and altered uterine myocontractility are well documented. Exacerbation of asthma is a risk in susceptible patients. Drug interactions do occur, with the action of oral hypoglycaemic agents being potentiated, warfarin binding being inhibited and the concomitant use of steroids reducing the effectiveness of salicylates.

3. Clinically useful agents.

- *Aspirin* is a salicylate and is an effective analgesic. It is relatively ineffective against the visceral pain in myocardial infarction and colic where the central effects of the narcotic analgesics are preferred. It is the best available anti-pyretic drug. It inhibits platelet aggregation via cyclo-oxygenase inhibition and is prescribed prophylactically in paediatric doses to patients at high risk of cerebrovascular accident (CVA).
- *Propionic acid derivatives* naprosyn, fenoprophen and ibuprofen are widely used in rheumatic disorders and acute gout. Acetates such as indomethacin, anthranilic acid derivatives such as mefanemic acid and oxycams such as piroxicam are all newer generation non-steroidal drugs. Although they are

the most potent available non-steroidals, pyrazole derivatives such as phenylbutazone are not widely used any longer as they have quite profound bone marrow suppression activity. Azopropazone remains useful as a potent anti-rheumatic agent. Diclofenal sodium is widely used in facial surgery.

- *Paracetamol* is a phenacetin derivative and not strictly a NSAID. It is available singly or as a combination with other analgesics. It does not have the same deleterious gastric side effects but it is hepato- and nephrotoxic in overdose.

4. Complications. The dyspepsia related to ingestion of the aspirin-like drugs can be prevented by concomitant use of sucralfate or misoprostol for the cytoprotective effect on the mucosa and mucous layer. H2 antagonists or omeprazole have been proposed for prophylaxis where NSAID prescription is essential.

Local analgesic techniques

The use of infiltration and regional local anaesthetic nerve blockade and treatment of chronic pain is a useful therapeutic manoeuvre. Postoperative use of infiltration for regional local anaesthetic techniques is of great benefit. It aids smooth recovery from anaesthetic, acts as an effective adjunct to other analgesic agents and permits cough and mobility after chest or abdominal wall surgery.

Epidural infusions of local anaesthetic agents can be used to control pain after laparotomy or harvesting bone from pelvis or ribcage. Continuous infusions are used in the post operative period. This technique may also be used to control the pain due to malignancy.

Adjuncts

- *Tricyclic antidepressants* are useful in some facial pain syndromes for both their peripheral analgesic and central mood alleviating effects.
- *Anticonvulsants* such as carbamezepine are helpful in facial tics and neuralgias.
- *Corticosteroids* have a systemic anti-inflammatory action which can be useful.

In *maxillofacial surgery,* very severe

postoperative pain is uncommon. Although in the immediate postoperative period the patient may require opiate analgesia, the demand for narcotics should not persist or remain severe. If this occurs, it is likely that surgical complications have supervened and require specific attention.

Non-pharmacological methods

The psychological component of pain-related behaviour should not be overlooked and the benefit of psychotherapy cannot be dismissed.

Acupuncture and alternative methods are postulated to induce the formation of encaphalin-like substances which are agonists at opiate receptors in the brain and spinal cord. The mechanism of action of TENS (transcutaneous nerve stimulation) and other such methods is unclear.

Surgical pain relief

Local phenolic injection, cryoneurolysis, rhizotomy, cordotomy, tractotomy, ganglion excision and nerve root section are neurosurgical options for treatment of intractable pain. Although occasionally used in trigeminal neuralgia, they are rarely used in other orofacial pain syndromes.

ANTERIOR OPEN BITE

Anterior open bite is present when the posterior dentition occludes with an adequate degree of function but leaves the anterior teeth unable to achieve interarch contact. The severity of the condition and the degree of functional impairment is very variable.

Aetiology

Habits and parafunction

Digit sucking in children is common and particularly damaging to the developing occlusion. Early cessation of such childhood habits will usually allow the anterior teeth to correct a degree of open bite. Prolongation of the habit may result in severe, potentially irreversible derangement of dental occlusion. Treatment to make the digit unpleasant tasting or 'gate appliances' to prevent ready access to the mouth have all proved of mixed benefit.

Pen or instrument sucking in adults can function as an orthodontic appliance and may lead to acquired anterior open bite. In adults, advice is the only measure likely to provoke cessation of the habit. Collateral damage to the teeth or anterior restorations may occur with this sort of habit.

Tongue thrusting may be primary (endogenous) or secondary due to a definable abnormality such as macroglossia. In some patients there is a definable syndromic association with macroglossia; Down's syndrome for example. In others there is no recognisable syndrome. Surgery may help with the secondary pattern but is of no benefit in endogenous tongue thrusting. Partial glossectomy or jaw osteotomies and muscle attachment repositioning have all been advocated but with doubtful long-term success.

Trauma

After severe midface trauma or bilateral mandible fractures, anterior open bite may result. Dentoalveolar maxillary fractures and fractures of mandibular angles are common causes. Fractures whose treatment has been suboptimal are more frequently complicated by acquired anterior open bite; rigid fixation placed without establishing the occlusion using temporary IMF is associated with an increased risk of this complication.

Orthognathic	Anterior open bite can be associated with either retrognathism or prognathism. It is often more difficult to identify in patients in whom the more severe abnormality is their antero-posterior jaw discrepancy. It is important to identify these patients as the correction of their antero-posterior deficit may require modification if simultaneous anterior open correction is to be performed.
Iatrogenic	After orthognathic surgery. Bimaxillary osteotomy may result in a degree of open bite due to technical problems with the surgery or inaccuracies in construction of the occlusal positioning wafers. Inter-arch elastics may correct slight discrepancies but severe errors may require revisional surgery.
Long face syndrome	There are a variety of facial syndromes, some of which may be associated with anterior open bite. The commonest pattern is the high Frankfort–Mandibular plane (FM) angle patient in whom the vertical vector of mandibular growth is greater than the autorotational element.
Craniofacial syndrome associations	Adverse skeletal patterns, macroglossia, maxillary alveolar clefts and neuromuscular incoordination all contribute to the production of anterior open bite in these patients. There are very many eponymous syndromes the most illustrative of which include Treacher Collins, Crouzen and Aperts syndromes.
ENT related	Immature or incomplete midface development with so called 'adenoidal' fascies may result in facial dysharmony and anterior open bite development. Mouth breathing is commonly associated and dental problems including excessive caries due to mouth drying supervene. Seasonal or perennial rhinitis with persistent nasal obstruction and consequent mouth breathing exacerbates such problems.

Management

Correction of underlying factors	Where possible, identification and correction of parafunctional habits, removal of adenoids and medical treatment of upper airway inflammation will benefit

some patients. Nasal surgery may be required. Where the aetiology is traumatic, correct management of fractures is preventative and where the patient is inherited from another surgeon, interval osteotomy will usually be required. Major craniofacial abnormalities require the joint consideration of the members of the specialist craniofacial team.

Analysis

Cephalometric and profile analysis are required to establish the severity of the condition and serial analyses will document progression and identify patients with progressive failure of mandibular growth. Surgical and orthodontic planning requires tracings and study models and sometimes digitised cephalometric plots and 3D imaging using reconstructed CT scans.

Orthodontic

Incisor decompensation may help but if the severity of open bite is more than a few millimetres, surgical correction is likely to be necessary. Dental intrusion or extrusion is not commonly associated with a stable result.

Orthognathic

Osteotomy planning may require sagittal split ramus with or without Le Fort I level maxillary osteotomy. Standard bimaxillary osteotomy often produces disappointing results for correction of anterior open bite. Arcing mandibular ramus osteotomies such as 'C', inverted 'L' or Trauner pattern procedures may be used and are preferable. Vertical subsigmoid osteotomy with or without bone grafting has its exponents.

Related topics of interest

Cephalometric analysis (p. 58)
Imaging (p. 206)
Osteotomies (p. 297)

Revision point

Pre- and postnatal facial growth

BENIGN DISEASE OF THE NECK

Benign masses in the neck present as swellings, infected lesions or with obstructive or pressure symptoms. Some benign neck masses are of thyroid origin. Others are congenital or developmental in origin. Neurogenic and vascular tumours occasionally present in the neck.

Congenital and developmental lesions

Dermoids and epidermoid cysts

1. Epidermoids are simple cystic lesions with keratinous contents.

2. True dermoids develop from anlage of skin appendages. They arise due to inclusion or implantation of epithelial cells.

3. Teratomatous cysts contain dervatives of ecto-, meso- and endoderm and may include keratin, nails, teeth, brain and vascular structures.

4. Clinical features. These lesions are usually painless swellings unless infected.

5. Treatment. Excision is curative.

Salivary cysts

1. Salivary gland retention or extravasation cysts are described. They typically arise in minor salivary glands. Cystic degeneration in the major salivary glands is described and usually occurs in sialectasis owing to chronic duct obstruction or chronic inflammatory destruction such as occurs in Sjogren's disease.

2. Presentation. Intermittent submucosal swelling and occasional discharge of 'salty tasting' salivary contents into the mouth.

3. Treatment. Excision is usually curative and requires the underlying gland tissue to be removed with the lesion.

Thyroglossal duct cysts

4. *Sublingual ranulae* may be intra-oral or plunging. Intra-oral lesions are excised via a floor of mouth approach removing the sublingual gland in continuity with the lesion. Transmylohyoid extension in a plunging ranula need not be excised if the affected gland is removed via an intra-oral approach but procedures for complete excision of these lesions via a combined intra-oral and submental incision are described. The need for the submental part of the operation is debatable.

1. *Embryology.* The normal thyroid gland develops from embryonic tissue at the foramen caecum at the tongue base. The thyroid primordium then descends from the primitive pharynx through the anterior neck to its adult pre-tracheal position. Remnants of this thyroid anlage may persist and such vestigeal tissue can remain along the path of descent. It is unusual for there to be significant functional thyroid tissue in such remnants.

2. *Pathology.* Seventy-five per cent are pre-hyoid. Ninety-five per cent are midline. Most occur in childhood or early adolescence. Spontaenous fistula formation is rare. Infected lesions occur and local infection may be the reason for a previously occult thyroglosaal cyst to become symptomatic.

3. *Presentation.* Ninety-five per cent as a painless midline swelling and 5% as an acute infected cervical lesion. Very rarely carcinoma ex cyst may occur with malignant tissue found in the excised tissue.

4. *Treatment.* If symptomatic, excision by Sistrunks hyoid splitting operation is curative.

Branchial cysts

There have been several theories to account for the pathogenesis of these lesions.

- *Branchial apparatus theory*, postulates that the branchial cyst arises as a remnant of the pharyngeal pouches or branchial clefts.
- *The cervical sinus theory*, suggests that the embryonic cervical sinus of Hiss is the tissue of origin of a branchial cyst.

- *The inclusion theory*, suggests that epithelial inclusions into cervical lymph nodes occur and subsequently act as foci for cyst formation. It proposes therefore that a branchial cyst does not arise from the branchial apparatus proper. This theory is the currently accepted one.

1. Presentation. Branchial cysts present in early adult life as a simple swelling or an acute infective episode. They are more common in men and a left side predominance is described.

2. Treatment. Excision via a peri sternomastoid dissection allows removal of the lesion.

3. Pathology. A squamous epithelial lining with cholesterol-rich fluid contents is typical. The high incidence of lymphoid tissue present in the wall tissue supports the inclusion theory of cyst formation.

Branchial sinus

This lesion occurs as a fistulous track passing from the tonsillar fossa to the exterior of the neck at the anterior border of the sternomastoid. A branchial sinus usually has a cutaneous tissue lining. Occasional openings into the cartilaginous external auditory meatus occurs. These lesions are considered to occur as an embyological remnant of the cervical sinus.

1. Presentation. Serous discharge onto the neck in a young child. Occasionally they present as a persistent aural discharge.

2. Treatment. Excision with preservation of the mandibular branch of facial nerve and hypoglossal nerve.

Lymphangiomas

Three types of lymphangioma are described: thin walled or simple lymphangiomas, cavernous lymphangiomas and cystic hygroma.

1. Pathology. The embryological origin of the head and neck lymphatic system is the jugular sac located on each side of the neck. This embryonic tissue is considered to be the tissue of origin of the cervical lymphangiomata.

2. Simple and cavernous types occur in lips, cheeks, tongue and floor of mouth. Fifteen per cent occur in the maxilla and the posterior triangle may be affected. There is no sex predominance. Most occur in childhood or early adult life.

3. Cystic hygromas occur most frequently in neonates and 75% present before the end of the first year of life.

4. Presentation. Cystic hygroma can cause obstetric complications with obstructed delivery of infant if large. They may present as an upper respiratory tract infection in a young child and the lymphadenopathy associated reveals the underlying lymphatic lesion. Tracheal compression with stridor, brachial plexus involvement with arm pain and sensory disturbance and intralesional haemorrhage may all occur.

5. Treatment. Excision is usually required. An extraoral approach is usually advised as clearance is difficult and recurrence is common.

Laryngocele

Laryngoceles are most common in the 5th and 6th decades and 80% occur in males. They must be differentiated from an enlarged laryngeal saccule. They may be external and present as a subcutaneous mass or internal in the vallecula. Laryngeal carcinoma may co-exist and is an important clinical association. Trumpet playing and 'blowing' hobbies or professions may unmask rather than cause laryngoceles.

1. Presentation. The usual features are hoarseness and neck swelling. Occasionally stridor and throat pain, snoring and cough also occur. Ten per cent present as infected pyoceles.

2. Treatment. Excision via partial laryngectomy.

Pharyngeal pouch

Pharyngeal pouches typically occur as pulsion diverticulea through Killian's dehiscence. Thought to be related to incoordination of swallowing the precise mechanism remains unclear. They are most common in the elderly population.

1. Presentation. Dysphagia, regurgitation of undigested food, halitosis, weight loss, cough, hoarseness and recurrent chest infections due to aspiration are all features. Barium swallow is diagnostic as the lesion fills readily and is outlined by the contrast medium. Oesophagoscopy is essential to delineate the opening of the pouch internally and to exclude co-existent carcinoma by endoscopic biopsy. Hiatus hernia often co-exists which suggests that an underlying upper gastro-intestinal tract motility disorder may account for the origin of the pouch rather its cause being a simple pressure or pulsion effect.

2. Treatment. Unless entirely symptom free or discovered as a coincidental radiographic finding, pharyngeal pouches should be excised. Surgical options include endoscopic diathermy, inversion with cricopharyngeal myotomy or excision.

3. Surgery. Preoperative oesophagoscopy permits packing with acriflavine gauze and passage of a nasogastric tube if required. Excision is performed via a collar incision and posterior oesophageal dissection permits repair of the pharynx with sutures or staples. Stapling the neck of the lesion and subsequent division to complete the resection is rapidly completed.

4. Complications. Infection, fistula formation, vocal cord paralysis and stomal stenosis may occur. Myotomy is associated with a lower complication rate.

5. Associations. Carcinoma ex-pouch. A rare lesion occuring only in long-standing pouches. It is associated with chronic irritation. Barium studies in a patient with worsening dysphagia and hoarseness may reveal a filling defect. MRI scanning may aid determination of the extent of the malignant disease in the neck. Pharyngectomy with reconstruction is usually required and the prognosis is poor.

Infective lesions

The common causes of infective swellings in the neck are inflammed lymph nodes and neck fascial space abscesses.

Cervical lymphadenopathy   Oral, facial, tonsillar, cutaneous and scalp lesions may all occur and result in the lymph nodes in the respective fields of drainage becoming inflamed, swollen and on occasions purulent. Acute toxaemic episodes may occur. Malignant disease in the head and neck may result in reactive cervical lymphadenitis as commonly as metastatic nodal disease. Other causes of cervical lymphadnopathy include toxoplasmosis, actinomycosis, cat scratch disease, brucellosis and infectious mononucleosis. Fine needle aspiration cytology will permit diagnosis and exclusion of malignancy.

Neck space infection   1.   *Ludwig's angina* arises due to a spreading cervical cellulitis. It may arise from an infective focus in the mandible, around the lower teeth or from an infected submandibular salivary gland or upper cervical lymph node. It constitutes a significant threat to the airway as laryngeal oedema may occur. High dose intravenous antibiotics are required and definitive treatment of the focus of origin should be planned as an interval procedure once the acute episode has resolved.

2.   *Cervical abscesses.* These may arise is association with oro-dental infection, submandibular space infection or partially treated Ludwig's angina. Foreign body implantation via the cutaneous or pharyngeal mucosa may lead to abscess formation and some micro-organisms may produce metastatic cervical abscesses. Early incision and drainage is required and high dose antibiotics are usually given to prevent spread across the fascial planes of the neck.

3.   *Tuberculous cervical adenitis (Scrofula).* With the recrudecsence of tuberculosis in the UK population this pattern of disease may be expected to become an increasingly common problem. A single enlarged cervical lymph node in a patient with tuberculosis requires investigation to establish its cause as

tuberculous lesions are often long-standing. Multiple nodes are often associated with discharging sinuses and antituberculous therapy is essential. Surgery carries a risk of fistula formation that is greatly reduced if antituberculous drugs have been commenced prior to operation. Treatment of close family members is advised.

AIDS

Head and neck manifestations of AIDS include tuberculous lymphadenitis, multiple parotid cysts, benign lymphoid hyperplasia, oral and pharyngeal Karposi sarcoma, multiple cutaneous lesions and aggresive pharyngeal and oesophageal candidiasis.

Neurogenic tumours

Neural crest tissues

Embryonic neural crest cells are the primordia of many tissues in the adult. Of interest in the head and neck are the Schwann cells, sympathetic ganglia and parasympathetic tissue, in particular the pressure receptors of carotid and vagal systems. Tumours arising in these tissues include the chemodectomas, Schwanomas, neurofibromas and ganglioneuromas.

Chemodectomas

These lesions are uncommon outside people living at high altitudes. The populations of the Andes or Mexico City exhibit a higher incidence therefore. Occuring late in life carotid body tumours present as slow growing painless upper neck masses. Some tumours occur as pulsatile pharyngeal lesions in the tonsillar region. Vagal paraganglionomata occur near the skull base. Pulastile tinnitus, deafness, worsening syncope and pharyngeal pain may be the presenting features. The malignant potential is greater in vagal lesions than with carotid body lesions. Angiography or duplex ultrasound scanning will diagnose the lesions and excision should be considered in the presence of pressure symptoms or where rapid expansion raises the suspicion of malignancy. Vasular shunting may be required to facilitate tumour removal.

Neuromas and neurofibromas

Neurofibromas present as slow growing masses in the neck or with pressure symptoms. Acoustic neuromas or schwanomas present as unilateral deafness and neurofibromas may form part of Von Recklinghausen's syndrome. In this condition café au lait spots and neurological lesions such as gliomas, ganglioma and menigiomas are described. The multiple endocrine syndromes in which neurofibromata occur associated with phaeochromocytomas and medullary thyroid carcinomas are well documented. Malignant change occurs in about than 10% of these tumours.

Vascular lesions

Haemangiomata. Cavernous haemangiomata may occur singly or as extensive interconnected multicentric lesions. MRI scanning and duplex ultrasound scanning both delineate and determine blood flow through the lesions. Radiological embolisation with or without excision is possible.

Related topics of interest

Malignant neck disease (p. 232)
Neck space infections (p. 270)
Vascular lesions of the head and neck (p. 423)

Revision points

Anatomy of the lymphatic drainage of the head and neck
Microbiology of the common head and neck pathogens

BLUNT TRAUMA TO THE HEAD AND NECK

Non-penetrating head and face injuries are common. In patients with very swollen and contused facial soft tissues, underlying facial bone fractures can sometimes be difficult to exclude. Vital structures such as eyes and facial sensation can be dysfunctional in the early post-traumatic period.

Perioral tissues

Facial lacerations can result from blunt trauma and should be closed primarily and early. Complex injuries around the lips, commisures and injuries in children are often better explored under GA than treated sub-optimally under LA in casualty.

Periorbital tissues

Periorbital contusions (black eye) are very common. Soft tissue loss due to shearing forces should be made good where possible but complex flaps should be avoided in the early stages. Tarsal plate injuries can usually be repaired primarily. Eyelid margins should be approximated accurately to minimize the risk of ectropion. Nasolacrimal system damage may resolve spontaneously but temporary epiphora is quite common.

Eye

Globe injuries. Corneal abrasions, conjunctival haematomata, hyphaemas and retinal detachments are all possible. Complete globe disruption is rare. Traumatic mydriasis and ophthalmoplegia is common. An ophthalmic surgical opinion is helpful and should be sought in the early post-traumatic phase.

Nose

Traumatic septal haemorrhage and epistaxis from mucosal tears associated with adjacent fractures may occur. Middle third facial skeleton injuries often result in antral mucosal tears and consequent per nasal haemorrhage. Cartilaginous septal and alar injuries are often missed. Fractures and columella dislocations if unrecognised may result in troublesome late nasal airway obstruction and the need for septoplasty. Nasal bone fractures are common. The commonest pattern is non-displaced comminution of the anterior part of the bony nasal capsule. Manipulation under anaesthesia (MUA) and simple reduction is adequate to manage such injuries. If more complicated nasal complex fractures are present, simple MUA is inappropriate and formal reduction is required. These injuries can be described according to various classifications. The most clinically useful describes three levels based on the plane of injury viewed from the coronal plane. Level 1 injuries are purely cartilaginous and can be managed by closure of soft tissue planes and approximation of cartilaginous margins. Level 2 injuries involve the protuberant part of the bony nasal skeleton and require reduction with or without nasal packing. Level 3 injuries involve the maxillary part of the nasal capsule, or the intranasal bones. Careful operative reduction of both bone and cartilage is required. Acute or immediate septorhinoplasty is currently advocated by many. When severe septal disruption has occurred, judicious resection or recentralising is required. Severely comminuted nasal bones may be associated with medial orbital rim fractures. Naso-ethmoid injury should be excluded.

Lips

Care with the mucocutaneous junctions and the philtrum of the upper lip is required to ensure good post operative cosmetics.

Ears

1. Pinna. Perichondrial haematoma may result in unsightly scarring and thickening (cauliflower ear). Immediate aspiration or drainage is required as prevention. Pressure bandaging is helpful and effective. Complete or partial avulsion by shearing, tearing or biting occur. Debridement, primary closure and achievement of skin closure are the initial surgical goals. Subsequent reconstruction including post auricular insertion of tissue expanders and fashioning of new cartilaginous skeleton may be required.

2. Otological. Tympanum perforation, canal laceration and ossicular chain disruption are all described. Petrous temporal bone fracture may occur in longitudinal or transverse directions. Post auricular bruising (Battle's sign) and CSF otorhoea may occur and are evidence of a severe insult. Pure tone audiometry within hours of the injury is essential as a baseline against which to monitor clinical progress and for purposes of medicolegal documentation.

Intra-oral

Contusions, lacerations and dental fractures or avulsions are all possible. Closure of soft tissues is required and completely avulsed teeth may be replaced in the alveolus and splinted *in situ.*

Calvarium

Closed head injuries with or without underlying skull fracture may occur.

1. Intracranial complications. Extradural haematoma with meningeal vessel tears may be related to adjacent fractures. Subdural haemorrhage related to minor head trauma in susceptible elderly or alcoholic patients. Early CT scan will exclude and determine those needing transfer to a neurosurgery unit for urgent surgery.

Neck

Direct blows, attempted strangulation and acceleration – deceleration (whiplash) injuries are common mechanisms of cervical injury.

1. Hyoid bone fractures are uncommon and may result in stridor and dysphagia.

2. Laryngeal cartilage injuries may result in airway occlusion due to anatomical disruption and oedema. Intubation or tracheostomy may be required as an emergency.

3. Cervical spine. Hard collar placement at the scene of injury is mandatory as are meticulous attention to the movement and transport of patients to hospital. Soft tissue ligamentous (whiplash) injuries are very common in road traffic accident (RTA) victims. Fractures are less common and may require surgical fixation.

4. Oesophagus and trachea. Disruption or rupture may occur although a severe insult is required and the other associated injuries may be incompatible with life.

Related topic of interest

Penetrating trauma of the head and neck (p. 305)

Revision points

Management of closed head injury
Glasgow Coma Scale

BONE GRAFTS

Autogenic bone transfer is quite commonly required in maxillofacial surgery. Reconstruction of cleft related defects, of the facial skeleton after ablative cancer surgery and after trauma are the most frequent reasons for bone grafting.

Sources of bone

1. Anterior superior iliac crest (ASIC). Cortical plate, chips or fragmented cortical bone or cancellous bone may be harvested from the ASIC. Cancellous harvest is required for closure of alveolar clefts, cleft related oronasal and oroantral fistulae. Cortical bone may be harvested in good quantity for a wide range of uses including atrophic ridge augmentation, sandwich ostetomies and impaction grafting into titanium mesh preformed trays in mandibular segmental reconstruction. The technique involves a 2–3 cm incision over the crest and dissection to the subperiosteal plane or subperichondrial plane in children. A 'coffin lid' elevation raised on the medial aspect permits access to the cancellous bone. Trephine excision is also possible. Cortical bone may be harvested from the outer table. Pre-excisional implantation of osseointegrated implants is possible. Closure in layers using a vacuum drain and infusion of bupivacaine for analgesia permits early postoperative mobilisation.

2. Posterior superior iliac crest (PSIC). A larger quantity of bone may be harvested from this site than ASIC. Its disadvantage is that intraoperative turning of the patient is required. Operative approach is similar to that described for ASIC harvest.

3. DCIA flap. Vascularised iliac crest bone may be harvested pedicled on the deep circumflex iliac arterial system. Muscle and skin are available and may be raised in continuity. The form of the anterior crest is near ideal for reconstruction of the mandibular angle.

4. Tibia. In children, cancellous bone may be harvested by trephine from the lateral aspect of the tibial plateau. Adequate quantities of bone for grafting a cleft alveolus are available. Early mobilization is possible and the morbidity of this approach is reportedly less than with an ASIC approach.

5. Calvarium. Calvarial bone may be used to reconstruct orbital floor defects, palatal dehiscences and if full thickness skull is harvested, segmental mandibular defects may be repaired. Pedicled calvarial bone grafts may be raised on a superficial temporal arterial pedicle with temporalis muscle. Calvarial bone fragments may be harvested also.

6. Fibula. A source of vascularized bone for free tissue-transfer as a myofasciocutaneous flap pedicled on branches of the anterior tibial artery. Preoperative angiography to demonstrate patent vessels in the peroneal and posterior tibial distribution with good distal run-off must be available. The bone harvested can be osteotomized to allow curvature appropriate for mandibular reconstruction.

7. Radius. The myofasciocutaneous free forearm flap is well described. A unicortical segment of radius may be harvested in continuity to provide vascularized bone. For mandibular reconstruction it is not as good as fibula or DCIA flaps. Radial fracture is a troublesome complication.

8. Scapula. Free scapula flaps permit harvest of appropriate shaped and textured bone for intraoral reconstruction. Skin, muscle and facia are also available in good quantities.

9. Rib. Rib may be harvested in continuity with a pectoralis major or latissimus dorsi flap. Its survival depends on the harvest of an adequate degree of muscle covering. Vascularized rib flaps may also be harvested.

10. Clavicle. The clavicular head of sternomastoid may be raised in continuity with a section of clavicle. Mandibular reconstruction is possible.

11. Perioral. Palatal and mental mandibular bone is available in small quantities for closure of small alveolar defects.

12. Prosthetic tissues and xenografts. Hydroxyapatite, reptilian kiel bone and lyophilized bone are all available but are less commonly used as the problems of infection and graft failure are high.

Uses

Alveolar bone grafts

Alveolar clefts may be grafted. Cancellous bone is required and all traces of cortical bone and cartilage must be removed. Impaction of grafted bone is performed by some and good adaptation to the cleft margins once dissected free of all soft tissue and scar tissue is necessary. Firm mucoperiosteal cover over the graft site must be achieved and various flap designs have been designed to ensure this. Most are modifications of the Burrion flap.The advantages of the grafted cleft alveolus are principally that of uniting of the cleft segments and provision of bone through which the permanent canine may erupt. Subsequent maxillary osteotomy is likely to be easier if previous bone grafting has been performed.

Fistulae

Oroantral fistulae rarely require bone grafting with the exception of cleft related fistulae. Many of these are post-palatal closure and closure of a residual communication is associated with a high rate of failure. Oronasal fistulae are almost all found in cleft patients. Grafting is often better performed using a soft tissue flap. Galeal flaps are often proposed for this role. Bone is less commonly required but clavarial bone is a useful source if required.

Mandibular reconstruction

Many methods of segmental reconstruction are described. Free or vascularized rib, clavicle, vascularized iliac crest, free fibula, corticocancellous fragments in titanium mesh or Dacron trays are all proposed.

Palatal resonstruction	Post maxillectomy reconstruction is debated as the classical rehabilitative treatment is obturation. The opponents of reconstruction suggest that tumour recurrence will be missed if the palatal shelf is reconstructed and the cavity is not readily visualized. Nevertheless bone grafts using calvarial or iliac bone are described. Vascularized bone is considered to be better than non-vital bone grafting.
Othognathic surgery	Augmentation genioplasty, sandwich osteotomies and onlay grafts are all described. Cortical bone blocks are used and harvested from iliac crest or outer table of skull.
Preprosthetic surgery	In preparation of the mouth for osseointegrated implants sinus mucosal lifts via a Caldwell Luc operation and submucosal grafting increases the effective depth of the maxillary alveolus and so permits implant placement where it would previously not have been possible.

Adjuncts

Analgesia	After harvest of iliac crest bone, the pain and morbidity can be considerable. Fan blocks using local anaesthetic or insertion of an epidural catheter into the wound for continuous infusion of local anaesthetic are good methods of pain control.
Biomaterials	Titanium mesh trays or Dacron for use of fragmented cortical grafts are described. Impaction grafting into preformed titanium mesh trays is becoming a popular technique in some centres.
Medical problems	Prevention of fractures with radial bone harvest and prevention of thromboembolic problems may be important depending on the preoperative medical status of the patient. Therefore TED stockings, anticoagulant use, limb splints, postoperative physiotherapy are all of use.

BONE LESIONS

Benign lesions

1. Exostoses or tori are common. They are non-neoplastic and usually well circumscribed localized bony overgrowths. They occur as single or multiple lesions distributed in a haphazard fashion. Typically they occur on the palate or in the lingual plate of the mandible.

2. Osteoma. An uncommon benign bony tumour, the osteoma is typified by neoplastic bony proliferation with mixed cancellous and cortical patterns or may be predominantly of one form or another. Normal bony architecture is well preserved, and some tumours are difficult to differentiate clinically and radiographically from exostoses or osteochondromas. Central osteomata occur on endosteal surfaces. The subperiosteal pattern grows on the outer or peripheral surface of the cortical bone. Multiple lesions affecting the jaws may represent Gardener's syndrome; the other features include impacted teeth, dermal fibromas, cystic change in the epidermis and pre-malignant intestinal polyposis. Central osteomata must be differentiated from fibrous dysplasia and focal sclerosing osteomyelitis.

3. Chondroma. A benign skeletal tumour characterized by the formation of mature cartilage. It is common in the chest wall and limb girdles. Chondrogenic tumours in the jaw are rare and more likely to be malignant than benign. In elderly patients they are usually painless, slow growing and solitary. In the mandible they are more commonly associated with condylar and coronoid processes; the site of bone formation in the child. Multiple enchondromatosis is known as Olliers disease.

4. Chondroblastoma. A benign tumour occurring in the epiphyses of long bones, it most frequently affects the lower limb. It is a tumour of adolescence and young adults and rarely affects the jaws; jaw lesions typically occur in the mandibular condyle. Although the tumour is benign it shows a marked tendency for local recurrence if excision is incomplete.

5. *Osteoblastoma.* A rare benign tumour of bone-forming tissues which occurs usually in children. The tumour may be painful, the bone is typically sclerotic and microscopically the tumour is vascular with abundant osteoblasts.

6. *Haemangioma.* Central haemangiomas do affect the jaws, albeit rarely, and cavernous haemangiomas in bone are well described. They are more frequent in the mandible than in the maxilla and can achieve quite a large size prior to presentation. Those that erode completely through the cortical plate may present as a pulsatile soft tissue swelling. They can be physiologically active with high blood flow rates, and if very large can consume a significant percentage of the cardiac output. Most lesions exhibit low perfusion pressure but bleed profusely if punctured. The treatment has been revolutionized in recent years with the advent of pre-excisional embolization under radiological control.

7. *Giant cell granuloma.* A lesion which tends to occur in the alveolar bone and adjacent soft tissues. There are several variants but most are rapid growing and initially appear neoplastic on clinical examination. They recur frequently after simple curettage and quite extensive removal is required in order to achieve satisfactory healing and resolution. There is a slight female preponderance and most patients are young. The mandible is affected, more commonly the maxilla. Bone is frequently eroded and teeth are loosened or exfoliated. Soft tissue may be infiltrated or destroyed. Anaesthesia or paraesthesia results from nerve involvement. Bone erosion may give rise to epulis formation and radiographically, bone destruction is haphazard, with ill-defined margins and the appearance of lobulation. Histologically, the tissue is very vascular, highly cellular with a rich stroma in which are found many multi-nucleated osteoclast-like giant cells. Haemorrhage into the lesion is common, and mitoses, although frequent, are not abnormal. Dystrophic calcification, squamous metaplasia and metaplastic ossification within the stromal tissues are all described.

The principal differential diagnoses include aneurysmal bone cysts, fibrous dysplasia and blastic tumours of bone or cartilage. The cause is unknown.

Malignant tumours

1. Osteosarcoma. Although the most common primary malignancy of bone, this lesion is still rare in the jaws. It is more common in the long bones. Jaw lesions typically affect patients in their thirties whereas it is a tumour of children in the long bones. There are reports of its occurrence secondary to irradiation and as a complication of Paget's disease. It is a rapidly growing tumour leading to pathological fracture and local tissue destruction. It is a mixed osteolytic and sclerotic lesion typically producing a 'sun ray' appearance on radiographs. There is a chondroblastic variant characterized by abundant cartilage formation and a reportedly better survival rate than for the more frequent osteosarcoma. The overall prognosis is poor. Haematogenous spread with early metastasis to the lungs is common and aggressive treatment with chemotherapy prior to salvage surgery is the treatment of choice currently.

2. Chondrosarcoma. Considerably more rare than osteosarcomata, this tumour shows a predilection for the anterior aspect of the maxilla. In mandibular lesions, pre-molar and angle regions are more usually involved. It is a tumour of older patients, and is quite variable in histological appearance; it may be rapidly growing and although it will metastasize it does so late in the course. Extensive local destruction will occur without radical excision. In spite of its tendency to metastasize late, it carries a poorer prognosis than osteosarcoma. There are several sub-types.

3. Metastatic deposits. The jaw bones are an uncommon site for metastasis, but when they occur they can arise from a wide variety of primary tumours. More common in the mandible than the maxilla, painful swelling and neurapraxias may be the presenting features. Loosening of teeth and pathological fractures may also occur. Secondary tumours may be osteolytic or sclerotic and most will arise from primaries in the breast, bronchus, colon, kidney and thyroid. Prostatic lesions typically produce sclerotic secondaries in bone.

Histiocytosis

1. Eosinophilic granuloma is a non-neoplastic destructive bone lesion whose aetiology remains uncertain. Cells of the mononuclear series, presumably Langerhans cells, are thought to be the tissue of origin and the lesion is rich in eosinophils. Painful bony destruction or pathological fractures occur, and constitutional symptoms such as a low grade flu-like illness with malaise, anorexia and pyrexia, recurrent otitis media and upper respiratory tract coryza are associated. Systemic disease or haematological abnormalities are not usual in this variant. In the jaws, eosinophilic granuloma invades marrow spaces, perforates cortices, erodes through teeth and involves soft tissues. Foci may be solitary or multi-focal. The multi-focal variety typically affects children in their first decade of life and more commonly occurs in flat calvarial bones.

2. Hans Schuller Christian syndrome. About 20% of patients with multiple eosinophilic granulomata progress to classical Hans Schuller Christian syndrome. Extensive bone destruction occurs particularly in the head and neck. Multiple punched out areas of bone destruction are characteristic on radiographs and microscopically the lesions are typically histiocytic with acidophilic cytoplasm. Cholesterol accumulations result in vacuolation in the macrophages. Multiple endocrine abnormalities occur; typically diabetes insipidus.

3. Letterer Siwe disease is the rarest of these histiocytic conditions and typically affects very young chidren. Hepatitis, generalized lymphadenopathy, purpuric skin lesions and destructive pulmonary disease is associated with the lytic bone condition. Constitutional symptoms may be severe and oral symptoms may be present, with non-specific ulceration, gingivitis and hyperplasia of the gingival tissues. Langerhans cells are present on microscopy in high numbers. Letterer Siwe disease is considered to be the most malignant form of histiocytosis X and carries a very poor prognosis.

Further reading

Hartman K. Histiocytosis X; a review of 114 cases with oral involvement. *Oral Surgery, Oral Medicine, Oral Pathology,* 1980; **49:** 38–54.

Verner J, *et al.* Osteosarcoma and chondrosarcoma of the head and neck. *Laryngoscope,* 1984; **94:** 240–2.

Related topics of interest

Calcium and metabolic bone disease (p. 41)
Granulomatous conditions (p. 171)
Odontogenic tumours (p. 285)
Vascular lesions of the head and neck (p. 423)

Revision points

Chondrogenesis
General features of benign tumours
Osteogenesis

BURNS

Facial burns may occur alone or in association with burns of the trunk, when the patient is upright and the flames travel upwards to the head, neck and scalp. Oral burns are uncommon injuries which present more frequently in children. Associated inhalation or smoke injuries may occur. Pulmonary, thermal or toxic damage may occur. In military injuries, hand and face flash burns may occur without burn injury to other parts of the anatomy due to the protective effect of combat clothing. Associated blast injury may occur if the mode of injury is an explosion rather than domestic fire. Paediatric burns may be associated with accidental or non-accidental injury.

Immediate assessment of the burned patient

Depth of burning

1.   *Superficial burns (syn; 1st degree burn)* are usually caused by non-boiling liquids, limited sunlight exposure and some chemicals. They are erythematous, wet, painful and may blister. They are very sensitive to pin prick testing. They heal well from underlying and marginal epithelial tissues with little scarring or cosmetic impairment. With the exception of simple analgesia, little active treatment is usually required.

2.   *Partial thickness burns (syn; deep dermal or 2nd degree burn)* are usually caused by scalds from boiling liquids, flame burns and contact burns. They are usually very painful, mottled in appearance and may blister. They are less sensitive to pin prick testing than superficial burns but are hyperaesthetic to cold and air currents if the patient is transferred with an exposed wound. These burns will usually heal spontaneously from surviving epithelial and dermal remnants. Hypertrophic scarring, contracture and poor cosmetics are major problems if the wound is not excised and grafted in the initial phase. Infection will impair healing and graft take.

3.   *Full thickness burns (syn; 3rd degree burn)* are caused by some scald injuries particularly in children and the elderly. Contact burns in unconscious patients and high voltage electrical burns can be full thickness. These burns are typically painless and appear dark,

sometimes charred and dry. They are typically insensate on pin prick testing. Untreated, they heal by slow secondary intention with much scarring. Epithelial appendages and skin adnexae are destroyed, which renders the injury relatively pain free. Some burns extend to the deep fascia and destroy muscle and muscle groups. Epithelialization occurs very slowly from the edges of the wound. Skin grafting will generally be required to speed healing and reduce scarring and contracture formation.

Extent of burning

The 'rule of nines' indicates the total body surface area affected by burn and accounts for surface area as a percentage; 9% each for arms and head, 18% each for legs, front and back of trunk, and 1% for the external genitalia. This scheme requires adjustment for children due to the relatively greater surface area of the head and face.

An alternative scheme uses the patient's palmar surface area as 1% and describes burn area as a multiple.

The calculation is important, as fluid replacement is calculated using the burn percentage as a basis.

Management

General

1. Airway management. Indications for airway support include deep burns of the face and neck, burns of the tongue and pharynx, stridor or hoarseness or near-encircling neck burns. Escharotomy may be required to permit airway protection from the inevitable oedema and to reduce the late threat to the airway due to scar contracture.

2. Restoration of the circulation. During the first 48 hours after a significant burn, the patient is hypovolaemic due to pericapillary tissue exhudation and tissue oedema. Surface fluid loss does occur but is a minor contributor to the demand for fluid replacement. Pulmonary oedema in the elderly and cerebral oedema in the very young are significant risks. After about 48 hours, the patient becomes diuretic and fluid replacement demands fall. Urinary catheterization is required and urine output should be maintained at 50 ml/hour. Adequate fluid replacement is monitored by documenting urine output, peripheral perfusion and temperature. A warm patient with full veins and good urine output has a better prognosis than one whose initial resuscitation is inadequate.

There are several published formulae to calculate the fluid, plasma and whole blood requirements all based on the extent of burn injury. For fluid replacement with colloid, the volume is calculated as half the product of body weight and percentage burn. The derived volume is given as colloid, usually human plasma protein fraction or salt-poor human albumin via IV infusion. The calculated volume is given three times in the first 12 hours, twice in the second 12 hours and once more in the third 12 hours after burning. If Hartman's solution is to be used, the volume calculation is based on Baxter Sire's formula of 4 ml per kg per percentage of burned area. This volume is given over 24 hours, half during the first 8 hours and half in the remaining 16 hours. All administered volumes should be adjusted in accordance with the patient's condition and monitored urine output. In an adult 15% burns or in a child 10% constitute indication for IV fluids. After 24 hours red blood cells may require replacement.

3. Analgesia. Opiates are often required in substantial doses. Regular parenteral or PCA infusions are necessary. Absorption via the IM route is unpredicatble. Mixed opiate and simple analgesic regimens are commonly used.

4. Associated injuries. Life-threatening injuries to thoracic or abdominal viscera require immediate attention. If they occur in association with extensive burn injury, survival rates fall significantly. Limb fractures and associated vascular injuries similarly require immediate reduction to prevent ischaemic damage to distal tissues.

5. Prevention of infection. Chemoprophylaxis does not completely eliminate the risk of bacterial sepsis, and may encourage the emergence of resistant strains or super-infection with *Candida* species. However, suspicion of Group A β-haemolytic streptococci is an indication for antibiotics. Staphylococcal infection may lead to septic or endotoxic shock. This complication is an ever present threat in burned patients. Early IV fluids, fresh frozen plasma and appropriate antibiotics are life saving. Early coverage of burns by temporary dressings or grafts may reduce the risk of septic complications.

6. Inhalation injuries. The effects of blast and smoke adversely affect the airway. Airway obstruction may occur and mucosal oedema may result in severe stridor due to supraglottic obstruction. Lower respiratory tract involvement may result in heat injury, and pulmonary oedema may be marked and respiratory distress severe and slow in onset. Facial singeing and carbonaceous deposits in the mouth, pharynx and in sputum are danger signs.

Burns are associated with an increased risk of adult respiratory distress syndrome (ARDS), and inhalation injury compounds this risk. Systemic sepsis, prolonged hypovolaemia or hypotension and muscle loss with or without myoglobinuria further exacerbate the condition. The role of systemic steroids in prevention of pulmonary oedema and alveolar atelectasis remains controversial.

Local

1. Dressings. The purpose of a dressing is to absorb the exudate from the wound and prevent infection. Topical antibiotics should be avoided, and a non-antibiotic agent such as chlorhexidine used instead. For the prevention of Gram-negative sepsis, 1% silver sulphadiazine (Flamazine) or aqueous iodine is used with occlusive dressing treatment. Biological dressings such as lyophilized pig skin may be used to provide an adherent collagenous dermal surface with a keratinized waterproof epidermis.

2. Primary excision. A better result may be obtained by excision of part or all of the burn, and grafting, between the 5th and 10th day post-burn. Some units advocate earlier excision. Tangential wound excision minimizes the amount of tissue excised and is consistent with good graft 'take'. Tangential excision can be used on the 3rd post-burn day and is most successful in areas of deep dermal burns that otherwise take at least 3 weeks to heal. Small 3rd degree burns and deep burns of the eyelids should be excised and grafted in the first week to prevent ectropion.

3. Exposure. An alternative method of treatment of partial thickness facial burns is to leave the wound 'open to the air'. Epithelialization is evident at 12 days.

Facial reconstruction

It is important to consider the aesthetic units of the face. Each cutaneous area is reconstructed by a single, separate graft or flap. There are many types and patterns of flap described for facial reconstruction.

1. Tissue-expanded visor flap may be used for severe post-burn scarring of the lower face. Post-burn facial resurfacing with a split ascending neck flap is also advocated by some units. This technique is good for cases of scars to the face with healthy neck skin and chest wall.

2. Primary pressure grafts may be used in early reconstruction of deep facial burns. This technique replaces burned tissue at an early stage with tissue which is normal in thickness and quality.

3. Free flaps. In modern reconstructive surgery, microvascular free tissue transfer may be proposed. It has a significant disadvantage because the prospective recipient vessels may be thrombosed or exhibit burn-related arteritis at a distance from the burn site.

4. Tissue expansion and transposition flaps. These techniques have been used in the late reconstruction of scarring and contracture.

Burns to the oral cavity

Problems

Males are affected more commonly than females. These burns usually result in a combination of flash and contact burn. Anatomically, the oral commisure and lips are involved more often than intra-oral tissues. Intra-oral burns most frequently affect the tongue.

In children, electrical burns due to biting through electrical cabling may affect developing tooth germs, are slow to heal and cause extreme cosmetic disfigurement. The late effects of oral electrical burns result in scarring, and the associated contracture in pre-adolescents may lead to reduced bimaxillary dimensions and worsening antero-posterior relations over time. Microstomia may be a disfiguring complication of severe burn injuries of the soft tissues of the face. Labial artery rupture may occur in about 25% of patients at about the 10th day post-injury.

Management

1. Conservative. Allows eschar to separate with healing by secondary intention, but scarring may be unacceptable even after quite small burns.

2. Interventional. Surgical excision of the wound after about 5 days of conservative care with skin grafting gives lesser problems in the months after burning.

3. Microstomia prevention devices. Static or dynamic intra-oral or extra-oral devices are described. External mouth spreaders used in the early postoperative period may reduce development of microstomia. The aim is to produce oral symmetry and reduce the number of surgical procedures needed. One technique using an intra-oral splint similar to an orthodontic retainer has been described .

4. Reconstruction. For minor burns, simple grafting may be all that is required. Physical manipulation and massage during scar maturation may help reduce contracture. In moderate and severe burns, more extensive reconstruction may be needed. Where intra-oral tissue loss has been excessive due to excision of burned tissue, vestibular or tongue flaps may be useful after eschar separation.

Related topics of interest

Revision points

ATLS principles
Fluids and electrolytes
Principles of resuscitation

CALCIUM AND METABOLIC BONE DISEASE

Calcium metabolism

Distribution

Ninety nine per cent of body calcium is skeletal. Plasma calcium exists in several states; a non-diffusible, protein or albumin bound fraction (40%), an ionised or free calcium element (approximately 50%), and the remaining 10% complexed to anions such as bicarbonate and phosphate. The protein-bound fraction is of little physiological significance. Total plasma calcium assays are corrected to account for variations and abnormalities in plasma albumin concentration. Automated biochemical analysis usually measures total plasma calcium. The normal range is from 2.20 to 2.70 mmol. Venepuncture performed with a tourniquet, with the patient standing, or following a meal, may all increase the measured concentration of plasma calcium.

Absorption

Calcium is actively absorbed from the duodenum by an ATP-dependent process regulated by active vitamin D, and passively absorbed in the jejunum. Ninety seven to 98% percent is reabsorbed in the proximal tubule of the kidney.

Vitamin D3

There are two sources, diet and cutaneous metabolism. Vitamin D is a steroid which is activated by UV light or produced from dietary vitamin D2. It is hydroxylated to 25 hydroxy-D3 in the liver and 1,25 dihydroxy-D3 in the kidney. It promotes mobilization of calcium from bone, increases gut calcium and phosphate absorption by inducing calcium-binding protein, and increases phosphate and calcium absorption in the kidney. The 24, 25 hydroxy form is the inactive moiety.

Parathyroid hormone (PTH) This is an 84-amino-acid peptide secreted by the chief cells in the parathyroid glands in response to increased serum calcium. It increases serum calcium by mobilizing calcium and phosphate from bone, increases the renal tubular resorption of calcium and reduces tubular reabsorption and increases secretion of phosphate, promoting phosphaturia. It also stimulates hydroxylation of vitamin D3 and thereby increases absorption of calcium from the gut. PTH stimulates osteoclastic bone resorption.

Calcitonin

This is a 32-amino-acid peptide produced by the parafollicular C cells in the thyroid. It is released in response to hypercalcaemia. It reduces plasma calcium by decreasing osteoclastic resorption and decreases calcium resorption in the kidney and absorption from the gut. Its precise role in human physiology is disputed.

Metabolic bone disease

Hypercalcaemia

Definition. A single plasma assay demonstrating a raised plasma calcium may not reflect a true and sustained hypercalcaemia. Spurious hypercalcaemia may be diagnosed from poor sample technique, in patients with hyperlipidaemias, myeloma or macroglobulinaemia. All these conditions give calcium assay results which reflect the relative expansion in the non-aqueous phase of the plasma and hence of the non-ionised part of the plasma calcium.

Causes. The most common causes of hypercalcaemia include malignancy (55%) and primary hyperparathyroidism (35%). Other causes include renal dialysis and transplantation, sarcoidosis, Vitamin D excess or abuse, milk alkali syndrome, immobilized Paget's disease, and William's syndrome. Endocrine causes include thyrotoxicosis, Addison's disease, acromegaly, phaeochromocytoma VIPoma, and multiple endocrine neoplasia. Drugs such as thiazide diuretics, lithium, and syndromes like familial hypocalciuric hypercalcaemia are documented aetiological factors.

Clinical features. About 50% of patients with hypercalcaemia are completely asymptomatic. Others have vague or non-specific symptoms including polyuria, thirst, weakness and lassitude. Gastrointestinal symptoms include constipation, anorexia, nausea and vomiting. Acute pancreatitis or peptic ulceration may occur. Depression is a common psychiatric manifestation of hypercalcaemia, but confusion, hallucinations or even coma are described. Musculoskeletal pain and weakness are thought to be due to disordered neuromuscular transmission and hyperreflexia occasionally occurs. Cystic bone disease and Brown tumours present in 10% of patients with primary hyperparathyroidism. Hypercalcaemia reduces glomerular filtration rate and tubular reabsorption of water. Dehydration and renal failure occur and exacerbate the hypercalcaemia. Symptoms of thirst and polyuria may result. Renal stones are a complication of prolonged hypercalcaemia and are found in up to 20% of patients with primary hyperparathyroidism. Nephrocalcinosis is found especially in primary hyperparathyroidism, sarcoidosis and the milk alkali syndrome. Ectopic calcification may also occur in soft tissues, blood vessels and the eye. Patients with underlying malignancy will often be symptomatic as a result of the tumour irrespective of the hypercalcaemia.

Hyperparathyroidism

Causes. Primary hyperparathyroidism is caused by overproduction of PTH usually by a benign parathyroid adenoma. Increased osteoclastic resorption produces osteopenia, osteitis fibrosa cystica (with marrow infiltration with fibroblasts). Brown tumours (with giant cells, red blood cells and haemosiderin deposition) and chondrocalcinosis. Skeletal X-ray films show osteopenia, ill-defined bone trabeculae and areas of radiolucency. Renal calculi are common.

Hypercalcaemia. Inappropriate raised PTH in simultaneously tested sample to hypercaemic assay, non suppressible during steroid suppression test. Parathyroidectomy is curative.

Secondary and tertiary hyperparathyroidism. Hyperplasia of the parathyroid glands is commonly associated with chronic renal failure. The chronic hypocalcaemia associated acts as a stimulus to parathyroid hyperplasia and hyperparathyroidism. Long term overstimulation of the parathyroid axis results in autonomous secretion of PTH is some patients; this is tertiary hyperparathyroidism. The life expectancy of patients with chronic renal failure has been dramatically improved by effective dialysis and transplantation, and consequently many patients now survive to suffer complications of hypercalcaemia. If medical treatment fails to control the hypercalcaemia, parathyroid surgery should be considered.

Diagnosis. A gross elevation of plasma calcium to greater than 4 mmol/l and elevation of serum alkaline phosphatase to twice the upper limit of normal are uncommon in primary HPT. Serum chloride, phosphate, chloride to phosphate ratio and acid-base balance have all been suggested as good discriminators of primary HPT from other causes of hypercalcaemia. None is specific. Immunoreactive parathormone (iPTH) assay is arguably the most useful distinguishing investigation. Activity of the parathyroid gland should be suppressed when hypercalcaemia is due to a non-parathyroid cause. iPH should be low or unmeasurable. Significantly elevated iPTH levels in a hypercalcaemic patient supports a diagnosis of HPT. Normal or moderately increased iPTH concentrations may be found in malignancy and familial hypocalciudic hypercalcaemia. Some carcinomas, particularly oat cell bronchial carcinoma, may produce ectopic or inappropriate PTH. Radiology of the hands for periosteal erosions and cysts and an intravenous urogram to detect nephrolithiasis and nephrocalcinosis may confirm renal complications of HPT. An isotope bone scan may demonstrate occult bone metastases. Steroid suppression and calcium infusion tests have been used, but neither reliably discriminates between HPT and non-HPT induced hypercalcaemia.

Localization of parathyroid adenomas. Arteriography has high false positive rates but selective central venous sampling may accurately localize more than 80% of tumours. Functionally abnormal parathyroid tissue can be localized by the use of an isotopically labelled substance incorporated actively into the secreted parathormone. Selenium has been investigated but this and many other isotopes are taken up both thyroid and parathyroid tissue. Dual isotope techniques have been described to overcome this non-selectivity. Thyroid tissue is first outlined by intravenous injection of technetium-99m. A bolus of thallium 201 is then given and is taken up both by thyroid and parathyroid tissue. The two images are recorded by gamma camera and the thyroid image subtracted from the combined image, leaving a parathyroid 'hot spot'.

Preoperative localization. Methylene blue or supra-vital staining has been shown to aid localization of the parathyroid tissue during surgery. Some normal parathyroid glands stain a pale green and diseased glands stain brown to black. The dye may produce alarming 'cyanosis' of the skin and mucous membranes and a discolouration of the urine. The technique is not completely reliable however.

Hypercalcaemia of malignancy

Hypercalcaemia in a patient with a malignancy implies presence of bony metastases, multiple myeloma or paraneoplastic humoural factor production by tumour cells. Biochemical evidence which suggest a malignant cause for hypercalcaemia includes a paraprotein presence on plasma electrophoresis, urinary Bence–Jones protein, suppressed or unmeasurable plasma PTH levels. Hepatic and bony metastases often induce elevated gamma glutamyl transferase levels. Any patient with a malignancy, whose general clinical condition deteriorates rapidly should have hypercalcaemia excluded because malignant hypercalcaemia often responds well to a treatment. It is uncommon in patients with head and neck tumours.

Medical management. Severe, symptomatic hypercalcaemia constitutes a medical emergency irrespective of the underlying cause. The most important step in treatment is careful rehydration. Intravenous normal saline titrated against central venous pressure is essential. Intermittent doses of frusemide prevent circulatory overload and increase urinary calcium loss by blocking distal tubular calcium reabsorption. Serum electrolytes and calcium should be measured frequently in the early stages of treatment.

Intravenous rehydration may reduce plasma calcium by up to 2 mmol/l in 24 h, although the maximum effect may take up to 72 h.

Patients with malignant hypercalcaemia may require specific treatment to lower serum calcium further and relieve symptoms. Limitation of oral intake of calcium is ineffective as patients with malignancy already have impaired calcium absorption. Glucocorticoids act by inhibiting osteoclastic bone resorption but have no effect in over 50% of cases and may take up to a week to be effective. Calcitonin has a similar action and also has a direct calcliuric effect on the kidney. Response is often incomplete and transient. Mithramycin, a cytotoxic antibiotic, is effective but its use is limited by toxicity. The diphosphonates inhibit bone resorption. Sodim etidronate is widely used.

Hypocalcaemia

Causes. Osteomalacia, rickets, hypoparathyroidism, renal failure, acute pancreatitis and hypomagnesaemia.

Clinical features. Hypocalcaemia presents with neuromuscular tetany, cataracts, prolonged QT interval and fungal hyponychia. In tetany, alkolosis must be excluded.

Hypoparathyroidism

Hypoparathyroidism may be primary as a result of thyroid surgery or may be pseudohypoparathyroidism, a rare X-linked recessive condition resulting in end organ receptor resistance to PTH. Short metacarpals and variable mental deficiency occur.

Renal osteodystrophy

Occurs due to insufficient phosphate excretion in chronic renal failure. Hypocalcaemia, and secondary hyperparathyroidism with poor phosphate excretion are typcial. One-alpha hydroxycholecalciferol is therapeutic.

Rickets and osteomalacia

Normal or raised bone volume but hypocalcified tissue is characteristic. Rickets is a childhood disease occurring before epiphyseal fusion. It is typified by long bone bowing, rachitic rosary, pathological fractures, Looser's zones and muscle hypotonia. Biochemical findings include elevated alkaline phosphatase, hypocalcaemia and low or low normal serum phosphate.

Vitamin D deficiency may occur due to dietary deficiency, inadequate sun exposure, malabsorption, renal impairement and chronic parenteral nutrition. Calcium and vitamin D supplements are used to treat this condition.

Vitamin D resistance is found in chronic renal failure (renal rickets), chronic hepatic disease and anticonvulsant rickets. Resistance to vitamin D metabolites occurs in vitamin D-resistant rickets or phosphaturic hypophosphataemic rickets, chronic acid–base disturbances and Fanconi syndrome.

Scurvy

Vitamin C deficiency results in deficient collagen production and osteoid synthesis. Connective tissues and bone growth are affected. Subperiosteal heamorrhages and subsequent pathological calcification is described. Tooth loss is pathognomonic.

Mucopolysaccharidoses

These are a group of rare genetic metabolic disorders. Glycosaminoglycans accumulate in tissues. Most are autosomal recessive. Hunter's and Hurler's syndromes are best described. The phenotypical effects are variable with most children exhibiting severe mental retardation and growth disorders.

Gingival hypertrophy, incomplete dental eruption, intrabony mucoid cysts and progressive fibrous dysplasia are characteristic.

Osteoporosis

This is a common age-related loss of bone mass and osteopenia. It is more common in women and is related to the higher incidence of femoral neck fracture in elderly females than males.

Type I osteoporosis is an oestrogen-dependent, post-menopausal loss of trabecular bone.

Type II is age-related and affects both trabecular and cortical bone to produce hip fractures. Risk factors include being Caucasian, smoking, excess alcohol intake and phenytoin ingestion (impaired vitamin D metabolism).

Secondary osteoporosis is caused by hyperparathyroidism, hyperthyroidism, Cushing's syndrome, malabsorption and malignancy. Physical activity and calcium help prevent fractures in type II osteoporosis and oestrogen–progesterone therapy is beneficial in type I if initiated within 6 years of the menopause. Other causes include osteomalacia, scurvy and marrow infiltrative disorders.

Biochemical indices are all normal in primary types.

Paget's disease

Paget's disease affects 3% of the population. It is typified by increased bone density. Increased osteoclastic resorption is accompanied by irregular bone formation with trabecular thickening, bowing and osteosclerosis. Increased skull diameters and hat size, deafness and high output cardiac failure may occur. Increased alkaline phosphatase and increased urine hydroxyproline are characteristic. Pathological fractures commonly occur. Calcitonin inhibits osteoclastic bone resorption and diphosphonates inhibit bone turnover. Osteosarcoma occurs in up to 5% of cases and carries a poor prognosis.

Osteopetrosis

Osteosclerosis and obliteration of the medullary canal due to decreased osteoclast function are characteristic. The most severe autosomal recessive form leads to hepatosplenomegaly, aplastic anaemia and the 'bone within a bone' appearance on radiographs. Bone marrow transplantation with transfers of osteoclast precursors, high dose calcitriol (1,25 dihydroxy-D3) and steroids may be helpful. The autosomal dominant tarda form (Albers–Schonberg) presents with generalized osteosclerosis but without haemopoetic disease.

CANDIDAL DISEASE

Candida albicans is a yeast-like fungus which invades epithelia in its hyphal form and induces epithelial proliferation and plaque formation.

Predisposing factors

- Defects in cell-mediated immunity (e.g. AIDS).
- Post-organ transplant immune suppression.
- Interference with normal microbial flora (antibiotics).
- Systemic corticosteroids.
- Idiopathic with no explanation for candidal infection diagnosed.
- Associated with the dystrophic effects of iron deficiency.

Clinical syndromes

1. Thrush (syn; acute pseudomembranous candidiasis). The creamy white plaques in infants and neonates due to poorly developed cell mediated immunity are well documented and self-limiting. In adults a predisposing factor should be sought and treatment aimed at its elimination. The plaque is easily wiped off leaving an erythematous base. Topical antifungals are effective. Dissemination is rare as a result of this form of candidiasis. Vaginal candidiasis and candidal balanitis can readily be transferred from the oropharynx and as a sexually transmitted infection. Concomitant oral and genitally applied treatment may be required.

2. Antibiotic-related stomatitis (syn; acute atrophic candidiasis). Prolonged use of broad spectrum antibiotics may depress the local microbial flora and encourage superinfection and overgrowth of fungal species such as *Candida*. The stomatitis associated with antibiotic use is commonly noted and is self-limiting once antibiotic drugs are withdrawn.

3. Denture stomatitis (syn; chronic atrophic candidiasis). The upper acrylic full palatal coverage pattern denture is a potent predisposing factor to proliferation of *Candida* on the fitting surface and the contiguous mucosa. A precisely demarcated inflammatory response is induced. Underlying haematology is usually normal, although pre-existing anaemia will exacerbate the condition. Immune status is usually normal. The clinical association with angular stomatitis is frequently noted. Correction of denture design, and treatment of the infection with topical antifungals is effective.

4. Angular stomatitis. This is closely associated with denture stomatitis. The overclosure of elderly dentures and the maceration of the lip commisures predispose to candidal infection.

5. Chronic candidal leukoplakia (syn; chronic hyperplastic candidiasis). One of the many causes of 'non-wipeable' intra-oral white mucosal patches. This lesion constitutes an example of the chronic mucocutaneous candidal lesions. Its aetiology is uncertain, and patients are usually entirely healthy otherwise. Heavy smoking may predispose, but the pre-malignant potential has been debated but never proven. The condition is usually chronic but self-limiting. It may be pre-malignant and vigilance is therefore required. Biopsy provides reassurance about the absence of dysplastic change.

6. Mucocutaneous candidal syndromes (CMCC). Although there are several established patterns, all the syndromes have some common features. These include persistent candidal infection resistant to antifungal therapy, an association with skin and nail involvement, with no tendency to disseminate beyond the mucous or skin surfaces even if cell-mediated immunity is defective (a rare problem). All are characterized by hyphal invasion, parakeratosis, acanthosis and chronic sublesional inflammation.
(a) *Familial CMCC.* Inherited as an autosomal recessive trait; dermal, ungual and oral plaques are usual. Some patients are sideropaenic, but cell-mediated immunity is usually normal.
(b) *Diffuse CMCC.* Exhibiting no characteristic pattern of inheritance, the oral lesions can be numerous and

widespread. They are warty in character (*Candida* granulomas) and can leave thick scars with severe disfigurement. Iron deficiency is common, and defective cell-mediated responses show selective non-response to candidal proteins *in vitro*.

(c) Candida *endocrinopathy syndromes.* Demonstrating autosomal recessive inheritance with multi-glandular deficiencies, these syndromes are treated by addressing the underlying endocrine condition. The commonest of these are hypoparathyroidism, and Addison's disease as part of the MEN2 or Sipple syndrome. The response to the candidiasis is very unpredictable, however. Topical ketoconazole or miconazole is the treatment of choice as an adjunct to the endocrine replacement therapy.

(d) Candida *thymoma syndrome.* The association of chronic candidiasis with myasthenia gravis in the presence of a thymoma has been noted. Treatment of the underlying acetylcholine esterase deficiency is required and the candidal disease requires antifungal therapy.

CARCINOMA OF THE ORAL FLOOR AND LOWER ALVEOLUS

Squamous carcinomas of the floor of the mouth pose different surgical problems depending on whether they arise laterally or anteriorly. Lateral tumours arise commonly in close proximity to the opening of the submandibular duct. Anterior tumours lead to a severe functional and cosmetic deficit if excised without appropriate reconstruction ('Andy Gump' deformity).

Lesions
Painless, non-healing ulcers are the commonest presentation. Exophytic lesions do occur. Late lesions may be painful due to local sepsis, inflammation or neural invasion. Non-squamous lesions account for less than 5% of oral floor tumours.

Spread
Spread into the tongue or distally toward the epiglottis may occur. Tonsillar fossa lesions may be oral floor in origin. Anterior tumours may invade via the submandibular duct system. All types may invade mandibular bone. In dentate patients, invasion via the gingival crevice may occur, and periodontal pockets with the associated bone destruction and loss of the lamina dura afford easier ingress of tumour into the cancellous space of the mandibular body. Bone invasion is nevertheless quite uncommon.

Lymph nodes
Lymph node metastasis is common. Upper deep cervical nodes and submandibular nodes are the first echelon nodes. The presence of lymph node micrometastases is variously estimated at 35–55% at the time of surgery for the primary tumour.

Surgery
Excision of the primary lesion is performed using the options of lip split and mandibulotomy as necessary. Excision with a good margin is essential, requesting frozen section if margin excision quality is in doubt. Mandibular bone is removed if suspicion of invasion is high. The lower border or buccal plate of the mandible can be left *in situ* to maintain mandibular continuity and minimize the defect. Rim resections or marginal mandibulectomy retain an intact mandibular arch, making it easier to restore function in the postoperative months.

Neck dissection

Neck dissection is planned to account for the clinical and radiographic status and TNM stage.

The surgical specimen is removed in continuity with the primary lesion where possible. Where reconstruction using free tissue transfer is planned, the dissection should preserve the internal jugular venous system to permit its use as recipient vein for the graft. The resection of the tumour should not be compromised to achieve this, however. If radical neck dissection is required, interpositional vein grafting of the vessels of the contralateral neck may be used for donor supply of blood to the free flap.

Reconstruction

1. Primary closure is occasionally possible, although tethering and drooling may occur due to loss of the gutter of the oral floor. If marginal mandibulectomy has been performed, primary closure is easier and less disabling.

2. Local flaps. If new tissue is required, local flaps such as nasolabial flaps based on the superior labial artery give good quantities of appropriate soft tissue.

3. Free flap placement. Typically, use of radial free forearm fasciocutaneous flaps give good quality soft, pliable tissue.

4. After segmental mandibular excision bone can be provided using a sternomastoid flap which includes clavicle, a pectoralis major myo-osseous graft harvesting fifth or sixth rib in continuity or with a trapezius pedicled or free flap raising the scapular spine. Free radial or fibula bone as part of a composite free flap is also possible. Extensive mandibular resection particularly involving the angle may be reconstructed using a free deep circumflex iliac arterial based composite flap.

5. Biomechanical implants using Dacron or titanium mesh trays with cancellous bone from the iliac crest are a reconstructive option.

Radiotherapy

Neck disease with histological evidence of extracapsular nodal spread or failed clearance at the primary resection margins may necessitate radiotherapy to the neck or oral floor. External beam therapy is preferred, although interstitial techniques have been used. Osteoradionecrosis of the residual mandible is likely to be severe with this latter technique.

The long-term problems and complications of endarteritis, xerostomia, osteoradionecrosis and second malignancies should be considered in planning radiotherapy.

Medical management

Nutrition

Preoperative feeding confers benefits. Complication rates particularly for wound breakdown and fistula formation are less in a normally nourished patient. Percutaneous endoscopic gastrostomy (PEG) insertion during the immediate preoperative weeks may be required.

Sepsis

Antiseptic mouthwashes and antibiotics may be required preoperatively.

Dental status

Diseased teeth should be considered for extraction preoperatively. The risk of osteoradionecrosis after radiotherapy is great if dental extractions are required post-treatment.

Endoscopy

Panendoscopy to exclude pharyngolaryngeal invasion or to identify second oropharyngeal primary lesions is required.

Radiology

Magnetic resonance imaging (MRI) scans to determine the degree of neck node metastases are required. Chest X-ray for pre-anaesthetic screening is commonly required as cancer patients are frequently smokers and suffer concomitant pulmonary disease. Pulmonary metastases may occur.

CARCINOMA OF THE TONGUE

Most tongue carcinomas are squamous lesions. Over half of all such lesions affect the anterior tongue and of these, 85% occur along the lateral border. Most patients are elderly, although a cohort have their primary lesions in the third decade. The latter group have a poor prognosis.

Spread
- *infiltrating lesions*; submucosal and transmuscular spread results in an indurated hard tongue
- *posterior lesions*; spread may involve the epiglottis and upper pharynx
- *lateral border*; the floor of the mouth and occasionally the mandible may be invaded

Lymph node involvement
Anterior lesions metastasize to the submental and lower deep jugular system of nodes. Posterior lesions spread to upper deep cervical nodes and tip lesions, and posterior third lesions may lead to early bilateral lymph node involvement.

Management

Diagnosis
1. Clinical. History and examination are essential to determine the general medical condition of the patient.

2. Radiographic. Plain films to exclude mandibular involvement and to plan neccesary dental treatment and mandibulotomy if required. Chest radiographs are essential, and MRI scanning of the tongue, floor of the mouth and neck are part of the preoperative management.

3. Tissue diagnosis. Biopsy of the intra-oral primary lesion and fine needle aspiration cytology (FNAC) of neck lesions are options. Upper aerodigestive panendoscopy and gastroscopy may be required if there is suspicion of a second primary lesion in the head and neck.

4. Doppler flow studies or limb angiography if free tissue transfer is planned as reconstruction.

Treatment

1. *Laser.* Excision of leukoplakia, dysplastic mucosa and T1N0M0 squamous lesions is possible.

2. *Excision. Tip:* V-shaped excision and primary closure is often adequate. Neck dissection may be required. T1N0 lesions on the lateral border or dorsum may be excised locally and closed primarily.

3. *Partial glossectomy.* Lateral border lesion of T1, T2 or small T3 size may be resected with a 1 cm margin. Perioperative frozen section may aid the decision about marginal clearance and the need for more extensive resection.

In lesions larger than T1 size, the defect cannot be closed primarily with satisfactory functional results. To prevent tongue tethering, new tissue is required. Pectoralis major flaps give good muscle volume if required, but are often too bulky for adequate function. Radial fasciocutaneous free flaps provide satisfactory pliable tissue.

4. *Subtotal or complete glossectomy.* For large tongue lesions, radiotherapy is less mutilating than surgery but is more debilitating.

Where surgery is contemplated or where previous radiotherapy has failed to gain local lesion control, radical glossectomy can be performed.

Laryngectomy and stoma formation may be required, to prevent salivary aspiration if posterior tongue tissue is removed. Reconstruction is often difficult. Pectoralis major flaps or similar bulky flap design is required, but functional results are often disappointing.

5. *Mandibulotomy.* Access to the posterior oral cavity and floor of the mouth is greatly enhanced by midline or paramedian mandibulotomy. Pre-section placement of plates and screws is advised.

6. *Neck dissection.* Clinically or radiographically positive evidence for involved neck nodes requires neck dissection. The pattern of neck dissection is required are a matter of controversy. In T2, T3 or T4 lesions with

nodes in the neck, the risk of micrometastases in the cervical nodes is greatly increased in proportion to increasing size of the primary tumour. Neck dissection should, therefore, usually be considered in the presence of large primary lesions. Functional neck dissection is required to preserve the venous drainage if microvascular anastomosis is planned.

7. Radiotherapy. Preoperative radiotherapy is becoming much less frequently the treatment of first choice in the UK. Postoperative radiotherapy can be used for the primary site if marginal clearance is incomplete, or for the lymphatic drainage field if extracapsular spread is evident on histological examination of the resection specimen.

8. Reconstruction. Axial flaps such as pectoralis major or latissimus dorsi may be used. Free radial forearm flaps are becoming the flap of first choice for reconstruction of the tongue.

9. Complications.

- *bleeding*
- *sepsis*
- *fistula formation*; if concurrent neck dissection is performed
- *poor speech, poor swallow and aspiration*
- *non-union*; at the mandibulotomy site
- *recurrence*; of the primary tumour or in the neck
- *post-radiotherapy complications*; osteoradionecrosis and xerostomia.

CEPHALOMETRIC ANALYSIS

Cephalometric analysis is the measurement of head and face dimensions from true lateral skull radiographs. This pattern of analysis is used in planning orthodontic appliance treatment and plotting for orthognathic surgery. Follow up films allow monitoring of treatment progress and results. For orthognathic surgery, the lateral cephalometric analyses may be inadequate if used in isolation. There are useful systems of profile analysis and frontal facial analysis which may contribute to the treatment plan.

Lateral skull cephalometry

1. Lateral skull radiographs are true laterals taken in a cephalostat in which the central X-ray beam passes through both external auditory meati. These landmarks should be superimposed on one another, ensuring that the transmeatal axis is the axis of the radiograph. Tracings are made with tracing paper and a pencil or by using a digitizer/computer/plotter system to detail the cephalometric points.

2. Lateral analyses. There are many systems. Down's angle documents the degree of protrusion or retrusion of the anterior segment of the maxilla in relation to the facial plane N–Po. It is measured as N–A–Po angle. Sassouni, Ricketts and Tweed all described different methods of tracings and analysis using true lateral skull X-ray films. Normal values for Caucasian races have been established, and Broadbent and others have detailed the linear measures of vertical heights and by derivation of facial growth in the vertical and A–P planes.

3. Cephalometric landmarks

* *A point,* point of maximum concavity of the anterior maxilla between ANS and maxillary crest
* *ANS,* anterior nasal spine
* *articulare (Ar),* point of intersection between mandibular ramus and temporal bone
* *B point,* point of maximum concavity of the anterior mandible between mandibular crest and pogonion
* *gnathion (Gn),* most anteroinferior point of the chin symphysis

- *gonion (Go)*, most posteroinferior point of the mandibular angle
- *menton (Me)*, most inferior point of the chin symphysis
- *nasion (N)*, anterior point of frontonasal suture
- *orbitale (Or)*, inferior point of orbital floor
- *PNS*, posterior nasal spine
- *pogonion (Pg)*, most anterior point of the bony symphysis
- *porion (Po)*, upper margin of the bony auditory meatus
- *pterygomaxillary (PTM)*, pterygomaxillary fissure
- *sella or S point*, centre of sella turcica
- *condylion (Co)*, uppermost point of condylar head.

The hard tissue outline is completed by tracing the maxilliary and mandibular outlines. The soft tissue profile including the glabella, subnasale, nasal tip, upper and lower lips and chin button is traced.

The following lines may then be drawn:

- *S–N*
- *S–Ar*
- *N–A and N–B*
- *Po–Or or FP (Frankfurt plane)*
- *ANS–PNS or MP (maxillary plane)*
- *Go–Me or MnP (mandibular plane)*
- *Long axes of upper and lower incisors*
- *OP (occusal plane).*

Measurements

Linear and angular measurements are taken from the tracing. Values differ according to races, age and sex, and standard tables of norms are available for most racial types. Some typical mean values for Caucasians are (degrees ± 1 SD);

SNA	81 ± 3
SNB	78 ± 3
ANB	3 ± 2
SN to MP	8 ± 3
SN to MnP	35 ± 4
FP to OP	8 ± 4
NS–Ar (saddle angle)	125 ± 4
S–Ar–Go (articular angle)	140 ± 5

Ar–Go–Me (gonial angle)	128 ± 7
Mp to Mnp	27 ± 4
UI to MP	109 ± 6
UI to LI	130 ± 6
LI to MnP	93 ± 6

Vertical measurements giving linear values are important and as useful as angular measurements.

1. Vertical linear measurements.

- *Vertical facial heights*; anterior and posterior dimensions can each be subdivided into upper anterior facial height and lower anterior facial height.
- *Dentoalveolar heights*;upper and lower and anterior and posterior dental heights are traceable.

Some typical values for mean linear cephalometric values in Caucasians (millimetres ± 2 SD)

- *TAFH*; total anterior facial height 124 ± 8. Equivalent dimension, (N–Me)
- *LAFH*; lower anterior face height is 55% ± 2% of TAFH, 68 ± 8
- *UAFH*; upper anterior face height is 45% ± 2% of TAFH, 56 ± 8
- *TPFH*; total posterior face height 79 ± 6. Equivalent dimension (S–Go)
- *LPFH*; lower posterior facial height 42 ± 2% of TPFH, 34 ± 5
- *UPFH*; upper posterior face height 58 ± 2% of TPFH, 46 ± 5.

The dentoalveolar segment of the film can be analysed to give a series of measurements of dental heights. Reference points on the occlusal planes are the incisal edges and the mesio-occlusal point of the first molar teeth, and perpendiculars are drawn to intersect the mandibular and maxillary planes.

- *LPDAH*; lower posterior dentoalveolar height 38 ± 3.
- *LADAH*; lower anterior dentoalveolar height 40 ± 2 (males), 44 ± (females).

- *UPDAH*; upper posterior dentoalveolar height 28 ± 3
- UADAH; upper anterior dentoalveolar height 33 ± 3.

In Caucasians, a typical overjet is 4 ± 2 mm, and a typical overbite is 4 ± 2 mm.

2. *Angular measurements.*
(a) *SNA and SNB.* The antero-posterior relationships can be measured by the angles of the facial planes to the skull base rather than linear AP dimensions. These angles illustrate the differences in facial form between races. In Caucasian patients an SNA of 81° and an SNB of 79° with an ANB difference of 2° is average. In Negro patients, 5° is acceptable, whereas in oriental patients 3° or less is normal.
(b) *Ao and Bo.* ANB differences can be inaccurate in short cranial base syndrome or where there is an abnormality of the pituitary fossa. The alternative method is not influenced by these difficulties. Perpendiculars drawn from A and B points to their intersection with the occlusal plane give a linear value in millimetres. This is an accurate reflection of the AP jaw relationship. As Ao is the reference point, the normal Ao–Bo for Caucasians is –1 mm ±1.
(c) *Incisor decompensation.* The angles subtended by the incisors to the maxillary and mandibular planes determine the degree of prognathism or retrognathism due to abnormal dental angulation. UI–MxP and LI–MnP angles are 109° ± 6 and 93° ± 6 respectively.

Profile planning

Although lateral cephalometry permits accurate tracing of skeletal points detailed determination of the facial profile is not routinely performed. Surgical planning requires attention to this facet of the patients preoperative records. As with lateral cephalometry, there are several described systems by which the profile analysis may be performed. Those of Steiner, Merrifield and Ricketts are well documented. All rely on the establishment of soft tissue points such as the nasal tip and soft tissue pogonion.

Full face analysis

1. Frontal views, both photographic and radiographic, allow assessment of vertical dimensions, orbital dystopia and intercanthal distance and facial symmetry. The analysis of facial symmetry is complex. Once again there are described systems of analysis including those of Sassouni and Ricketts. The important points in all such analyses include determination of real or apparent asymmetry. Apparent asymmetry will disappear when mandibular displacement and posturing is corrected. Real asymmetry will be unaffected.

2. Vertex views permit delineation of orbital recession or proptosis and nasal capsule asymmetry.

Treatment planning

Templates such as the Bolton standards can be superimposed on the tracings manually or by computer. Different standards to account for racial differences are available. Predictive tracings and surgical planning are closely allied, and the final treatment plan is based on the predictions of outcome derived from manual tracing and photomontage or from computer-aided prediction.

Clinical diagnostic aids include the grid pattern protractor–ruler designed by McEwan and Martin.

1. Photocephalometrics. Surgical plans may be made by superimposing lateral cephalometric tracings on to photomontages in identical orientation to the X-ray film. The facial analysis is performed using the radiographs and any necessary movements made on the photomontage.

2. Plaster model surgery. Movements planned on the photographs are performed on articulated plaster study models. Once completed, acrylic splints for intra-operative use may be made.

3. Computerized and digitized plots. The ability to store initial co-ordinates and progress data for each patient over a period of time facilitating a collection of digitized data for future audit and research purposes is valuable.

4. *Modern imaging methods* include computerized tomography (CT) scanning with three-dimensional (3D) reconstruction and allow both visualization in real time and hard copy to be generated. Laser tracings and 3D reconstructions based on such plots allow very accurate soft tissue profile and full facial views to be digitized and measurements to be taken. They are expensive methods and not in wide use as yet.

Further reading

Harris and Reynolds. *Fundamentals of Orthognathic Surgery.* London: W.B. Saunders and Co, 1991.

Related topics of interest

Osteotomies (p. 297)
Presurgical orthodontics (p. 311)
Symmetrical facial disproportion (p. 372)

Revision points

Facial growth
Head and neck radiology

CLASSIFICATION OF HEAD AND NECK TUMOURS

The TNM system as recommended by the International Union against Cancer (UICC) is a method of describing the anatomical extent of malignant disease based on the clinical assessment of three elements: tumour (T), nodes (N), metastases (M).

Measurements are taken at the greatest dimension of the tumour or nodes and the extent of each parameter is scored. For each parameter, there are numerical options, higher numbers indicating more advanced disease.

General rules
- cTNM; clinical description based on preoperative assessments.
- pTNM; postoperative assessment including histopathological data.

Uncertainty about T, N or M classification should permit a case to be allotted the lowest possible category. In patients with multiple primary tumours affecting a single organ, the highest T category should be used. In synchronous bilateral primary lesions in paired organs, each lesions should be classified separately. In head and neck lesions, this primarily affects thyroid cancers.

Associated descriptors
These include 'r' and 'C' and 'R' factors. 'r' factors signify recurrent disease and are appended to standard TNM notation.

- C1 classification based on clinical and simple radiological assessment
- C2 classification based on special radiological, nuclear medicine and endoscopic investigations
- C3 evidence from biopsy or cytology
- C4 evidence from definitive surgery and histopathological examination of resected specimens
- C5 evidence from autopsy.

Residual disease index ('R' factor) details the presence or absence of disease after definitive treatment.

- RX residual disease cannot be assessed
- R0 no residual disease

- R1   evidence of microscopic residual disease
- R2   evidence of macroscopic residual disease.

TNM system

T primary tumour

- TX   primary tumour cannot be assessed
- T0   no evidence of primary tumour
- Tis   carcinoma *in situ*
- T1   2 cm or less in maximum diameter
- T2   2–4 cm in maximum diameter
- T3   > 4 cm in maximum diameter
- T4   tumour invades adjacent structures.

Radiographical, clinical or scintiscanning evidence of invasion through the cortical bone all suggest that the tumour must be classified as T4.

N regional lymph nodes

- NX or pNX   regional lymph nodes cannot be assessed
- N0 or pN0   no regional lymph node metastases
- N1 or pN1   metastasis in a single ipsilateral lymph node, 3 cm or less
- N2 or pN2   metastasis in a single ipsilateral lymph node, 3–6cm or in multiple ipsilateral lymph nodes, none more than 6 cm or in bilateral or contralateral lymph nodes, none more than 6 cm
- N2a or pN2a   metastasis in a single ipsilateral lymph node, 3– 6 cm
- N2b or pN2b   metastasis in multiple ipsilateral lymph nodes, none more than 6 cm
- N2c or pN2c   metastasis in bilateral or contralateral lymph nodes, none more than 6 cm
- N3 or pN3   metastasis in any lymph node, more than 6 cm.

M distant metastases

- MX   presence of distant metastases cannot be assessed
- M0   no distant metastases
- M1   distant metastases present.

M1 disease can be classified further according to affected distant sites. For example, pulmonary metastases would be noted as M1 PUL.

Stage grouping

Disease staging is a derived single digit composite numerical index based on all the factors assessed in the TNM, radiological and pathological assessments.

In head and neck cancers stage grouping is determined as follows;

- Stage 0   Tis   N0   M0
- Stage I   T1   N0   M0
- Stage II   T2   N0   M0
- Stage III   T3   N0   M0
  -    T 1 -3   N1   M0
- Stage IV   T4   any N   any M
  -    any T   N2 or N3   M0
  -    any T   any N   M1

Specific head and neck sites

Oral cavity

Applies to carcinomas of the vermilion surfaces of the lips and oral cavity. Anatomical subsites are:

- lips
  - upper lip vermilion surface
  - lower lip vermilion surface
  - commissures.

- oral cavity
  - buccal mucosa
  - upper alveolus and gingiva
  - lower alveolus and gingiva
  - hard palate
  - tongue
  - floor of mouth.

Oropharynx

- Anterior wall (glossoepiglottic region)
  - base of tongue and posterior one-third of tongue
  - vallecula.
- Lateral wall
  - tonsil
  - tonsillar fossa and faucial pillars
  - tonsillar folds and sulci.

- Posterior wall
- Superior wall inferior surface of soft palate uvula.

Nasopharynx
- Postero-superior wall; extends from hard–soft palate junction to skull base
- Lateral wall
- Inferior wall; includes upper surface of soft palate
- *Primary malignancies*

> T1 tumour limited to one subsite of nasopharynx
> T2 tumour invades more than one subsite of nasopharynx
> T3 tumour invades either nasal cavity or oropharynx
> T4 tumour invades either skull or cranial nerves.

Hypopharynx
- Post-cricoid region (pharnyx–oesophageal junction)
- Pyriform fossa
- Posterior pharyngeal wall
- *Primary malignancies*

> T1 tumour limited to one subsite of hypopharynx
> T2 tumour invades more than one subsite of hypopharynx or an adjacent site, without fixation of hemilarynx
> T3 tumour invades more than one subsite of hypopharynx or an adjacent site, with fixation of hemilarynx
> T4 tumour invades adjacent structures.

Maxillary sinus

Ohngren's line: defined as the plane which passes through the inner canthus and the mandibular angle and which divides the upper jaw into the supero-posterior structures (suprastructure) and the infero-anterior structures (infrastructure). The suprastructure includes the posterior bony wall and the posterior half of the superior bony wall. The other bony walls belong to the infrastructure.

Primary malignancies

- TX Primary tumour cannot be assessed
- T0 No evidence of primary tumour
- Tis Carcinoma *in situ*
- T1 Tumour limited to the antral mucosa with no erosion or destruction of bone
- T2 Tumour with erosion or destruction of the infrastructure including the hard palate or the middle nasal meatus
- T3 Tumour invades any of the following: skin of cheek, posterior wall of the maxillary sinus, floor or medial wall of orbit, anterior ethmoid sinus
- T4 Tumour invades the orbital contents or any of the following:
  cribriform plate,
  posterior ethmoid,
  sphenoid sinuses,
  nasopharynx,
  soft palate,
  pterygomaxillary or temporal fossae,
  base of skull.

Salivary glands

The classification applies only to carcinomas of the major salivary glands, that is parotid, submandibular and sublingual glands.

Tumours arising in minor salivary glands are not included in this classification but are classified according to their anatomic site of origin.

Further reading

TNM Atlas : Illustrated Guide to the TNM/pTNM Classification of Malignant Tumours, 3rd Edn, 1992

CLEFT LIP AND PALATE

This is the one of the commonest group of congential malformations affecting the head and neck. The spectrum of disease severity is wide, with defects such as bifid uvula and submucous cleft of the soft palate representing the most minor forms. Isolated cleft lip, either unilateral or bilateral, affects approximately 1:1000 live births in the UK. There is an association of cleft lip with clefts of the primary and secondary palate, and many of the syndromes of the head and neck have palatal or facial clefts as part of the symptom complex.

Incidence data

The frequency of the different patterns of cleft lesions against the 'live births' rate is illustrated below.

- cleft lip   1:1000
- cleft palate (isolated) 0.45:1000
- complete cleft   1:1800
- submucous cleft   1:1200
- bifid uvula   1:100

Aetiology

1. Family history. Cleft lip is commonest in the mongoloid and asiatic races and relatively rare amongst negros. There is a slight male preponderance and unilateral clefts are more common than bilateral. In cases of isolated cleft palate there is a female:male ratio of 3:2. In cleft palate patients where the cleft is not an isolated defect, genetic studies have revealed that a definable family history is available in about 12–20% of cases. Twin studies demonstrate that the twin sibling of an affected child is also affected in 30–50% of monozygotic twins and in about 5% of dizygotic pairs.

2. Family studies. First-degree relatives of an affected child exhibit a recurrence risk of 30–50 in 1000 live births whereas second- and third-degree relatives have a risk the magnitude of which appears to decay exponentially in proportion to the closeness of the family relationship with the patient. The risk to a subsequent child or sibling in a family with one affected infant is about 2.5% in unilateral and 6% in bilateral cleft lip and palate.

3. Demographic factors. Although some reports cite social class, birth rank or order, maternal age or season of conception as significant, there appears to be no consistent pattern with aetiology of clefting in children.

4. *Other factors.*

- *Intra-uterine posture and moulding* is strongly implicated in the Pierre–Robin syndrome. Nursing in the prone position helps to reverse some of the adverse effects of the intra-uterine environment, allowing the tongue to fall forwards away from the palatal defect.
- *Many drugs* such as anticonvulsants (e.g. phenytoin) and anxiolytics (e.g. diazepam) have been linked with cleft syndromes.
- *Infections* such as rubella, toxoplasmosis and syphilis have all been associated with cleft formation in the infants of infected mothers.
- *Diet,* vitamins and minerals have been variously cited as preventative.

Applied anatomy

1. *Upper lip.* The orbicularis oris muscle, the skin and vermillion lip border all require surgical correction as all exhibit defective development.

2. *Nose.* Nasal orifices and associated cartilages are affected and the columella is shortened. The damage to the philtrum and Cupid's bow requires correction. In bilateral clefts, the prolabium contains the midline vascular pedicle and the normal upper lip anastomosis is missing. Compensatory inferior turbinate hypertrophy is usual and adversely affects the airway function.

3. *Maxilla.* Skeletal development on the cleft and non-cleft sides often differs in rate and volume of bone production. This results in the formation of a major and minor segment. Maxillary arch width, incisor formation, eruption and angulation are all affected, and compensatory changes occur in the dental arch in an attempt to overcome these.

4. *Pharynx.*

- *Soft palate.* Levator palatini and the lateral musculature exhibit disorders of function, and the most pronounced effect is velopharyngeal sphincter incompetence and nasal speech.

- *Eustachian tube* and the tensor palati insertion to the palate is lost, resulting in tubal occlusion and secretory otits media.
- *Passavants ridge* is often hyperplastic as a compensatory mechanism.

5. *Teeth.* There are many possible, sometimes complex, dental developmental abnormalities. The commonest forms include absence, enamel hypoplasia and dental ectopia.

6. *Ear.* Eustachian tube dysfunction improves to a degree with palatal surgery. However, grommets are almost always required in cleft palate patients.

Treatment planning

The detailed schedule is very variable between different specialist centres, but the following is a close approximation for most centres.

Birth	Initial assessment
	Pre-surgical orthopaedics (controversial)
3 months	Primary lip repair
9–18 months	Palate repair
2 years	Speech assessment
3–5 years	Lip revisional surgery
8–9 years	Initial interventional orthodontics in preparation for alveolar bone grafting
	Continuing speech therapy
10 years	Alveolar bone grafts
12–14 years	Definitive orthodontics
16 years	Nasal revisional surgery
17–20 years	Orthognathic surgery
	Advanced conservation treatment

Aspects of surgery

1. *Flaps.*

- *Lip repair* performed usually during the first year of life. Very many patterns of primary lip repair have been described. The earliest recorded describe a 'straight line' closure with excision of the sides of the cleft and suture of the defect. The Millard rotation–advancement technique is very widely used worldwide, and the functional repair of Delaire is gaining popularity.

- *Palate repair* requires attention to the nasal floor, the soft palate and the hard palate. The von Langenbeck pattern closure or one of its modifications is common as is the palatal push back operation. The von Langenbeck technique involves elevation of lateral palatal flaps from the lateral aspects of the defect which is closed by inward rotation of the flaps so developed. It is possible to repair the nasal aspect of the cleft and a vomerine mucosal flap is commonly used for this. The palatal side of the defect is repaired by some using a push back technique where the mucosal flaps raised are sutured in a more posterior position with the anterior aspect of the palatal wound left to granulate. The intention is to increase the antero-posterior length of the palate. Its value remains debated.
- *Velopharyngeal incompetence.* Tongue flaps and posterior pharyngeal flaps are described.

2. Alveolar bone grafts. Closure of secondary clefts, alveolar clefts, oronasal fistulae and preparation of the mouth for later osseointegrated implants can be achieved by this operation. The primary importance of this procedure is to encourage eruption of the permanent canines. The iliac crest or tibia are the usual donor sources of cancellous bone.

3. Orthognathic surgery. Once the adolescent rapid growth phase is past, the correction of maxillary hypoplasia and class III malocclusions, common amongst treated cleft patients, can be undertaken. Early palatal closure is good for development of normal speech, but most operations described are associated with some degree of interference with midface growth. The rate of osteotomies performed in patients with repaired palatal clefts reflects in some measure the quality of the technique used to repair the palate in childhood. Other jaw disproportions and facial asymmetry can also be corrected in the same way as for non-cleft patients.

4. Nose. Correction of the columella, alar cartilages and bony nasal skeleton is often required. Rhinoplasty is increasingly common in adult cleft patients.

Orthodontics

The range of malocclusions which present in cleft patients is similar to that for non-cleft patients. They have problems in addition with missing teeth, crowding, maxillary hypoplasia and retrusion and poor transverse maxillary width. Primary corrective surgery, although it closes the defects, can severely limit subsequent facial growth. Third World experience demonstrates the beneficial effect of allowing facial growth to proceed to adulthood without childhood surgery to close the defects. Scar tissue and fibrous bands deform the maxillary dental arch even further.

1. Malocclusion

- *Skeletal base.* There is a tendency toward a class III skeletal base pattern, and cross-bites are common.
- *Dental ectopia and delayed eruption* are common, especially adjacent to the cleft, as are gemination and dilaceration.
- *Soft tissue activity.* Upper lip and tongue activity are important in maintaining any cleft closure.
- *Arch form.* Rapid maxillary expansion is often required to correct the extreme palatal arch narrowing common in cleft patients.

2. Pre-surgical orthopaedics. In infants with bilateral clefts and a pronounced prolabium or in wide unilateral clefts with a pronounced and forward major segment, preoperative orthopaedics may aid subsequent closure of the lip defect. However, it remains a controversial subject.

3. Feeding appliances. Palatal obturation or construction of feeding appliances to permit bottle feeding is sometimes required during infancy.

4. Deciduous dentition. Little active treatment is required and exhausts tolerance for later, more important appliance therapy. Treatment to aid normal speech development is the exception.

5. Mixed dentition. Early correction of dental class III malocclusion and cross-bites is commenced.

6. Permanent dentition. Most major orthodontics and pre-orthognathic orthodontics are performed during this phase.

Restorative dentistry

Prosthetic work, careful restorative work during childhood and osseointegrated implants in adulthood all constitute part of the comprehensive service which may be required by cleft patients. It should be the goal that all surgery design to treat the cleft defects in these patients should reduce or obviate completely the need for prosthetic, orthognathic or restorative dental surgery later in life. In few patients is the surgery performed in childhood the complete solution however. In residual oronasal fistulae and in patients otherwise unsuitable for surgery, obturators may be required.

Speech therapy

Both the anatomical defects and the functional, muscle imbalance require ongoing help from speech therapy services. Excessive nasality in speech due to an ineffective nasopharyngeal sphincter and the inability to produce adequate oral air pressures result in difficulty with fricatives and plosives. Nasal resonance, palatal dysfunction and midfacial hypoplasia all contribute to speech difficulties.

Prosthetic aids are available. However, early palate closure remains the single most effective measure for ensuring normal speech development.

Research

Prenatal diagnosis and intra-uterine surgery have all been the subject of experimental work. Little clinical use is made of such techniques as yet.

CLEFT LIP DEFORMITY

The treatment of cleft lip deformities has evolved with surgical advances. The deformity is a complex one, the unilateral cleft arguably being more complex than a bilateral lesion.

Lip clefts may be complete or incomplete. Simonart's bands are fine slips of tissue bridging the cleft in severe, incomplete lesions.

Surgical goals

- closure of the cleft
- apposition of the skin, orbicularis oris and mucosa
- preservation of normal form for philtrum and Cupid's bow
- scar positioned along a natural skin line or crease
- normal eversion of the vermillion border
- functional symmetry of upper lip
- construction of nasal floor and vestibule
- establish symmetry of alae and length of columella
- no interference with facial growth.

Lip closure timing is determined by the age and medical status of the infant. Satisfactory weight gain and growth is associated with low surgical morbidity. The presence of other congenital abnormalities needs careful consideration in planning of timing of lip closure. Most primary lip closure is performed with the patient between 3 and 6 months of age.

Feeding In the neonate, feeding is essential to permit adequate weight gain preoperatively. Various modifications to bottle teats are available. Palatal clefts pose a greater problem than isolated lip clefts.

Counselling Careful discussion with parents is essential. Genetic advice and discussion of plans for surgery and treatment sequence are important. Discussion with older siblings may be required. The team approach to management is introduced, and warnings about the need for speech therapy, grommets and multiple surgical procedures over forthcoming years are given.

Pre-surgical orthopaedics Much less popular than previously. It is not important unless an alveolar or palatal cleft is present in association with the lip cleft. Control of a protrusive prolabial segment to permit easier lip closure may be needed. Future maxillary growth may be impeded due to greater tension in subsequent lip repair if pre-surgical orthopaedics is used.

Clinical records Photographs are important.

Lip surgery

Lip adhesion Not commonly performed today. Apposition of incised edges of the cleft was performed without flap design or elevation. Definitive lip closure was often required subsequently.

Definitive repair
- Straight line (Rose–Thompson, Mirault, Blair Brown)
- Rectangular flap (Le Mesurier)
- Triangular flap or 'Z' plasty (Tennison, Randall, Skoog)
- Rotation advancement (Millard)
- 'Functional' (Delaire)

In modern practice, the Millard rotation advancement is very common. It is associated in many cases with columella shortening and an apparently higher rate of lip revisions in adolescence. The Delaire operation is gaining popularity.

Early nasal surgery

Alar cartilage Early correction of flattened, displaced alar cartilages should be considered. An alar rim incision is used and the alar cartilage is dissected free. Cartilage grafts may be used and suspensory sutures used to impose a correct form on the freed tissue.

Primary cleft nose repair The option to undertake nasal correction at the time of primary lip repair is an issue for cleft surgeons. Several techniques have been developed, including those of Salyer and Blair Brown. Most patients require revisional nasal surgery in early adulthood. The advantage of early correction therefore appears in doubt.

Secondary surgery

Scar revision

Skin scars may hypertrophy, contract or spread with facial growth. Revision may be required. Excision and simple or 'Z' plasty closure once growth is near completion is often of benefit.

Muscle revisions

If primary lip closure has resulted in less than optimal muscle position or fibre bunching, correction may be required. Lateral segment muscle excess is the commonest secondary deformity. Straight line primary closure appears to offer little muscle correction and is associated with a high number of patients requiring secondary correction.

Secondary lip deformities

Most techniques are associated with some degree of philtrum deformity and columella shortening. Lip and nose correction will attempt to correct these deformities. Physiological positioning of the orbicularis oris sphincter associated with columella lengthening and alar correction may be performed together. An overtight upper lip may require attention. Abbe flap in-rotation using the lower lip as the donor is widely used to increase the upper lip length. The reconstruction of an aesthetically pleasing philtrum where the primary lip repair has failed to achieve it is possible using an Abbe flap.

Rhinoplasty

Should not be required frequently in isolated cleft lip patients.

Osteotomy

There should be no requirement for midface osteotomy after isolated cleft lip correction.

Osseointegrated implants

If alveolar clefts are associated with missing dental units, in late adolescence implants may be considered.

Further reading

McCarthy (ed.) Embryology of the head and neck. *Plastic Surgery,* Vol. 14. Cleft lip and palate. 1990: WB Saunders, pp. 2451–95.

CLEFT PALATE SURGERY

History

Unlike repair of clefts of the lip, the development of techniques for surgical palate closure has been slower. Obturation has been performed down the centuries principally driven by the need to treat acquired clefts due to syphillis or gunshot wounds. There are a number of classical operations described by Roux, then Von Langenbeck followed by Veau and then Wardill and Killner. Each added refinements and modifications to what had been described previously. Lateral osteotomies, lateral relieving incisions and wide subperiosteal undermining were described by various authors during the early part of the 19th century. The early 20th century saw many modifications of flap design, palatal push-back procedures and the later years were typified by detailed studies into the muscular anatomy and design of functional palate repairs. Alveolar bone grafting has been developed in conjunction with the functional pattern palate repair procedures.

Speech versus facial development

It was realised quite early by many surgeons that the significance of early palate closure on normal speech development was very great. The problem of impedance of normal midface growth and development as a result of these childhood operations was a major handicap however. This clinical conundrum remains one to be faced by modern specialist cleft surgeons.

Classifications

There are many systems of classification of palatal clefts. The simplest is that of Veau in which four groups are described.

- Soft palate cleft only.
- Complete palatal cleft without alveolar involvement.
- Complete unilateral cleft palatal and alveolus.
- Complete bilateral cleft of palate and alveoli.

Submucous clefts and bifid uvulae are indicative of a risk of hypernasality of speech if adenoids are removed without appreciating the association of the condition of the velum.

Feeding

Feeding a cleft palate infant requires intensive nursing and training of parents. Modifications of standard feeding techniques including nursing position, spooning and frequent small feeds and early introduction to semi-solid diets decrease the fatigue of relatively futile prolonged suckling. Many cleft palate infants are slow to thrive but gain weight nevertheless. Weight gain is important as general anaesthesia in small infants is more hazardous. This is less of a problem with modern advances in neonatal anaesthesia however.

Speech

Misarticulation, hypernasality, and nasal escape all contribute to the poor intelligibility of individual words or phrases. Early palate closure is the single most important aspect of treatment to ensure development of near normal speech. A speech therapist is an essential team member.

Dental and orthodontic

Only clefts affecting the alveolus have direct deleterious effects on the development of normal occlusion. Palate closure produces scarring and growth retardation which may as a consequence impair normal dental occlusal development. Orthodontic maxillary arch expansion, and correction of crowding and dental malalignment is important. Preparation for alveolar bone grafting usually requires some degree of arch expansion.

Otology

Most cleft palate children have significant eustachian tube dysfunction, chronic middle-ear effusions and infections, and may suffer significant conductive hearing impairment. A few are permanently hearing impaired. Most require insertion of grommets. Syndromic patients with palatal clefts may have more complex otological problems and occasionally sensorineural pattern deafness.

Surgical techniques

Double 'Z' plasty

Soft palate 'Z' plasties are prepared, one in the oral mucosa and the other in reverse direction in the nasal mucosa. The levator palati is included the posteriorly based flap in each of the 'Z's and once repaired these transposed muscle bearing flaps add strength to the repair. The hard palate is repaired with a vomer flap in most cases. These techniques were popularised by Furlow and separately by Randall *et al.*

Vomer flap

Mucosa covering the vomerine bone is elevated, turned down and sutured to the contralateral shelf across the cleft. The oral mucosa is raised from both palatal shelves and closed across the vomer flap repair. This is a method of hard-palate repair.

Von Langenbeck operation   This is the classical hard-palatae repair. The oral mucosa on each side of the cleft is elevated supraperiosteally. The nasal mucosa is elevated subperiosteally and repaired across the cleft. The oral mucosal flaps are developed freeing the greater palatine vessels fully. The flaps are advanced across the defect and closed. Usually this requires lateral relieving incisions bilaterally. A granulating area of palatal bone remains exposed over the lateral relieving incisions.

Wardill–Killner Veau   As velopharyngeal incompetence (VPI) may result from palate closure, many operations incorporating an element of 'push-back' have been described. The Wardill–Killner Veau operation is a modification of the von Langenbeck in that the midline incisions and lateral relieving incisions are converted to bilateral flaps leaving intact, unraised anterior palatal mucosa. The flaps are posteriorly based pedicled on the greater palatine vessels and the levator muscles are raised separately from the mucosal flaps. The muscles are turned from their oblique fibre orientation to cross the cleft at right angles and are repaired in this new position. The mucosal flaps are approximated across the cleft, the 'push-back' is performed and the midline repair completed with the new palatal length planned as sufficient to overcome any tendency towards postoperative VPI.

Functional   There are several functional pattern repairs described. The best known in recent years is that of Delaire. All functional repairs involve more extensive dissection of the abnormally positioned and orientated musculature which is then restored to a more 'normal' orientation. Mucosal flaps are designed to cover the muscle repair. Good quality long-term data about the alleged long-term benefits over the more established types of repair are not yet widely available.

Postoperative care   Feeding can commence with 12 hours of surgery, IV fluids may be required initially and antibiotics are advised in the early hours after surgery.

Complications

1. Bleeding can be a signficant problem in cleft palate surgery and blood loss in small infants is a particular hazard. Good intra-operative control is essential

2. Airway maintenance may require a nasopharyngeal airway for 12 hours postoperatively

3. Dehiscence and oro-nasal fistula occasionally occur. Late closure may be necessary but has a higher failure rate than initial palate closure. Bone grafting is helpful.

Acquired clefts and fistulae

Tumours, trauma particularly gunshot wounds, granulomatous disorders such as syphillis or sarcoidosis and failed repairs of congenital clefts may all cause late presenting palatal clefts. Treatment of any underlying active disease is required and the techniques of flap development and grafting appropriate to childhood cleft surgery find use in adult surgery. Galeal flaps are useful in both hard and soft palate repairs in adults.

Related topics of interest

Cleft lip and palate (p. 69)
Cleft lip deformity (p. 75)
Syndromes of the head and neck (p. 377)

Revision points

Embryology of palate development
Anatomy of the velar musculature

COMMON MEDICAL PROBLEMS

The range of medical problems with which patients present is predictably wide. However, there are a small number of very common clinical conditions and intercurrent treatments which pose management problems in surgical practice.

Anticoagulants

The indications for use of medium- or long-term oral anticoagulants include previous deep vein thrombosis (DVT) or pulmonary embolus, chronic atrial fibrillation (AF), prosthetic heart valves, coronary artery bypass graft (CABG), unstable cardiac dysrhythmias, polyarteritis nodosa, mitral valve disease, including congenital prolapse. Pulmonary hypertension, cardiomyopathies and post-infarct structural abnormalities such as ventricular aneurysm may also need anticoagulation. The problems for surgeons are principally the disordered blood clotting and drug interactions. Control of warfarin therapy requires dose adjustment based on periodic estimations.

Minor oral surgery may be performed when the INR is approximately 2.0. Local control of haemostasis is required. Atraumatic surgery, use of oxycellulose and careful suture placement will usually control postoperative haemorrhage. In patients with prosthetic cardiac valves, where the INR should remain above 2.5 or in the region of 3.0, stopping warfarin tablets for the necessary 2 or 3 days prior to surgery is ill advised. Planned admission is arranged and formal heparinization by continuous infusion is commenced on the day that oral anticoagulant is stopped. The effective period of activity if oral warfarin is used lasts for about 3 days. The plasma half-life of heparin is less than 30 minutes. In the immediate preoperative hour, the heparin is stopped and surgery is then performed. Immediately postoperatively, both heparin and oral warfarin are recommenced. Heparin infusion is discontinued 24 hours after recommencing formal warfarinization.

Drug interactions of importance include diazepam and the related benzodiazepines, cotrimoxazole and alcohol.

Hypertensive patients

These patients are principally at risk from post-general anaesthetic cerebrovascular haemorrhage and myocardial ischaemia. Optimized antihyper-tensive therapy should be instituted by the physicians or GP prior to surgery. Those patients currently on antihypertensive treatment may require surgery under local anaesthetic.

Endocarditis risk

This is a risk if there is a history of previous rheumatic fever. In the developing world, rheumatic disease is much more common than in the UK. All patients with prosthetic cardiac valves, congenital cardiac abnormalities, persistent septal defects, patent ductus arteriosus or ventricular aneurysms are considered to be at risk of infective endocarditis. Whether atrial septal defect poses a risk remains in doubt. In-dwelling central catheters increase the risk, and IV drug abusers are at risk from tricuspid disease particularly due to fungi. All such patients require high dose antibiotic prophylaxis before oral surgery and head and neck surgery for malignant disease. The recommended protocols are updated regularly and should be consulted for up to date details of antibiotic regimens.

Antibiotic cover

There are other groups who require antibiotic prophylaxis preoperatively. The immunocompromised or immunosuppresed and those with low leukocyte counts due to disease or chemotherapy are examples. Urinary catheterization, urological surgery, gynaecological investigation carry a risk of infective endocarditis. Haemodialysis patients and those with severe or extensive skin disease are at risk. By contrast, prosthetic joints, ventriculoperitoneal shunts, and maxillofacial or orthopaedic plates and screws probably do not pose a risk.

Steroid cover

Medical uses of oral steroids are many. They include treatment for asthmatics, atopic patients, some connective tissue diseases and those undergoing chemotherapy for malignant disease. These patients all require supplemental high dose corticosteroids perioperatively whether the planned surgery is minor or not and irrespective of the mode of anaesthetic used. Hydrocortisone exhibits ideal bioavailability for this use, and a dose at least twice that of the hydrocortisone equivalent of the patient's normal daily prescription is required. Prevention of Addisonian hypotensive crisis is the goal. This is a risk if the normal stress-induced release of adrenocortical steroids is suppressed by feedback inhibition due to the prescribed medication. The hydrocortisone supplement replaces the required enhanced corticosteroid levels in anticipation of the surgical stress.

Diabetic patients

The term diabetes mellitus (DM) describes a class of diseases characterized by a chronically elevated blood glucose concentration, often accompanied by other clinical and biochemical abnormalities. The diabetic state may vary in its expression from being totally asymptomatic to rapidly lethal, and this range is largely related to the degree of defect in insulin production or insulin action.

The prevalence of diabetes mellitus in industrialized countries is approximately 3–4%, and about 10% of all diabetics are insulin-dependent.

1. Type 1 diabetes carries the implication of an autoimmune pathogenesis. Possession of the major histocompatibility complex (MHC) specificities HLA DR3 or HLA DR4, is often associated with the presence of circulating islet cell autoantibodies. However, severe ketosis-prone, C-peptide-negative diabetes may occur in the absence of these characteristics. Presentation of IDDM depends on the degree of insulin deficiency. When this is severe, hyperosmolality and hyperketonaemia develop rapidly with dehydration, nausea and vomiting, and sometimes with abdominal pain, stupor and coma. With a more sub-acute onset, symptoms and signs include polyuria and polydipsia, weight loss in spite of polyphagia, fatigue and weakness, paraesthesias, pruritus and visual disturbances.

2. Type 2 diabetes is probably best defined as all patterns of diabetes that are not type 1 (with the exception of gestational, malnutrition-related and 'other types' of diabetes). There is good evidence that NIDDM emerges from a background of cell membrane resistance to insulin and that the function of the insulin receptor may be disordered.

- Genetic factors: underlying genetic susceptibility appears to play an even more important role in NIDDM than in IDDM.
- Environmental factors: obesity is a major environmental factor capable of unmasking an underlying NIDDM susceptibility. Physical inactivity is also thought to contribute to NIDDM, perhaps by diminishing the responsiveness of tissues to normal concentrations of insulin. In many obese people, high circulating insulin concentrations and reduced insulin receptor numbers are found, though it is unclear which occurs first and the nature of their interrelationship.
- Haemochromatosis is associated with diabetogenesis.

3. NIDDM in young people (maturity onset diabetes of youth – MODY). NIDDM in young people probably includes several subtypes. It appears to exhibit a dominant inheritance pattern in some families, and other families seem less liable to microvascular complications than in other diabetes types.

4. Malnutrition-related DM (MRDM). There are two subtypes, *fibrocalculous pancreatic diabetes (FCPD)* and *protein-deficient pancreatic diabetes (PDPD).* These types exhibit a high prevalence in tropical developing countries (e.g. India, Indonesia and Africa), and clinical features include severe symptoms in young people without ketosis. Pancreatic calcification occurs in the FCPD subtype.

5. Impaired glucose tolerance (IGT). The justification for distinguishing IGT from normal glucose tolerance is based on long-term follow-up results which show that, annually, only 2–4% of patients in this group deteriorate to unequivocal diabetes. There is a comparable likelihood that some will revert, apparently spontaneously, to normal tolerance.

In pregnancy, IGT should be taken seriously and treated as gestational diabetes. The risk of developing clinically significant diabetic retinopathy in patients with IGT has been shown to be negligible over periods of up to 10 years. However, individuals with IGT, like those with unequivocal NIDDM, show a doubling of the risk of coronary heart disease and stroke.

Diabetes in surgical patients

The important issues are to determine the patient's fitness for anaesthesia, to decide details of anaesthetic management and establish the extent and severity of microvascular disease if microvascular anastomoses are planned.

Local anaesthesia No need to starve therefore no requirement for interruption of normal glycaemic management.

General anaesthesia

1. Diet-controlled diabetes.

- minor surgery; starve normally
- major or prolonged surgery; pre-operatively starve and cover with IV dextrose and insulin infusion during the operation.

2. Oral hypoglycaemics.

- minor surgery; stop long-acting drugs 24–48 hours prior to surgery. Starve normally.
- major surgery; stop long-acting drugs 24–48 hours prior to surgery. Starve and cover with IV dextrose and insulin.

3. Insulin-controlled.

- minor surgery; omit morning insulin and starve. IV insulin regime may be required.
- major surgery; starve and cover with IV Alberti regimen or a similar alternative.

4. Alberti regimen.

- 10% dextrose intravenous infusion
- 10 IU soluble insulin per 100 ml
- 10 mmol KCl

Frequent glucose and electrolyte estimations permit independent variation of the IVI constituents according to the ongoing biochemical picture.

Oral contraceptive pill

The increased risk of perioperative thromboembolic complications is well documented. In maxillofacial surgery these problems are only of concern in multiple trauma patients and malignancy. Short operations on the upper parts of the body and face carry little risk. Where previous history of thromboembolic disease is present, judicious use of graduated compression stockings and subcutaneous heparin or enoxapyrin is adequate.

Intercurrent medication

There is little indication in maxillofacial surgery for interference with the patient's normal drug regimen. The risk of drug interactions should be considered and recent antibiotic prescription and allergies should be documented.

COMPLICATIONS

Morbidity and mortality are a feature of surgical problems and treatment. Audit is a feature of daily surgical practice and serves to document rates of complications from different treatments and attempts to offer an approach to prevention of future similar problems.

Risk factors

Although all anaesthetics and all operations carry a risk of complications, the risk of problems varies significantly with the patient's age and general preoperative condition.

Age

Extremes of age pose physiological problems.

1. In infants, body weight, pulmonary maturity and intravascular volume all pose particular difficulties if anaesthetics or surgery are required. Increased age and nutritional status with the associated increase in body weight determines the quantity of brown and subcutaneous fat deposited and, as a result, the ability of the infant to withstand the catabolic post-operative state more easily. Thermoregulation is poorer in infants, and the margin of error with blood loss and fluid replacement is narrower than in adults. Wound healing and resistance to infection are better in the more mature infant.

2. The elderly withstand surgery less well due to the high incidence of concurrent disease and medication. Co-existent cardiac, peripheral vascular, respiratory and malignant disease all predispose to increased complication rates in this age group. Cerebrovascular disease increases significantly with increased age, and the risk of postoperative myocardial infarction is much greater.

Obesity

The greater the degree of obesity, the greater the attendant risk of haematoma and wound infection, respiratory complications including atelectasis and chest infection, venous thrombo-embolic problems and postoperative mobility. Diabetes, ischaemic cardiac disease and occlusive peripheral vascular disease are more common in obese patients.

Cardiovascular status

1. Postoperative myocardial infarcts (MIS) pose a risk to the elderly and those with pre-existing coronary artery disease. Surgery after MI carries a risk of a second MI which is proportional to the time between the first MI and the operation. Anaesthetic within 3 months of an MI is associated with a 75% incidence of second MI in the immediate postoperative period. This statistic reduces with a greater delay in surgery so that at 6 months post-MI the risk of second MI is 55%, between 12 and 24 months after MI it is 24% and once 3 years have elapsed it reduces to 2%.

2. Dysrhythmias. All carry a risk of MI and embolic disease postoperatively. Medical control greatly reduces the risk but does not completely abolish it. AF is common and is frequently associated with postoperative cardiac and peripheral vascular complications.

3. Cardiac valve disease. The risk of infectious endocarditis requires prophylactic antibiotics perioperatively, and, in patients who have had a valve replacement, the problems include the very common incidence of dysrhythmias, lifelong warfarinization in addition to the endocarditis risk.

4. Hypertension. Although not markedly associated with cardiac complications, hypertensive patients are significantly more at risk of cerebrovascular events than if normotensive.

Respiratory disease

1. Upper respiratory tract infections, if present in the immediate preoperative period, greatly increase the risk of chest infection after the anaesthetic.

2. Asthmatics. Reversible airways disease responds well to pre-induction bronchodilation but the patient may be taking steroids with the attendant risks. The risk of bronchospasm is greater in the atopic asthmatic, and the anaesthetic hazard should, therefore, be noted.

3. COAD. The poor gas exchange, arterial hypoxaemia and underlying poor medical state of many of these patients predisposes to severe respiratory problems postoperatively. These include chest infections, difficulty weaning off ventilation, and risk of concomitant ischaemic cardiac disease

4. Smokers. Smoking increases the risk of lung and cardiac complications many fold. This factor is additional to the effect of smoking on the incidence of many cardiac, respiratory, metabolic and neoplastic disease processes.

5. Combined cardiac and respiratory disease. The effect of combined cor pulmonale and ischaemic cardiac disease is associated with a high mortality; some reports estimate a mean mortality rate of about 50%.

Liver disease

1. Jaundice. Preoperative jaundice is a significant risk factor for poor postoperative wound healing, disorder coagulation and abnormal drug metabolism. The infection risks are significantly increased due to greater bleeding into the tissues, haematoma formation and wound infection. The reticuloendothelial cells exhibit impaired function, and the incidence of Gram-negative endotoxaemia is greater. 'Hepato-renal syndrome' or acute tubular renal failure secondary to preoperative hyperbilirubinaemia is well documented. The effects of endotoxaemia, disseminated intravascular coagulation (DIC), microembolic effects on the renal circulation and hypoperfusion of the renal vascular bed all contribute. Fluid replacement and appropriate antibiotic prophylaxis are partially protective.

2. Diabetes. Apart from the metabolic disorders well documented for diabetics, the increased risk of poor wound healing, sepsis, peripheral vascular disease and thromboembolic complication should be considered.

Drugs

1. Corticosteroids. These agents are commonly used and may be associated with increased local infection rates and a risk of Addisonian hypotensive collapse unless adequate preoperatove replacement is made.

2. Warfarin. The INR should be documented and the warfarin dose adjusted or stopped as appropriate for the operation planned and the underlying condition. It may be necessary to admit the patient for formal heparinization prior to surgery.

3. Cytotoxic agents. Impaired marrow function results in decreased white cell and platelet counts. Dysfunctional wound healing and cell-mediated immunity are common in these patients unless surgery is timed appropriately and antibiotics are give perioperatively.

Disease-related factors

Soft tissue facial trauma

This may result in damage to essential nerves and vessels. Midface lacerations potentially damage branches of the facial nerve and the parotid duct, and control of haemorrhage may be as damaging if inaccurately applied. Soft tissue avulsion around the eyelids may result in ectropion or loss of functioning lip tissue in perioral trauma. Scarring may result and, in some patients, keloid development follows.

Fractures

1. Nasal bone fracture results in haemorrhage, sinus suffusion and airway obstruction due to oedema, fragmentation and depression of the nasal complex.

2. Zygomatic and orbital floor factures result in infraorbital numbness, diplopia and gaze palsy if inferior rectus entrapment occurs, coronoid impingement and periorbital eccymosis. The most serious but uncommon complication is retrobulbar haematoma.

3. Paediatric condyle fractures. Intracapsular fractures pose a risk of long-term growth disturbance if the growth centre is damaged. Hemifacial asymmetry may result.

4. *Mandible fracture.* Occlusal dysharmony, airway, swallow and sublingual haematoma may result. Inferior alveolar numbness may be associated.

5. *Maxilla fracture.* Bilateral periorbital eccymoses, occlusion of the upper airway if the fracture segment is depressed down the inclined plane of the cranial base and occlusal dysharmony may result.

Trauma to vital structures

1. *Eye.* Traumatic hyphaema, lens dislocation and retinal detachments may occur. Subconjunctival haematoma and severe globe disruption are possible.

2. *Ear.* Perichondrial haematoma may result in 'cauliflower ear'. Avulsion of the pinna and lacerations may occur. Tympanum rupture and perforation are described, as are temporal bone fractures.

3. *Larynx and hyoid.* Fractures of these structures pose a threat to the airway.

4. *Intracranial.* Fractures, mass lesions due to expanding haematomas and cerebrospinal fluid (CSF) leakage are the main problems.

Malignancy

1. *Local or primary lesion.* Pressure symptoms, local ulceration, sepsis, inflammation, neurogenic pain and major blood vessel erosion are common problems.

2. *Neck disease.* Swelling, pressure symptoms on the trachea or major vessels, sepsis, pain and carotid arterial rupture may all occur.

3. *Metastatic.* Lung secondary deposits occur typically in adenoid cystic carcinomas. Adenocarcinomas of the salivary or upper gastrointestinal (GI) tract may metastasize to the liver. Bone metastases in thyroid lesions are described.

4. *Paraneoplastic*

Clefts

The problems associated with cleft lip and palate and the surgery performed to correct the defects include fistula formation, impairment of facial growth, speech defects, abnormal swallow, malocclusion, obligate mouth breathing with mucosal drying and poor caries state. Conductive deafness is almost universal, and grommets are required to overcome the Eustachian tube dysfunction in most patients.

Anaesthetic

Local anaesthetic
- Needle fracture
- intravascular injection
- haematoma
- failed analgesia.

General anaesthetic
- Premedication
- induction
- muscle relaxation
- intubation
- conscious level
- drug reactions.

Sedation
- Depth of sedation
- reversal
- airway and respiratory depression risk.

Problems may also occur with epidurals, PCA and adjuncts.

Surgical

Pyrexia
- Pulmonary atelectasis
- transfusion related
- urinary tract infection
- URTI
- infection
- septicaemia
- wound infection
- failure of flaps
- MI
- DVT/pulmonary embolism (PE)
- organ failure
- central pyrexia
- malignant hyperthermia

Immediate	• Haemorrhage
	• surgical errors
	• drains and catheters
	• analgesia.
Intermediate	• Pain
	• haematoma
	• local sepsis
	• tumour recurrence
	• wound failure
	• impaired function
	• psychological and appearance.
Late	• Contracture
	• swallow
	• speech
	• mastication
	• cosmetics
	• psych.
Procedure specific	• Dentoalveolar
	• trauma
	• tumour excision
	• reconstruction of flaps/grafts
	• orthognathic
	• cleft.

COSMETIC FACIAL SURGERY

Patient demands for cosmetic surgery are increasingly common. The most frequent complaints include requests for surgical alteration in the nose, wrinkle reduction, excision of facial skin redundancy and lip revision. More major facial disharmony results from jaw disproportion or post-cleft surgery. Scar revisions are sometimes required.

Clinical problems

Trauma

Facial trauma may result in fractures and the need for operative reduction. The outcome may produce less than acceptable cosmetics. Nasal injuries are a common focus of requests for post-traumatic revision. Fractures of the zygoma may be missed and provoke requests for late treatment. Mandibular fractures, if misdiagnosed or mismanaged, may result in anterior open bite or malocclusion. Rhinoplasty or facial osteotomies may be required for late correction in patients after facial trauma.

Soft tissue trauma results in scarring, and even careful wound debridement and closure may result in a requirement for scar revision. Loss of intra-oral tissue results in a variety of functional deficits, including speech, swallowing and mastication. Poor cosmetics is commonly associated.

Malignancy

Excisional tumour surgery results in major facial defects, and reconstructive surgery to replace excised bone, bulk and mobility of oral and facial tissues is required. Bone grafts restore facial contours. Soft tissue or skin cover using distant skin of similar texture and adnexal concentration is variously available from the volar surface of the forearm, chest and flank walls and lower limb. Random, axial and free vascularized tissue may be used. Revisional surgery may be required after initial reconstruction. Scar revision, excision of subcutaneous bands after neck dissection and radiotherapy, closure of persistent mucocutaneous fistulae and vestibuloplasty are all options. Dental implant insertion and restoration of the dentition often produces improvement in facial form and contour.

Closure of palatal defects after maxillectomy may improve both function and facial aesthetics.

Cutaneous malformations

Cutaneous haemangiomata, neurofibromas and moles may induce requests for removal. Excision and biopsy of lesions which are clinically suspicious for malignancy and planned closure of the resultant defect may require transposition or rotational flaps for adequate coverage. Pigmented lesions may be removed, sequentially if necessary, by laser. Haemangiomata are sometimes very extensive, and excision is hazardous due to the complex vascular anatomy. Angiography and embolization is a preferable technique to primary excision.

Acne and facial skin infections

Chronic, low-grade skin infections can be very disfiguring. Once the active phase is resolved (and this may be prolonged), dermabrasion may be a useful technique to improve severely scarred skin contours. Laser resurfacing is a newer treatment modality.

Tatoos

Excision by surgical means or using a laser technique for removal is possible.

Skeletal base disproportion

In association with soft tissue or skin surgery, underlying facial skeletal diatheses may require correction. Orthognathic surgery should be considered prior to facial soft tissue surgery.

Results of early cleft surgery

Scar revision, lip nose correction and rhinoplasty are often required in late adolescence or early adulthood.

Congenital abnormalities

Aural tags, pinna clefts, facial clefts and neck webs may require excision and reconstruction. Cleft lobes of pinnae are amenable to rotational or 'Z' plasty correction. Closure of facial clefts requires the expertise of a craniofacial surgical unit.

Acquired facial skin defects

Brow ptosis, facial skin ageing and wrinkle deepening, ectropion and enotropion are problems of the ageing face.

Baldness

Alopecia may have an underlying autoimmune basis or may be related to use of cytotoxic therapy. Idiopathic 'male pattern' baldness appears to have no readily definable biochemical abnormality. Surgical ingrafting of hair follicles or follicle-bearing skin is sometimes advocated.

Techniques

Scar revision

Excision of keloids, 'Z' plasties, 'W' plasty and local flaps all have the effect of disguising unsightly facial scars. Avascular scar excision is required prior to revision.

Embolisation

For cutaneous haemangiomata, embolization under radiological control is effective but carries with it the attendant risks of major vessel occlusion and cerebrovascular infarct.

Laser ablation

Tatoos are amenable to removal by this means.

Dermabrasion

Traumatic dirty facial abrasions after moped accidents have high levels of road surface embedded superficially. Dermabrasion is effective in removal and allows healing of the skin surface without the inevitable tatooing that would result without thorough cleansing. Severe acne-related scarring may also be reduced by this means.

Collagen augmentation

Improvement in upper lip prominence is possible by subcutaneous injection of collagen, but very frequent repeat injections are required. Surgical means of vermilion advancement may be more appropriate.

Liposuction and liposculpture

Performed via puncture incision, suction lipectomy removes excess subdermal fat. If applied to heavily jowled neck tissues or marked dewlaps, significant recontouring can be achieved. Combination with formal facelifting operations may be required. Repeat surgery may be necessary.

Rhytidectomy

This means literally 'wrinkle removal'. There are several approaches. The superficial musculoaponeurotic system (SMAS) is key. The incision is usually placed in a pre-auricular skin crease and in the hair line post-auricularly. The dissection is performed in the supra SMAS plane. This preserves the branches of the facial nerve which lie immediately deep to the SMAS. Sub

SMAS face lifts are also described. Treatment of the SMAS layer involves either plication, or partial excision and closure of the space so created.

Blepharoplasty

Correction of periorbital skin wrinkling and orbital fat herniation through the tarsal plate of the lower eye lid. Upper and lower eyelid operations are well described. Excision of subdermal fat, correction of orbital fat herniation and plication of the skin and muscle layers form the elements of the operation.

Pinnaplasty

Correction of prominent ear lobes or pinnae is often requested. The most effective technique involves a post-pinna approach with perichondrial dissection anteriorly and posteriorly. Scoring and folding permits creation and maintenance of an antehelical fold; the most commonly absent of the pinna features. Pressure bandaging is applied for 5–7 days as perichondrial heamatoma formation is likely to lead to unsightly hyperplastic pinnea or 'cauliflower ears'.

Brow lifts

Performed via an eyebrow or mid brow incision or via an endoscopic approach, brow ptosis may be improved. Frontalis plication may be required.

Facial reanimation

Tendon transfer, 'sling' and suspensory procedures are all described in the treatment of the residual deformity after chronic facial nerve palsy. Free innervated muscle transfer, interpositional sural nerve grafts or cross-over innervation is used with some success. Oculoplastic surgery may be required to correct the eyelid problems which are associated with long-term facial nerve weakness.

Orthognathic surgery

Osteotomy may greatly enhance facial aesthetics and should be completed before final soft tissue cosmetic surgery. The associated orthodontic, prosthodontic and dental aspects of facial cosmetic surgery should not be neglected.

CRANIOFACIAL ASYMMETRY

Facial asymmetry can arise owing to hemi-hyperplasia or hypoplasia of growth centre tissues during the early years of life. It may be gross and rapidly progressive or slow and not striking in its aesthetic effects. All congenital growth disturbances should cease by the end of adolescence and if possible surgery should be delayed until this point. Very obvious, rapidly progressive lesions or those causing marked psychosocial distress should be considered for earlier surgery.

Laterality

1. Structural and functional differences in laterality are common observations amongst a wide variety of animals. In humans, handedness reflects behavioural differences which have corresponding structural asymmetries of brain tissue associated. It is a normal state in humans. Early development of handedness in human infants may suggest a neurological disorder such as cerebral palsy.

2. Normal variations in tooth crown size, limb size and foot size may be apparent on close measurement if not actually on casual observation. The obvious pathological laterality present is conditions such as trisomy 21 and limb reduction defects may be an accentuation of this effect.

3. Normal asymmetries related to the topography of non-paired structures such as liver, spleen and stomach may be disturbed in *situs invertus* where the organs are orientated in an exact mirror image of the normal anatomical arrangement.

Lateralized defects

The severity of lateralized defects is related in part to the stage of development during which the causative factors are most active. Early embryopathies may be inconsistent with life whereas later fetal disruptions may be disfiguring but otherwise consistent with adequate function.

Some definitions

1. Malformation. A morphological defect which arises owing to an intrinsically abnormal developmental process. Cleft lip deformity and hemifacial microsomia are examples of such defects.

2. Deformation. A morphological abnormality due to non-disruptive mechanical forces which perturb an otherwise normal developmental process. Uterine limitation of fetal movement and oligohydramnios contribute to this sort of abnormality which typically present as abnormal moulding of the limbs. The cleft palate in the Pierre Robin sequence is likely to arise owing to the severe micrognathia and poor mandibular intrauterine growth, but where the tongue attains near normal volume and impedes normal closure of the palatine shelves.

3. Disruption. A morphological defect which arises owing to breakdown in a previous normal process or which interferes with normal developmental progress or intrauterine growth. Amniotic bands are a good example and can be very disruptive. Rare facial clefts and limb amputations can result.

4. Syndromes. Recognized association where multiple congenital malformations occur affecting embyologically non-contiguous tissues. Good examples include cleft lip and palate when associated with genital or limb abnormalities. Some authors distinguish regional complexes from syndromes where the clinical associations involve related but embryological contiguous tissues. The long face syndrome or plagiocephally–torticollis syndromes illustrate.

Some causes

The causes are many and include gene mutations, embryopathies, amniotic bands, craniosynostoses, hamartoses, infection, tumours, fibrous dysplasia and childhood trauma.

Embryopathies and asymmetry

1. Eye. Unilateral microphthalmia or anophthalmia. Tessier clefts involving a single eye brow (type 10 cleft) prosencephalic cyst with disruption and displacement of normal eye development.

2. Nose. Heminasal aplasia, skin tags, pit and dimples, anomalous nasal bone, cribriform plate and septal skeletal development. Proboscis and holoprosencephaly are rare and usually midline rather than lateralized.

3. Ear. Accessory auricles, pits, dimples, positional defects such as low set ears in chromosomal syndromes (Potter's syndrome).

4. Mouth. Dental supernumeries, ectopic dental tissue and supernumery teeth occur. Supernumery stoma and associations with nasal and ocular abnormalities are to be expected with major oral malformations.

5. Tessier clefts. A comprehensive descriptive system for documenting craniofacial clefts. The system relates the cleft to the saggital midline and assigns a type number. Cleft types can be described within the Tessier system depending on the tissues involved; bone, skin, mucosa and major organs.

Craniofacial or hemifacial microsomia

This term has many synonyms but essentially denotes a pattern of growth inequality of widely varying severity between the two sides of the face, mouth and cranium. Associated soft tissue defects usually occur and the defect can have dramatic functional and aesthetic effects.

Hemi-hyperplasia

Clinically distinguishable subgroups of lower facial hyperplasia are noted. Asymmetric mandibular prognathism, condylar hyperplasia and generalized mandibular enlargement may be distinguished. These conditions may occur in isolation or as part of a more widespread dysmorphic tendency. Some abnormalities associated with hemifacial hyperplasia include skin pigmentation and telangectasia, syndactyly, talipes, hip dysplasia, scoliosis, cerebral hemiatrophy with mental deficiency or epilepsy, congenital cardiac defects, medullary sponge kidney, hepatic focal nodular hyperplasia, hypospadias and cryptorchidism, clitoromegaly, tracheo-oesophageal fistula, umbilical hernia and strabismus. Orodental abnormalities may include dental size disturbances, dental malformations, eruption date disturbance and macroglossia. The aetiology may involve chromosomal disturbances and there are well documented associations with Sturge–Weber syndrome and the Beckwith–Wiedmann sequence.

Hemi-hypoplasia

Multiple tissue types may be involved and aural, oral and mandibular growth centres are characteristically affected. There are several well established variants including the Goldenhar sequence. This involves ocular, vertebral and auricular abnormalities. The causes of hemifacial hypoplasia are many and include chromosomal abnormalities and many putative environmental agents such as thalidomide and retinoic acid given during pregnancy.

Branchial arch syndromes

First and second arch syndromes exhibit variable degrees of disturbed development in the ear, midfacial, infratemporal and mandibular anlage. There are severe forms and forme fruste or microexpressed phenotypes. An experimental model to explain these defects demonstrates the effect of haematoma formation associated with the embryonic stapedial artery on the genesis of hemifacial microsomia. The relevance *in vivo* remains unclear.

Hemiatrophy

Romberg's syndrome is a slowly progressive hemifacial atrophy which most commonly affects the left side and which is ultimately self limiting in most patients. Associated abnormalities include skin pigmentation, Jacksonian pattern epilepsy, periorbital fat atrophy with resultant enophthalmos. Circumscribed alopecia on the affected side is common and muscle atrophy affects the periorbital tissues, tongue and upper lip.

Classification

There are several systems for classifying the diverse defects causing hemifacial microsomia. Harvold *et al.* proposed the following:

- 1a   unilateral underdevelopment affecting ocular tissue typically;
- 1b   as 1a but with microphthalmos;
- 1c   bilateral asymmetric patterns;
- 1d   complex patterns but without limb or frontonasal defects;
- 2   associated with limb defects;
- 3   fronto-nasal defects with hypertelorism or with ocular dermoids, vertebral, cardiac or renal defects;
- 4   Goldehar type with ocular dermoids and upper eyelid colobomata.

Grading systems to document severity and assist with surgical planning are described. Mandibular aspects are described according to Pruzansky in three grades. Grade 1 is limited to size defects, Grade 2 to size discrepancy and distortion and Grade 3 forms exhibit ramus loss or severe hypoplasia.

Mandibular asymmetry

True mandibular asymmetry may occur in isolation or in association with more widespread hemifacial asymmetry. Apparent mandibular asymmetry may present but exhibit normal mandibular topography on investigation.

Causes

1. True. Developmental and syndromic; infection; tumour; trauma; ankylosis; idiopathic.

2. Apparent. Unilateral facial paralysis, muscle asymmetries, tumours.

Management

Assessment and full clinical records are essential. Timing and sequence of surgery are determined by patient preference and unit policy.

Surgical corrections

Specific surgical planning is required for each of the following parts of the facial skeleton, dental abnormalities, occlusal cant, mandibular ramus, mid-face skeleton, cranium.

Surgical options include

Onlay (bone, cartilage, alloplastic tissues), osteotomy, distraction osteogenesis, free tissue transfer, intraoral reconstruction.

CRANIOFACIAL DIAGNOSIS AND ASSESSMENT

Craniofacial conditions may be congenital or acquired. The primary group are uncommon and constitute the complex craniofacial deformities and syndromes. Acquired lesions are usually the result of trauma or tumour surgery and the need for reconstruction after ablation of malignant disease.

Primary craniosynostoses

1. *Vault craniosynostoses.* Simple, if a single suture is affected, or complex, if multiple sutures are affected.

2. *Simple craniosynostoses.* Sagittal craniosynostosis result in scaphocephaly, unilateral coronal craniosynostosis in plagiocephaly, metopic craniosynostosis in trigonocephaly and lambdoid craniosynostosis in posterior plagiocephaly.

3. *Multiple, non-syndromic craniosynostoses.* Bicoronal sutural craniosynostoses lead to brachycephaly.

4. *Multiple, syndromic craniosynostoses.* Complex deformities result, for example clover leaf skull deformity.

5. *Multiple, pan craniosynostosis.* Very complex deformities may result.

Craniofacial synostosis

- Crouzon's syndrome
- Acrocephalo-syndactyly
- Apert's syndrome
- Saethre–Chotzen syndrome
- Pfeiffer's syndrome
- Carpenter syndrome.

Secondary craniosynostoses

(a) Shunted hydrocephalus
(b) Microcephaly

- congenital
- acquired, for example cerebral atrophy.

(c) Storage disorders

- Hurler's syndrome
- Morquio's syndrome.

(d) Metabolic disorders

- rickets
- hyperthyroidism.

(e) Haematological disorders

- polycythaemia vera
- thalassaemia.

(f) Drug teratogens

- diphenylhydantoin
- retinoic acid.

Orbital dystopia

(a) Horizontal: hypertelorism
(b) Vertical: unilateral defects result in different orbital floor levels.
(c) Complex defects.

Meningo-encephaloceles

(a) Sincipital

- fronto-ethmoidal
- interfrontal
- craniofacial.

(b) Basal

- nasal
- midline
    palatal
    sphenoidal
    ethmoidal.

(c) Parietal
(d) Occipital

Craniofacial clefting syndromes

Tessier delineated a complex classification to describe craniofacial clefts. This system integrates topographic description and clinical observation with underlying skeletal disturbances. The orbit, nose and mouth are key landmarks through which the craniofacial clefts follow defined axes. In Tessier's system, the clefts are numbered from 0 to 14, with the lower half of the numbers representing the facial clefts and the higher numbers their cranial extensions. Multiple and bilateral clefts can occur in the same patient.

Secondary craniofacial defects

1. Trauma. Cranio-orbito-naso-ethmoidal-maxillary injuries involving need for craniotomy and neurosurgical assistance.

2. Craniofacial pathology. Benign and malignant tumours arising in the cranium or orbit or adjacent ethmoid sinuses. Tumours whose excision is facilitated by a combined craniofacial and subcranial approach.

3. Non-neoplastic craniofacial pathology.

- Fibrous dysplasia
- neurofibromatosis
- vascular anomalies
- osteopetrosis
- dermoids.

Assessment

1. History. Medical, obstetric, family and social histories are important. In an older child, history of specific or progressive functional deficits is important. In particular, cognitive and intellectual development, vision and hearing and socialization are essential parts of childhood and development, and deterioration may constitute an indication for urgent treatment.

2. Clinical examination.

- Skull shape and size
- cranial base
- orbits and eyes
- midface and nose
- mouth and palate
- dentition and occlusion
- lower face.

3. Details of associated anomalies.

- Neck and cervical spine
- shoulder girdle
- palate
- hands and feet.

4. Multidisciplinary liaison. Ear, nose and throat (ENT), ophthalmology, psychiatry, neurology, clinical genetics. Anaesthetic assessment is planned early as an outpatient.

Investigations

1. CT or MRI scan of head and face including 3D reformatting or production of milled 3D models is possible and may aid surgical planning. These investigations may require general anaesthesia or sedation in young children.

2. Plain radiographs of skull, chest, hands and feet are used to monitor progression of the defects. Lateral cephalometric and PA views of the skull and facial bones and OPG document dental development and jaw relationship defects.

3. Radionucleotide scans permit assessment of active bone growth and the time of growth cessation in adolescents.

4. Clinical photographs.

5. Functional tests. Electroencephalograph (EEG) and sleep studies and an electrocardiograph (ECG) may also be required.

6. Blood transfusion. Cross-matching is essential in major craniofacial operations.

Neurosurgical aspects

1. Monitoring of intracranial pressure. A transcranial transducer is fitted under a brief general anaesthetic.

2. Blood flow studies are undertaken in some patients and lumbar pressure measurements may be helpful.

3. Control of hydrocephalus. CSF shunting procedures may be required urgently when the presence of significant hydrocephalus is recognized. Shunting procedures may be deferred until after early vault expansion surgery to gain maximum benefit from the increase in skull volume.

Indications for urgent treatment

1. Signs of mental retardation or progressive deterioration in cognitive function not related to detectable structural brain defects are important determinants of the need for early operation.

2. *Impairment of vision* including papilloedema, severe exorbitism and the need for ocular protection due to inadequate lid closure, and dislocation of the globe with corneal ulceration all constitute ophthalmic demands for urgent surgery.

3. *Respiratory difficulties.* Impaired airway function or airway volume reduction, midface hypoplasia or choanal atresia are anatomical reasons for early intervention. Obstructive sleep apnoea is a functional indication.

4. *Absence of skin cover* occurs sometimes in children with encephaloceles.

5. *Haemorrhage.*

Elective surgery indications
- Gross anomalous development of skull and facial structures
- orbital deformity and resulting dystopia
- midface, nasal capsule or maxilla deformity
- mandibular jaw deformity may include asymmetry.

Localized functional deficits arising from these deformities may be present.

Associated problems
- Cleft lip and palate
- syndactyly
- palpebral ptosis and squints
- residual nasal deformity
- pinna and ear defects.

CRANIOFACIAL INJURIES

Patients with major head and facial injuries require immediate assessment and resuscitation. Other non-facial injuries may take precedence and may pose a greater immediate threat to life. Attention to airway patency, oxygenation and cardiovascular status precedes any attention to specific injuries.

Thoracic and abdominal wounds may produce life-threatening haemorrhage and require aggressive resuscitation and immediate surgery irrespective of the demands otherwise imposed by a concomitant head injury.

Head injury

Assessment of the severity of neurological injury is required. Conscious level, pre-traumatic amnesia, focal neurological signs and evidence of local or regional head or facial trauma are documented.

Minor degrees of brain injury are self-limiting and full recovery can be expected. Severe injury due to shear, stretch or crush of axonal tissue may occur.

Secondary brain injury due to cerebral oedema, mass effect and hypoxia are more damaging in many patients. Immediate status and post-traumatic progress is monitored using the Glasgow Coma Scale (GCS).

Skull X-rays exclude calvarial fractures, and a CT scan is required in the diagnosis of evolving neurological deficit. Neurosurgical intervention may be required for depressed skull fracture or deteriorating neurological state or conscious level.

Skull injury

Soft tissue injuries

1. *Contusions* should be examined carefully to exclude underlying fracture.

2. *Lacerations* should be closed primarily. If an underlying fracture is present, a compound injury is diagnosed. Immediate skin closure is required and neurosurgical referral instituted.

Fractures

1. *Frontal fractures.* These result from direct blunt trauma or assault. They are less common in the UK than before seatbelt wearing for vehicle occupants was mandatory. They may be linear, complex or exhibit depressed segments. Observation and GCS monitoring only may be required. If fracture reduction is required, a

bicoronal subperiosteal flap is the best approach. Fixation with low profile microplates is required.

2. *Frontal sinus.* Repair of the walls may be required. CSF leak via the frontonasal duct perinasally may occur. Obliteration cranialization or exenteration of the sinus may be required. Mucocoel formation may result. Bone or hydroxyapatite may be used to obliterate.

3. *Fronto-orbital fractures.* Where superolateral orbital rim or roof fractures are present, a combined neurosurgical and maxillofacial approach is often required. Bicoronal flaps give good access. Neurosurgical closure of the dura and evacuation of the haematoma should be performed in conjunction with reconstruction of the orbital skeleton. Ophthalmological injuries require appropriate treatment. This may be delayed until after the primary surgery to permit assessment of visual function.

4. *Naso-ethmoidal fractures.* These are complex injuries. Medial orbital walls, medial canthus and canthal ligamentous attachments should be examined. Traumatic telecanthus may result from canthal ligament rupture or detachment. Anterior and posterior ethmoidal vessels may require ligating, and concomitant nasal capsule injuries require reduction. Ocular injuries may occur. Anosmia may be a persistent post-traumatic problem due to damage to the olfactory apparatus. Nasal architecture damage can result in chronic nasal airflow obstruction.

The medial bicoronal brow or mid frontal endoscopic brow approach can be used.

Reconstruction may use calvarial bone or titanium mesh.

5. *Squamous temporal fractures.* Middle meningeal arterial haemorrhage imposes an increased risk of acute extradural haematoma formation. Depressed fractures are uncommon. High parietal fractures are more common. Venous sinus haemorrhage and dural tears are a risk. Ventricular injuries are more common in

children, the elderly and alcoholics. Neurological sequelae are very variable. Scalp injuries bleed briskly and should be closed primarily.

6. Zygomatic arch. Fractures of the arch are very common. Isolated injuries present most frequently. As part of a more severe or complex pattern of craniofacial fractures, arch reduction should be considered as part of treatment planning.

7. Petrous temporal. Horizontal or transverse and longitudinal patterns of fractures are described. CT scanning is required for diagnosis. Clinical signs include bloody otorrhoea, haemotympanum and positive Battle's sign. Pure tone audiometry is essential to document baseline hearing status and to permit monitoring of recovery of middle ear function.

8. Occipital. These are relatively uncommon fractures associated with severe head trauma and often with major head injury. Cerebellar trauma and posterior fossa haematoma are uncommon. Upper cervical vertebral injury should be excluded.

Complications
- Neurological damage
- secondary neurological damage
- haematoma formation and mass effects
- CSF leakage
- post-traumatic epilepsy
- meningitis
- ocular and hearing dysfunction
- poor post-fracture cosmetics.

Penetrating skull injuries

Calvarial fractures are very frequently associated. The risk of intracranial complications is higher than with closed injuries.

Dural tears
Associated with CSF oto- or rhinorrhoea, many are self-limiting and the CSF leak stops spontaneously.

In cases where a leak is persistent, surgical closure may be required. The bicoronal approach allows dural repair from above with or without muscle grafting.

Ascending meningitis is a risk with open dural injuries.

Haemorrhage

Intracerebral haemorrhage is associated with primary brain injury if a shearing force is applied to the skull.

Arterial tears result in brisk bleeding. Penetrating injuries do present a risk of clot accumulation even though the calvarial tables are breached.

Damage to venous sinuses may be catastrophic or self-limiting.

Cerebral oedema

Primary brain injury, hypoxia and sepsis all contribute.

Coning of the cerebellar tonsils across the foramen magnum and temporal unci across the tentorial hiatus are catastrophic. Dexamethasone may be preventative and IV mannitol infusions are a temporary holding measure to permit safe transfer to theatre.

Ventricles

Penetrating injury occasionally occurs. Pressure monitoring is a useful measure in both open and closed head injuries.

Principles of management

- CT scan
- intraventricular pressure monitors
- antibiotics
- anticonvulsants
- surgical access
- arrest of haemorrhage
- repair dura
- evacuate blood clots
- reduce fractures
- fix with microplates or titanium mesh.

CRANIOFACIAL SURGERY – PRINCIPLES

Craniofacial surgery is concerned with the treatment of patients with rare and complex congenital or acquired anomalies which together affect the head, upper face and jaws. Tessier developed and enunciated the principles of a radical surgical approach aimed at the total correction of the deformity in a limited number of operations. Better results with fewer major complications are achieved by this approach. Tessier also demonstrated the value of a multidisciplinary approach.

A craniofacial service should provide full assessment facilities including advanced imaging techniques. It should include the surgical capabilities necessary for the treatment of patients with severe congenital, traumatic or tumour-related combined deformities involving all or a major part of the cranial, facial, nasal and orbital regions. Long-term follow-up and audit are essential elements of this service.

Some surgical principles

- The facial skeleton remains viable even if stripped of much of its periosteum. It is possible to expose almost the whole craniomaxillofacial complex without detriment to the subsequent healing process.
- With the exception of the orbital foramenae, the whole craniomaxillofacial complex can be osteotomized and repositioned.
- A bitemporal or bicoronal flap is the most commonly utilised type of access for all intracranial and most subcranial procedures.

Indications for surgery

Congenital deformities; trauma; disease (neoplastic, non-neoplastic).

Timing of surgery

Advantages of early surgery (during growth phase)
- Stimulation of soft tissue development.
- Early aesthetic and functional improvement is achieved.
- Positive psychological effect on both parents and child and peer acceptance and normal assimilation into society is promoted.
- Reduction of intra-cranial pressure, prevention of visual problems and encouragement of normal mental, psychological and behavioural development.

	• Establishment of satisfactory craniofacial form and correction of an unusually shaped head and face and prompt treatment of restricted airway in cases of severe maxillofacial retrusion is possible.
Disadvantages of early surgery	• Possible untoward effects of early surgery on subsequent facial growth. • Difficulty in predicting final facial form with early surgery. • A more predictably stable result with less likelihood of relapse and multiple procedures is possible if surgery is performed at the end of growth phase. • Blood loss and fluid balance can be difficult to monitor and adequately control especially with major surgery in small infants.
Factors which have contributed to advances in craniofacial surgery	• The excellent healing potential of the craniofacial skeleton. • Innovative surgical techniques and instrumentation. • Advances in paediatric anaesthesia techniques. • Advances in radiological and imaging techniques.
	Craniofacial surgery carries a degree of risk. The determinants of risk include
General medical status of patient	• The presence of co-existing major systemic disease. • Poor nutritional status or failure to thrive. • Age, gestational maturity and physical size of patient are important.
Specific respiratory difficulties	Airway obstruction may be a significant problem with: • naso–maxillary and midface hypoplasia; • structural deformity of naso pharynx; • choanal atresia; • tracheal ring defects; • upper tract infections.
Associated congenital anomalies	Cardiac, renal, cleft lip and palate, and skeletal abnormalities all increase the potential for operative complications.
Severity of specific cranial deformity	The important factors are: • number of sutures involved in craniostenotic process;

- presence of raised intra-cranial pressure;
- anatomical abnormalities and defects of the cranial base;
- localized skull irregularities and cranial bone defects, for example, 'copper beating';
- presence of structural defects of brain or meninges;
- presence of intra-cranial vascular anomalies.

Social factors

Attention to the psycho–social condition of the patient and to the support available is essential. The factors of note include:

- patient cooperation and understanding;
- ethnic and language difficulties;
- unfavourable psychological status of patient;
- parental cooperation and understanding;
- home conditions;

Surgical approaches

Incisions

A bicoronal scalp flap or unilateral fronto–temporal scalp flap are standard modes of access for most craniofacial operations. In addition access to the inferior aspect of the orbit, nasal capsule, zygomatic arch and oral cavity may all be required. Transconjunctival, blepharoplasty, standard infra-orbital, paranasal, and intra-oral incisions may be used in conjunction.

Osteotomies

There are many patterns of osteotomy described and each has its specific uses and many have modifications. Strip craniectomy, parasagittal craniectomy, cranioplasty, floating forehead, fronto-orbital advancement, fronto-cranial remodelling, transcranial Le Fort III, subcranial Le Fort III osteotomies may be planned.

Orbital dystopia and hypertelorism may require Tessier or Converse procedures.

Fixation

Transosseous wires, bone plates and screws, titanium mesh and absorbable suture material all have uses.

Halo frames, bone pins and external fixation may all be required. Intra-oral fixation with arch bars, orthodontic appliances and preformed splints may be placed.

| **Harvesting bone grafts** | Sources include: |
| | |

- calvarial;
- iliac crest;
- rib;
- bone slurry from cranial bur holes.

Dural repair

Prevention of postoperative CSF leak is essential. Dural repair by direct suture, pericranial patch or fascia lata patch is sometimes necessary.

Other procedures

Rhinoplasty; tarsorrhaphy; cranioplasty (correction of defects in skull contour with alloplastic materials including titanium mesh or plates) are sometimes performed.

Long-term morbidity

- Ischaemic tissue loss affecting calvarial bone or scalp.
- Cranial nerve damage.
- Peripheral nerve damage.
- Infection of bone.
- Infection associated with bone plates or transosseous wires.
- Sinus disease; frontal sinus mucocele, chronic maxillary sinusitis or surgical ciliated cyst formation.
- Naso-lachrymal duct damage.
- Velopharyngeal incompetence.
- Unacceptable scars; wide scars, hair loss in relation to scar, hypertrophic or keloid scars.
- Graft donor site morbidity.
- Loss of grafted materials.

Related topics of interest

CUTANEOUS TUMOURS OF THE HEAD AND NECK

Keratoses

Seborrhoeic keratoses   Very common, elevated plaques. Superficial scaling may be present. There is no premalignant potential. Excision for cosmetic reasons may be required.

Actinic keratoses   Sun exposed skin areas are at risk. Wart like growths these lesions occasionally become inflamed. Scale is typical and may be marked and hyperkeratotic. Patients most at risk include fair skinned persons and those whose occupation entails high sunlight (UV) light exposure. Incidence is higher in fair skinned Caucasians. These lesions are considered to be premalignant. Excision biopsy is required. Epithelial dysplasia may progress to squamous carcinoma. Treatments of the keratosis have included shave excision, cryotherapy, and topical antimitotic agents such as 5 fluorouracil.

Basal cell carcinoma (BCC)

The most common skin malignancy. Risk factors include light skin colour, excess UV exposure, scars and immunocompromise results in a more aggressive clinical course when BCC occurs. The precise relationship between duration of sunlight or UV exposure and BCC incidence is unclear. BCCs are locally invasive and rarely metastasize. One per cent are infiltrative and perineural spread is described.

Types of BCC   *1. Fibro-epitheliomatous.* Raised, firm and erythematous.

2. Morpheic. Almost exclusively affects facial skin. Yellow plaques with poorly defined margins. The most aggressive type.

3. Nodulo-ulceratrive. Most common. Telangectatic, nodular becoming necrotic and ulcerated centrally. Border increasingly raised and rolled.

4. Superficial. Predominantly truncal lesions. Eczematous, indurated and erythematous.

5. Pigmented. Similar appearance to ulcerative type. More deeply pigmented.

6. Gorlin–Goltz Syndrome. Basal cell neavus syndrome. Autosomal dominant condition with increased risk of BCCs and multilocular keratocysts of the jaws. The greatest incidence of BCCs occurs between the ages of 20 and 40 and the number of lesions is very variable. Careful follow up and early excision of lesions is required as they can be very destructive if untreated.

Management of BCC

- Early diagnosis.
- Excision and histological confirmation of diagnosis.
- Cryosurgery, electrofulguration and topical chemotherapy have all been used.
- Radiotherapy is effective.
- Recurrence rates at 5 years are reported as 7.7–10% for cryosurgery and excision, respectively. DXT results in a 8–9% 5 year recurrence rate.
- *Mohs micrographic surgery.* Effective in reducing recurrence rates in surgical excision. Involves accurate delineation of surgical excision site and intra-operative frozen section followed by precisely guided re-excision.

Keratocanthoma

Clinically resembles a squamous cell carcinoma (SCC). Rapidly enlarging smooth, domed, keratinized, verrucous nodules. They attain maximum dimensons in 2–3 months and growth then slows or ceases. Involution occurs after several months. Occasionally central facial lesions are aggressive and multiple lesions may reflect a propensity for deep invasion or metastatsis. Excision is curative.

Squamous cell carcinoma (SCC)

The second most common cutaneous malignancy after BCC. It occurs most frequently in elderly males. It accounts for 20% of all skin tumours and about 90% of these affect the head and neck.

Aetiological factors
- UV exposure.
- Chemical exposure (coal tar, soot, petroleum derivatives).
- Immunosuppression.
- Advanced age.
- Papilloma virus infection (role uncertain).

Prognostic factors
- Anatomic site.
- Precise histology.
- Tumour size and depth of invasion.
- Immunological status (severe impairment results in increased risk of multiple primaries and a poor prognosis).
- Bowen's disease; intradermal SCC. Superficial plane of spread. Thirty per cent become invasive SCC. Excision should be radical.
- Recurrence rate increased in lesions of ear, lip, temporal skin, chronic skin lesions, ulcers, burns and scars.

Treatment
- Wide local excision.
- Deep clearance may be required.
- En bloc nodal excision may require neck dissection.
- Reconstruction with local or distant flaps if extensive resection has been performed.
- Adjunctive radio or chemotherapy may be required but its role depends on tumour site, size and differentiation.

Melanoma

Risk factors

1. Prolonged UV or sunlight exposure. Worse if excessive UV exposure occurs in early childhood or if associated with severe or repeated sunburn injury.

2. Pre-existing pigmented lesion. Seventy to 75% of head and neck melanomas arise in a pre-existing mole.

3. Race and complexion type. Fair skinned Caucasians are most at risk.

4. Age. Melanomas are more common after the fifth decade although this picture is changing with increasing incidence of this tumour amongst younger people.

5. Immunosuppression.

Subtypes of malignant melanoma

Lentigo maligna. Affects the sun exposed head and neck typically in older patient. Ninety per cent of these lesions occur on the face and neck. Initially macular hyperpigmented area becoming nodular once invasion has occurred.

Superficial spreading melanoma. Less common on the head or neck these lesions more commonly occur on the back or lower limb. Irregular shaped macular lesions.

Nodular malignant melanoma. Typically a blue black nodule affecting the trunk or face.

Acral lentiginous melanoma. Uncommon in the head and neck. Hands and feet typically involved with a deeply melanotic mixed pattern macular and nodular lesion.

Mucosal melanomas. These lesions behave in a more aggressive fashion than cutaneous lesions and have a poorer prognosis. They are less common, exhibit a slower rate of nodal metastasis and frequently spread to distant sites before diagnosis of the primary lesion.

Clinical features

Clinically suspicious pigmented lesions

- Altered skin sensation (pain or itch are important).
- Diameter increasing (lesions greater than 1cm diameter are suspicious).
- Irregular margins.

- Colour variegation.
- Inflammation.
- Bleeding or crusting.
- Satellite lesions.

Physical signs

In addition to the lesion which may be noted by the patient, regional lymph nodes may be enlarged. Extensive lymphadenopathy is described but malignant melanomata often metastasize before extensive lymph node disease is clinically apparent. The tumour has a predilection for liver and pulmonary tissue and secondary deposits are common in these sites. Neural tissue is quite frequently involved in head and neck lesions; cerebral metastatic deposits are well documented.

Histological diagnosis

1. *Biopsy* is required either by excision or punch biopsy. Marginal incision biopsy is acceptable in very large lesions but scrape or shave methods are not. No estimation of lesion thickness and extent of deep invasion can be made from such samples.

2. *Breslow thickness* records the depth of tumour invasion in millimetres from the granular layer of the epithelium to the deepest extent reached by tumour cells. It corrrelates with prognosis.

3. *Clark levels.* A similar index of depth of melanoma invasion which correlates with prognosis.

- Level 1 Intra-dermal neavus or *in situ* melanoma.
- Level 2 papillary dermis invaded.
- Level 3 papillary dermis breached but reticular dermis not invaded.
- Level 4 reticular dermis invaded.
- Level 5 subdermal fat invaded.

Treatment

1. *Surgical excision of the primary lesion* is the treatment of choice. Wide excision with a 1 cm margin is usually planned for tumours with a Breslow thickness of less then 2 mm. Thicker lesions require wider excision but extension of the resection margins beyond about 3 cm is not effective in improving life expectancy. In the head and neck, the proximity of vital structures such as eyes may limit the extent of resection,

although radical surgery is possible if it is considered a likely curative option.

2. Regional lymphadenopathy. Cervical lymph node biopsy, if positive for malignant melanoma usually requires a radical neck dissection to be performed. Some reserve radical neck dissection for extensive neck metastatic disease and with an isolated cervical node demonstrating melanotic deposits, a functional dissection is performed. Radiotherapy for neck disease may be helpful, particularly if extracapsular spread of tumour has been demonstrated histologically.

3. Distant metastases. The use of radiotherapy, systemic chemotherapy or immuno-modulation with BCG serial vaccinations remains of uncertain benefit for most patients. Occasionally multiple excisions may be performed but the survival rates are not significantly improved.

Sarcomas

Skin adnexae and the underlying connective tissues may be the sites of cutaneous sarcoma formation. More superficial lesions have a slightly better prognosis than deeper adnexal lesions. Fibrosarcomas, angiosarcomas and Kapsosi's sarcomas affecting head and neck skin are all described.

Related topics of interest

Head and neck oncology – biological aspects (p. 178)
Head and neck oncology – principles of patient management (p. 184)

Revision point

Anatomy and histology of skin and mucosa

CYSTS

A cyst is a pathological cavity whose contents may be solid, fluid or gaseous but not formed due to an accumulation of pus and whose lining if present may consist of an epithelium. This is a comprehensive definition based on that of Kramer (1974).

There are several theories about the mechanism of development of jaw cysts but none is entirely satisfactory. For intrabony cysts to expand, production of prostaglandin-like mediators (previously termed osteoclast-activating factors; OAFs) is important, but the role of increasing hydrostatic pressure in the cavity is less clear. For fissural or soft tissue cysts, the role of epithelial inclusions or cell remnants remains unclear. The role of embryological remnants in branchial cysts is not currently thought be important, but involutional changes in a cervical lymph node are believed to be responsible for the formation of these lesions.

A clinical classification is required, and the most widely used is the one proposed by WHO.

Classification of jaw cysts

Epithelial cysts can be developmental in origin or related to an inflammatory focus. Those of developmental origin can arise from odontogenic or non-odontogenic tissues.

Odontogenic developmental cysts

1. *Keratocysts*. These lesions occur most frequently in the mandibular ramus. They are typically multi-locular and have a tendency to recur after excision. A good margin of bony clearance is therefore required. Clinical and histological differentiation from ameloblastoma is necessary, as the latter lesion is much more locally destructive.

2. *Dentigerous or follicular cysts*. These cysts are fairly common and arise from the follicle of an unerupted tooth. They can become very large before presentation. Bony expansion may occur. Removal of the involved tooth and cyst enucleation is usually curative.

3. *Eruption cysts* in infants may delay eruption of the underlying tooth, and simple 'de-roofing' will expose the tooth to permit eruption.

4. *Gingival cysts* in both children and adults occur.

5. Calcifying odontogenic cysts are rare lesions, but enucleation is thought to be adequate treatment.

Non-odontogenic developmental cysts

The fissural cysts, so called, occur occasionally and must be differentiated from inflammatory dental cysts arising from the adjacent teeth. They include globullomaxillary cysts, nasopalatine cysts, nasolabial cysts, median palatine and median mandibular cysts.

Inflammatory cysts

Chronically infected teeth may progress to formation of apical or lateral radicular cysts. If cystic tissue is left *in situ* after tooth removal, it may reform and present as a residual cyst. Enucleation is curative.

Non-epithelial and bone cysts

These include simple bone cysts and haemorrhagic bone cysts.

Cysts of the other orofacial tissues

Skin cysts such as dermoids, salivary gland cysts and inclusions such as Stafne cavities are all well described. Neck cysts such as branchial, thyroglossal and cystic hygroma are all developmental in origin, although they may present later in life. Antral cysts are easily missed but may present with displacement of teeth. Cystic tumours are documented in the head and neck, parasitic cysts occur but are rare.

Pseudocysts

Encephalocele and *meningocele* occur and represent herniation rather than true cyst formation. They may be mistaken for cyst cavities if an extensive fluid or CSF filled sac is present.

Salivary extravasation cysts and mucous retention cysts are common, as are false cysts whose lining is attenuated, compressed gland tissue rather than true capsule and whose contents are composed of saliva.

There are other classifications of jaw cysts which take more account of the other features in cyst pathology such as the luminal production of keratin, ossification, multiloculation and whether there is any metabolic derangement associated with their formation or presentation.

Differential diagnosis

The important diagnostic features include dental and periodontal conditions, clinical and X-ray evidence of bone expansion or lysis, systemic upset and results of baseline biochemistry. Tissue diagnosis, initially from aspiration cytology and later from microscopic examination of surgically excised tissue completes the diagnostic picture.

Teeth   Periodontal destruction and tooth movement are typical of cyst behaviour. Root resorption occurs occasionally. Dead and discoloured tooth may be associated with a chronic inflammatory apical cyst. Root displacement due to cyst enlargement occurs and root resorption may be associated with locally destructive odontogenic lesions or secondary metastatic disease from distant malignancy.

Bone   Bone lysis and intrabony cyst enlargement occur due to production of prostaglandin-like mediators such as OAF. The source of the OAF and related mediators is probably the cyst lining. Expansion in cysts with no defined lining remains difficult to explain.

Mucosa   Mucosal attenuation and thinning may occur adjacent to a rapidly expanding jaw cyst. Intramucosal cysts occur. Mucous retention or extravasation lesions are examples. Excision is curative. Rarely, mucosal hyperplasia, hyperkeratosis or ulceration may occur in association with an underlying cystic lesion.

Skin   Skin cysts may be epidermal, deep dermal or formed in the underlying connective tissues. Infected cysts present by inflamed swelling on facial skin or purulent discharge on to the face.

Antra and sinuses Polyps and mucoceles are common. If excision is planned, a Caldwell Luc approach is usually required although an endoscopic approach may equally permit complete removal of such lesions.

Lymph nodes   Cysts are not typically associated with cervical lymphadenopathy unless chronically infected or cystic neoplasms. Whether branchial cysts arise as a result of cervical node degeneration remains to be fully determined.

Syndromes	Kartageners (ciliary immotility syndrome) and Gorlin Goltz syndromes are associated with frontal sinus expansion and mucocele formation and keratocyst formation respectively.

Treatment

Medical measures	Investigation of plasma calcium and phosphate is important in assessment of odontogenic keratocysts.
Marsupialization	A technique rarely used in practice today. It was previously thought appropriate for treatment of antral and some types of dental cysts. Enucleation or excision is preferred in modern practice.
Enucleation	This technique involves removal of the cyst lining and permits histopathological diagnosis.
Excision	Appropriate for treatment of large mandibular keratocysts particulary after local recurrence after enucleation. These lesions may require treatment by block excision, or more radical surgery if the risk of recurrence is considered significant.
Reconstruction	Reconstruction may become an issue if resection of an extensive cystic lesion has been required. Cancellous bone grafting to the cyst cavity or bone grafting for mandible reconstruction may be planned. Biomechanical or prosthetic materials may be used. These may include titanium mesh and, later, osseointegrated implants. Free vascularized tissue transfer is occasionally a suitable option if composite bone and soft tissue reconstruction is required.

Further reading

Kramer I. Changing Views on Oral Disease. *Proceedings of the Royal Society of Medicine,* 1974; **61:** 271–76.

Pindborg J. and Kramer I. Histological Typing of Odontogenic Tumours, Jaw Cysts and Fluid Lesions, World Health Organisation, Geneva.

ENDOSCOPY

Techniques to visualize the upper aerodigestive track and related structures have developed rapidly. Diagnostic and therapeutic uses may be made of this technology. Arthroscopy of the TMJ permits examination and operation.

Instrumentation

1. Simple endoscopy. Indirect laryngoscopy using long-handled laryngeal mirror and head light. Very useful technique for visualizing root of tongue, epiglottis, valleculae, pyriform fossae and supraglottic larynx. Routine part of systematic head and neck examination.

2. Fibre-optic endoscopy. Operates using principle of total internal reflection to ensure image transmission. The essential features of any fibre-optic endoscope include

- coherent fibre bundles for high-quality visual image transmission.
- non-coherent fibre-optic bundles for light transmission.
- a lens system near the eyepiece of the instrument.
- a proximal control system to manoeuvre the tip of the instrument and also to control suction and air–water flow.
- channel for passing air or carbon dioxide and water down the instrument.
- channel for suction which doubles as a biopsy channel.
- wire guide incorporated to control tip movement.
- cladding, consisting of a flexible, jointed construction, covered by a tough outer vinyl sheath.

3. Rigid endoscopy. Operating by principle of total internal reflection to produce image transmission, rigid fibre-optic glass rods require multiple lens systems to produce a clear view. The image is magnified and rectified, the primary lens is situated near the tip and the relay lens system is in the eyepiece. TMJ arthroscopes require continuous irrigation and multiple percutaneous ports. Viewing ports at different angles from 0° to 70° or 90° are available. Similar rigid rods are used for purposes of FESS.

4. Non-fibre-optic systems. Pharyngo-oesophagoscopy is possible using straight non-optically enhanced rigid endoscopes.

5. Light sources. Powerful halogen illumination is required by most fibre-optic systems.

6. Operating endoscopy. Biopsy, brushings and scrapings for cytology and foreign body extraction is possible. Suture placement, injection techniques and a variety of operative procedures are performed via endoscopic access. Laser transmission via fibre-optic cables is possible. This is the basis of minimal access surgery. It is not frequently used in head and neck surgery.

7. Visual enhancements. Microscopy, photography, video presentation and recording are all possible. Television screening of endoscope generated images are a good method of permitting the surgeon a more comfortable view of the operative site and students to gain a more instructive view.

Clinical uses

1. Fibre-optic nasendoscopy. Performed pernasally. Mucosal anaesthesia is obtained using cocaine or lignocaine spray. Superior laryngeal nerve infiltration may be used in preference. A fine endoscope is passed giving a narrow field of view but permitting simple examination to be performed as an outpatient. A wide variety of indications for this examination now exist. These include assessment of mucosal lesions from nose, nasopharynx down to supraglottic larynx, assessment of palatal and pharyngeal wall function in cleft patients, assessment of treatment and oncological condition in head and neck cancer and performance of Mueller manoeuvre in patients with obstructive sleep apnoea.

2. Pharyngo-laryngoscopy. Direct, rigid endoscopy. Requires GA. Difficult in patients with limited head extension. Good views of pharynx and larynx are obtained due to wide field of view. Operative correction of many vocal cord or laryngeal lesions is possible. Removal of polyps and nodules, injection of Teflon into vocal cords, stricture dilatation and preoperative packing of pharyngeal pouches are all readily performed.

3. Oesophagoscopy. Rigid oesophagoscopy for assessment of dysphagia, retrieval of foreign bodies and biopsy of upper luminal mucosal lesions may be performed. Lower oesophageal examination is more commonly performed by flexible gastroscopy as part of an upper gastrointestinal examination.

4. TMJ arthroscopy. Indications include internal joint derangements, arthritides and after condyle or joint trauma. Contraindications include periarticular sepsis and severe ankylosis. Performed under GA by preference although the technique is possible under LA. Both joint compartments may be examined. Inferolateral, anterolateral percutaneous or endaural puncture gives access to the upper compartment. The lower compartment is not routinely entered due to the risk of condyle and meniscal damage. Irrigation and manipulation is possible under arthroscopic visualization and requires separate portals.

5. FESS. Access to the paranasal sinus system via a Caldwell–Luc puncture or via the inferior meatal route is routinely performed. Diagnosis of mucosal lesions is readily achieved. More complex manipulations in ethmoid and frontal sinuses require middle meatal access.

6. Endoscopic cosmetic surgery. Brow lifts have been performed by endoscopic means. Percutaneous puncture from a lateral approach is required.

Related topic of interest

Functional endoscopic sinus surgery (FESS) (p. 161)

FACIAL NERVE

Anatomy

The seventh cranial or facial nerve is almost purely motor. It has sensory (visceral afferent) and parasympathetic (visceral efferent) fibres of the nervus intermedius associated with it. It may be described in several segments.

- Brain stem nuclei: *the motor nucleus* lies in the mid pontine section of the brain stem. Fibres from this structure pass posteriorly and cranially to loop around the abducens nucleus before traversing the brain stem anteriorly passing medial to the pontine part of the trigeminal nucleus.

  The superior salivatory nucleus is the origin of the parasympathetic fibres serving the submandibular glands and the lacrimal gland.

  The nucleus of tractus solitarius receives taste impulses from the anterior two-thirds of the tongue via the chorda tympani nerve.
- Meatal: *from the brain stem to the internal auditory meatus* fibres of facial nerve and nervus intermedius travel together.
- Labyrinthine: internal auditory canal to facial hiatus of fallopian tube.
- Tympanic: *from the geniculate ganglion to pyramidal process* of the middle ear. Greater petrosal nerve, stapedial nerve and chorda tympani all arise from the nerve at this part.
- Mastoid: *from the pyramidal process to stylomastoid foramen,* no branches arise.
- Extracranial: *from the stylomastoid foramen via squamotympanic fissure* the motor nerve traverses the parotid gland to reach the muscles of facial expression.

  Extracranial branches. The patterns are very variable but typically the fibre distribution is *temporal* to frontalis, and orbicularis oculi, *zygomatic* to the lower orbital muscles, *buccal* to the lateral nasal muscles, buccinator and upper lip, *mandibular* to the perioral muscles and lower lip, and *cervical* to platysma.

Embryology

The facial nerve is the nerve to the second branchial arch structures, in particular to the muscles of facial expression. The chorda tympani is the pre-trematic nerve between the first and second arches.

Functions

Nervus intermedius

1. Taste. The sensory part of the nerve subserves taste from the anterior two-thirds of the tongue, impulses being relayed by the chorda tympani to the nucleus of tractus solitarius. Cell bodies from these fibres lie in the geniculate ganglion. Taste sensation arising from the posterior tongue and pharynx is relayed via the glossopharyngeal nerve to the same nucleus.

2. *Tears.* The presynaptic parasympathetic fibres travelling in the nervus intermedius traverse the geniculate ganglion without synapsing and emerge as the greater superficial petrosal nerve. These fibres join the sympathetic fibres of the deep petrosal nerve and form the nerve of the pterygoid canal. They synapse in the sphenopalataine ganglion to provide postganglionic fibres to the lacrimal glands. The central nucleus for these fibres is the superior salivary nucleus in the lower pontine part of the brain stem.

3. *Saliva.* The presynaptic parasympathetic fibres traverse the geniculate ganglion without synapsing and emerge with the taste fibres as part of the chorda tympani. They synapse in the submandibular ganglion for secetomotor supply to the submandibular and sublingual glands. The central nucleus for these fibres is the superior salivary nucleus in the lower pons.

Reflexes

1. *Stapedial reflex and auditory acuity.* The nerve to the stapedius permits moderation of the intensity of sound transmitted across the ossicular chain. It may enhance reception of low-intensity sound and protect the cochlea against damage due to very high intensity sounds.

2. *Corneal reflex.* The efferent limb of the blink reflex initiated on touching the cornea is mediated by facial nerve fibres. Unilateral loss of blink suggests a lower motor facial nerve lesion, whereas bilateral blink failure suggests a lesion affecting the ophthalmic division of the trigeminal nerve.

Sensation

It is probable that a few cutaneous sensory fibres from the external auditory meatus are present in the facial nerve. Geniculate ganglion herpes may therefore present in this area.

Motor

1. *Motor fibres* for posterior auricular nerve supplying occipitalis and periauricular muscles and the nerve to stylohyoid and posterior belly of digastric arise immediately peripheral to the stylomastoid foramen.

2. *Pes anserinus*. The motor branches to facial expression muscles divide within the parotid gland.

Facial palsy

Clinical problems include exclusion of facial weakness in patients with mild idiopathic facial asymmetry and localization of neurological lesions where true facial paresis is demonstrated.

Facial asymmetry

True congenital causes of asymmetry must be excluded. Where mild soft tissue asymmetry is present, forehead and periorbital wrinkles and the nasolabial fold give some indication of the underlying muscle tone.

Patterns of facial weakness

Laterality and level are important clinical features.

1. *Upper motor neurone lesions* (supranuclear lesions) will produce lower facial weakness. The weakness does not affect the forehead which has bilateral cortical representation. The neurological lesion is contralateral to the lower facial weakness. The causes include vascular events, tumours and demyelination. Bilateral upper motor neurone (UMN) lesions are rare and some are likely to be fatal.

2. *Lower motor neurone lesions* (nuclear and infranuclear lesions) produce full ipsilateral hemifacial weakness including the forehead. They may be unilateral or bilateral. The causes of bilateral LMN facial nerve lesions include pontine vascular events, demyelination, tumours and abscess formation. Moebius syndrome may be a cause; it is a rare congenital agenesis of the facial and abducens nuclei. Guillain–Barre syndrome and rarely Bell's palsy may occur bilaterally. Muscle diseases, including dysptrophia myotonica and myasthenia gravis may also be causative.

Unilateral facial paralysis	*LMN lesions* of this type are a common clinical presentation. Differentiating nuclear from infranuclear lesions depends on the presence of other neurological signs. Contralateral limb weakness suggests a pontine level lesion and therefore a nuclear facial nerve lesion. Cerebello-pontine angle lesions typically affect multiple cranial nerves as well as producing hyperacusis and disturbances of lacrimation, taste and salivation. Lacrimation is affected in a proximal lesion of the facial canal but is spared in a more distal lesion. Salivation and taste are affected by all facial canal lesions. Facial level lesions affect only muscle function, leaving lacrimation, salivation and taste intact.

Causes

1. Idiopathic

- Bell's palsy
- Melkersson–Rosenthal syndrome.

2. Traumatic

- Temporal bone fractures
- Birth trauma or forceps delivery injuring the pre-auricular tissues
- Facial contusions or lacerations
- Penetrating wounds to the face in the parotid region
- Iatrogenic injury including neurosurgical procedures and after parotidectomy.

3. Infection

- Herpes zoster otticus (Ramsey Hunt syndrome)
- *Otitic infections*; otitis media with effusion, acute suppurative otitis media, mastoiditis, chronic serous otitis media, malignant otitis external (*Pseudomonas osteomyelitis*)
- Specific infections; tuberculosis, Lyme disease, AIDS, infectious mononucleosis.

4. Neoplasia

- Cholesteatoma
- glomus jugulare or tympanicum
- carcinoma (primary or metastatic)
- facial neuroma

- acoustic neuroma or Schwannoma
- meningioma
- leukaemia or leukaemic deposits.

5. Metabolic

- Pregnancy
- Diabetes mellitus
- Sarcoidosis (uveoparotid fever)
- Guillain–Barre syndrome
- Autoimmune disorders.

Investigations

1. Blood samples. Baseline haematology and biochemistry.

2. Imaging. MRI is preferred. CT scans of the internal auditory meatus (IAM) have largely superceded IAM tomography. Plain radiographs demonstrating middle ear structures may be obtained.

3. Audiometry. Pure tone audiometry (PTA) is widely used as a diagnostic aid. Charting of acoustic reflexes and calorimetry may be useful in the demonstration of acoustic neuromata.

4. Schirmer's test. Lacrimation may be examined by this technique which detects volume and rate of tear production by absorption on to a soft paper strip placed in the lower conjunctival fornix.

5. Electrophysiology. Nerve excitability tests, electromyography and electroneuronography may all be performed if required.

Some specific conditions

Bell's palsy

This condition represents about 50% of all facial palsies and is considered to be an acute demyelination characterized by viral prodrome (sometimes) and delayed onset of unilateral loss of facial expression, hyperacusis, loss of taste and difficulty chewing. Ten per cent of patients have a positive family history and

10% suffer recurrent episodes. Idiopathic Bell's palsy is less likely if trauma has occurred, if multiple cranial nerves are involved, if there are signs of neoplasia, if viral vesicles are present or if the paresis is slowly progressive or very chronic. Pregnancy and diabetes may predispose. The commonest complication of Bell's palsy is corneal dryness and scarring due to inadequate eyelid closure. A synthetic tear film may be of help if prescribed. Treatment with steroids remains controversial but is commonly given in spite of the doubts about the long-term benefits. Surgical decompression at the level of the facial canal is also performed occasionally.

Infection

Ramsey Hunt syndrome is caused by geniculate ganglion herpetic infection. Facial and pharyngeal vesicles may present as part of the prodrome. Underlying malignancy, immunocompromise or AIDS may predispose. Antiherpetic agents, including acyclovir, are often beneficial.

Traumatic or iatrogenic

Any injury with penetrating facial trauma or temporal bone fracture may be associated with a dense facial nerve palsy. Mastoid, tympanum or parotid gland surgery may be causative.

Neoplastic

A facial paresis which is slowly evolving, associated with other focal neurology, facial twitching, multiple cranial nerve deficits or with chronic Eustachian tube dysfunction suggests a possible malignant cause. A neck or parotid mass or history of previous head or neck malignancy is suspicious.

Treatment and rehabilitation of long-term facial palsy

Trauma

Surgical exploration of wounds acutely or ideally after an interval may permit microneural repair or reanastomosis.

Otological

Decompression or mastoid exploration may reduce the pressure effects of perineural oedema and permit the condition to resolve.

Orofacial

Tendon transfer or tendon sling procedures can ameliorate the effects of facial palsy on the eyelids and cornea. Problems due to oral commisural weakness cause speech defects, swallowing difficulties and drooling. *Prosthetic aids,* slings and denture modifications reduce the effect of chronic paresis on facial contour.

Oculoplastic   Gold weights inserted into the eyelid margins permit augmentation and improve palpebral closure.

Facial reanimation surgery   Microvascular surgery permits free tissue transfer of vascularized and innervated musculature. Cable grafting using sural nerves or cross-over facial nerve grafting may be performed.

Involuntary facial movements or 'tics'

There are many patterns of involuntary facial movements.

Blepharospasm and hemifacial muscle spasm are quite common. If intracranial arterial aneurysm and nerve compression is occurring, neurosurgical decompression may be of benefit. Demyelination may be causative. The idiopathic pattern is commonest. *Botulinus* intramuscular injections are occasionally beneficial.

Drug-induced dyskinesias are common in the elderly on long-term phenothiazine drugs. This form is largely irreversible.

Disseminated demyelination or malignancy may cause myokymia, particularly in the mid or lower facial musculature.

FISTULAE

A fistula is an anomalous communication between two epithelial lined surfaces such as two hollow visci or a hollow viscus and the exterior body surface. There are several types of fistula. They may be pathological in origin. They may arise as a complication in the postoperative or post-radiotherapy phase of treatment. The third sort of fistula is a planned iatrogenic one.

Pathological fistulae

1. Iatrogenic. Fistula formation after neck dissection, where extensive primary malignancy has also been resected and peristomal fistulae are well described. Salivary fistulae, in particular parotid fistula after gland excision are difficult to treat and occur in about 0.5% of parotidectomies performed for tumour.

2. Developmental. Thyroglossal fistulae and branchial remnants can persist into early adulthood and may require excision if they become infected. Cleft palate children often have wide oro-nasal fistulae. These may also occur after palate closure.

3. Inflammatory and neoplastic. Orocutaneous fistulae can form spontaneously from a focus of chronic sepsis or tumour deposit. Actinomycotic fistulae and tuberculous or scrofulous fistulae are rare examples.

4. Arterio-venous. Pathological shunts can occur in many regions of the vascular tree. In the neck, post-surgical or post-radiotherapy arterio-venous (AV) fistulae can occur. Carotico-cavernous fistulae causing pulsatile, tender unilateral proptosis are also described but are rare.

5. Other systemic fistulae. Encountered include urinary, gastrointestinal and aorto–enteric types. Cutaneo–intestinal fistulae can be of the high output type and protein and calorie requirements can be very great necessitating parenteral feeding until closure occurs.

Planned iatrogenic fistulae

1. Tracheostomy. A surgical portal into the upper airway can be performed as a lifesaving emergency measure or as part of a planned surgical procedure. Post-laryngectomy tracheostomes are examples of permanent fistulae.

2. *PEG*. Percutaneous endoscopic gastrostomy is a straightforward means of introducing a feeding portal into the stomach wall.

3. *Feeding jejunostomy*. A useful technique in pharyngeal surgery where a gastric 'pull up' has been performed making a PEG inappropriate.

4. *Vascular shunts*. In excision of carotid body tumours or in neck dissection to clear disease intimately related to the carotid system, insertion of a vascular shunt may be required.

Surgical closure of head and neck fistulae

1. *Most fistulae will close without the need for surgery.* Relief of distal obstruction to allow fistula closure is a surgical axiom and in the case of mucocutaneous fistulae between mouth or pharynx and neck the use of a temporary non-oral route of feeding is necessary. Good nutrition with adequate supply of calories and nitrogen are essential to ensure sound closure of the fistulous track.

2. *Where surgical closure is deemed necessary,* excision of the fistulous track and grafting of healthy tissue into the site is essential. In the neck, axial flaps such as a pectoralis major may be required to give sufficient bulk of healthy vascularized tissue. Free flaps may be used but carry a significant risk of failure as the conditions predisposing to fistula formation are also those associated with flap failure. Sepsis, poor vascularity and residual malignant disease are the principle problems.

3. *On occasions,* the patient may be best served by accepting the presence of the fistula, as quality of life in terminal illness may be better served by avoidance of further surgery.

4. Oro-antral and oro-nasal fistulae are usually iatrogenic or postoperative in origin. Oro-antral fistulae may occur after removal of maxillary posterior teeth and will often close spontaneously. Surgical closure may be required in some patients. Oro-nasal fistulae are commonest in cleft palate patients. Surgical closure is often required.

FIXATION

Fracture healing requires all bone segments to be held without movement relative to one another in good anatomical position. Mobility at fracture sites will result in an increased risk of fibrous union. Good fixation results in new bone formation in the form of a callus, which is slowly remodelled to restore adult pattern bone with near normal contour if the reduction has been adequate.

Metabolic aspects of fracture healing are important, particularly in maxillofacial injuries as feeding is often difficult. Some degree of weight loss is usual in patients, which suggests that protein and calorie intake is insufficient for normal maintenance requirements. The higher demand during the healing phase after a bone fracture further exacerbates this deficit. Protein, calories, minerals and a normal endocrine environment are essential.

In orthognathic surgery, the principles of fixation are essentially those of fracture management.

Principles

Fixation may be rigid, semi- or non-rigid and be placed internally or externally. Accurate apposition, good angulation and occlusion, absence of soft tissue interposition and reduction of deforming or shear forces across the fracture are important to ensure sound bony union. Soft tissue cover, of both skin and mucosa should be established as early as possible and is essential where internal fixation is used.

Techniques

Splints

1. Dental methods. Adhesive dental materials acid-etched on to teeth may aid stabilization of dento-alveolar fractures. This pattern of fixation has little application in definitive fracture management.

Acid-etched brackets and arch wires have a role in stabilization after orthognathic surgery, in particular after segmental osteotomies.

2. Arch bars. Malleable arch bar material can be fashioned at operation, or preoperative impressions may be taken and custom-made arch bars prepared. Interdental wiring for fixation of the arch bar is required.

3. Full coverage acrylic splints. Using hard, impact-resistant acrylic, a cemented splint can be made to a dental impression. They are most useful in dento-alveolar injuries and segmental osteotomies. Oral hygiene is often difficult once the splint is *in situ*.

Wiring

1. Direct wiring. Interdental wires (eyelets and Leonard buttons) for stabilization of small dento-alveolar fragments may be used. Intra-osseous wires such as upper border or lower border wires are well described for mandibular fractures.

2. Peralveolar wiring. An effective means in the maxilla for securing splints, but less useful in the mandible. This is inserted by hole preparation and passing the wire loaded on to an awl.

3. Suspension wiring. Transzygomatic, frontal, pyriform fossa wires are used to maintain the vertical position of fracture segments and are wired into an arch bar or cleat-bearing splint.

4. Circumferential wiring. Circum-mandibular wires passed around the lower border of the mandible in the submucosal plane may be used to secure an acrylic or Gunning pattern splint.

5. Intra-osseous wires. Kirschner wires are inserted with a power drill in the long axis of a bone. They have several uses, including management of edentulous fractured mandible, transfacial fixation of zygomatic complex fractures and in condylar neck fractures. Encircling wires may be used to secure a 'K' wire.

IMF

1. Intermaxillary or maxillomandibular fixation. Stability of fracture segments can be achieved by placing the teeth in normal occlusion and using the dental interdigitation to ensure a good functional position.

2. Extra-oral craniomandibular fixation. This requires use of a halo or box frame to unite a comminuted maxilla fracture between the upper facial skeleton and the intact or already repaired mandible. Although the popularity of internal microplating systems has eclipsed the use of this technique, it remains a safe method of management of complex maxillary injuries.

The principle objections to fracture treatment using any method where mouth opening is not possible include potential risk to the upper airway, reduction in tidal volume, temporomandibular joint (TMJ) stiffness and risk of ankylosis, weight loss and poor patient acceptance.

External fixation

This technique involves insertion of transcutaneous bone pins placed bicortically and aligned appropriately. Once *in situ,* these pins may be rigidly united with universal joints and locking bars or fast-setting acrylic. A safe method of fracture treatment in military settings, it also finds application in the management of infected fracture sites or as part of treatment of an infected non-union.

Internal fixation

Rigid osteosynthesis is the most modern development in maxillofacial trauma surgery. Titanium plates and screws have superseded the stainless steel variants, and many patterns and sizes are now available. Good surgical exposure of the fracture site is required and therefore, open reduction is inherent in the technique. Accurate adaptation of the plate to the cortical surface and accurate angulation of the screw long axis is required. All drilling requires good water cooling, as bone overheating results in bone necrosis, infection and plate failure. Kits designed specifically for cranial, orbital and mandibular fixation are all available. Plates may remain *in situ* indefinitely unless the patient experiences pain or ulceration of the overlying soft tissues. If this occurs, and it is uncommon, removal of the screws and plates is performed.

Screws alone: bicortical and lag screws may be used without an associated plate. The commonest application of this technique is fixation of the mandibular angles after saggital split osteotomy, and this requires the use of three such screws per side.

Biodegradables

Research continues into the development of a useful biodegradable or resorbable rigid internal fixation system. In theory this should overcome the limitation of leaving residual foreign bodies in the tissue once fracture healing is complete.

Cranial level fixation
Haloframes, box frames, Mount Vernon frames and Levant frames all represent examples of cranial level fixation and each may be used with maxillary or mandibular arch bars, in conjunction with internal fixation or internal suspension wiring. Traction wiring may be used in conjunction.

Non-fixation methods
Fractures whose position is functionally good and which are non-mobile, where TMJ function is likely to be compromised by prolonged fixation or where extensive surgery is required for fixation in a patient for whom a major operation is not appropriate may all be managed conservatively. The most common fractures managed in this manner include unilateral mandibular condylar neck fractures, favourable mandibular angle fractures and non-impinging zygomatic arch fractures. Patients whose fractures are not treated by active intervention should be followed up closely and treated more actively if the clinical picture changes.

Revision points

Fracture healing
Wound healing
ATLS principles
Management of the multiple traumatised patient

FRACTURES OF THE MANDIBULAR CONDYLE

Paediatric

Trauma involving the osteogenic centre can result in growth disturbance, hemifacial asymmetry, ankylosis and severe psychological disturbance. Early childhood and adolescence are important periods, as, in the first, taunts and verbal cruelty from peers are common and, during the latter, heightened sensitivity and self-awareness coupled with perceptions of deteriorating aesthetics during the years of normal facial growth may severely impair normal psychological maturation.

Where condyle fractures occur, they may be extracapsular injuries to the neck or intracapsular 'burst'-type injuries. This latter pattern is described most frequently as occurring in small infants. Non-accidental injury (NAI) should be excluded.

Adult

Falls on to the chin or blows directed axially can result in bilateral condylar neck fractures in adults. Guardsman's fractures involve a parasagittal mandibular fracture in addition. They are uncommon injuries. Unilateral condylar neck fracture may present as an isolated injury or in association with a contralateral body fracture. Complex patterns of injury may present, with fragment displacement into the external auditory canal or middle cranial fossa. Fracture dislocations may occur. Neurovascular complications are uncommon as a result of the injury but may occur as a result of open surgical reduction.

Management

1. Unilateral. Analgesia, soft diet and early mobilization will resolve most such injuries. In some patients, a short period in arch bars and light IMF or with elastic traction may be required for analgesia and to re-establish the occlusion. Prolonged immobilization is associated with post-traumatic TMJ joint stiffness and an increased risk of ankylosis. It should therefore be avoided. Surgery is sometimes required in unilateral injuries. Late post-traumatic TMJ dysfunction syndrome may occur, and such patients may require condylotomy, condylectomy or joint replacement if the condylar head becomes osteoarthritic.

2. Bilateral. IMF is often required with or without a posterior occlusal wedge to prevent condylar neck shortening and traumatic anterior open bite. Early mobilization is important once IMF is removed. Anterior and lateral open bite is common. Surgery is sometimes necessary, but there is little consensus about the precise indications for operative treatment in condyle fractures. Where surgical reduction is planned, most maxillofacial surgeons would elect for open operation on the worst side. This approach to the problem inevitably entails a more difficult reduction, but it is considered that the final occlusion is more harmonious and the mandibular ramus heights achieved closer to the patient's pre-traumatic state.

Pre-auricular incision similar to that for open TMJ surgery is usually employed, and an additional submandibular or Risden pattern incision may be required. Sufficient condylar neck exposure is required to permit placement of plates or wires. The minor fragment is often deeply placed, and disimpaction or reduction is frequently difficult. Fixation may also be achieved with K wires or with external fixation. Unilateral operation converts the bilateral injury to a unilateral one; the patient is thus more amenable to conservative treatment. Few surgeons advocate bilateral operation. Subsequent surgery for painful or arthritic TMJs is occasionally required.

Intracapsular

These injuries are almost unique to childhood, and expectant management and regular growth monitoring and charting are required. Costochondral grafting may be required to provide replacement osteogenic potential at the condylar centre. Prevention of acquired hemifacial microsomia or post-traumatic facial asymmetry may be possible by this method. Surgical recontouring in early adulthood may also be required.

Distraction osteogenesis, onlay grafts with alloplastic tissues or autogenous bone and, recently, free tissue transfer of fat or vascularized bone have been performed with varying degrees of success.

Late surgery

Joint surgery, orthognathic surgery or osteotomy for treatment of facial asymmetry may be required. TMJ ankylosis may require excision and insertion of a synthetic or alloplastic membrane to prevent re-ankylosis. Many materials have been used in the formation of such a barrier; muscle and Silatic sheets, for example.

Complications

(a) Joint stiffness and limited mouth opening. Early mobilization, limited use and duration of IMF and provision of training aids in the early rehabilitation phase (e.g. tongue depressor sticks as incisal separators) will reduce these problems.

(b) Ankylosis. More often a complication of missed intracapsular fractures. Commoner amongst non-Europeans. Excision with or without joint reconstruction is required. Prosthetic TMJ arthroplasty is possible, but currently available proprietary systems are associated with problems and a high failure rate.

(c) Occlusal derangement. Anterior and lateral open bites are common as a consequence of the injury or failed surgery. IMF may prevent if used in the acute phase.

(d) Growth disorders. Facial asymmetry can result from missed or untreated intracapsular fractures in children.

Surgical complications

Haemorrhage, sepsis, plate failure, facial nerve palsy and Frey's syndrome are described after open exploration.

FRACTURES OF THE MAXILLA

Classification

The French anatomist René Le Fort (1901) classified experimentally induced midface fractures in human cadavers and described them in three groups. Le Fort I maxilla fractures are low level dento-alveolar fractures. They may be segmental or exhibit detachment of the whole upper alveolus from the facial skeleton. Le Fort II fractures are pyramidal injuries involving the medial orbit and orbital floor bilaterally, with the fracture lines running postero-inferiorly across the midface ultimately separating the upper alveolus from the facial skeleton with the nasal capsule as part of the fracture segment. Le Fort III fractures are high level injuries involving the orbital walls above the level of the floor and extending laterally to the zygomatic regions. They are serious injuries. More recently, several different clinical classifications have been described. In one such, Rowe subdivided middle third facial injuries into lateral and medial types, amongst which he advised separate detailed descriptions of each component of the fracture.

Surgical anatomy

1. Skull base angle. This lies at approximately 45° to the horizontal with a forward and downward aspect viewed from the profile and front respectively. It is phylogenetically old, consists of dense endochondral bone which is an effective barrier to fracture unless very severe force is applied.

Fractures of the midface bones occur with much lesser forces and the facial skeleton is readily detached from the cranial base and displaced down its 'inclined plane'. Cranial base fracture, if present, suggests a very severe injury and is evidenced by CSF leakage from the nose or external auditory meati, post-auricular bruising (Battle's sign) and subconjunctival haemorrhage.

2. Orbits. The orbital walls are quite commonly damaged in midface trauma. The inferior rim and floor may be comminuted in lateral injuries. The lamina papyracea of the ethmoid bone, part of the medial wall, is readily fractured in compressing globe injuries. Severe trauma may produce blindness by direct optic nerve damage or by secondary injury due to compression of the optic nerve from a retrobulbar haemorrhage.

3. Maxillary antra. Comminution of the antral walls is common in midface injuries. Reduction in radiological volume, fluid collections, epistaxes, infra-orbital and upper dental nerve numbness are all well-described features. Orbital fat herniation can occur.

4. Nasal capsule. Isolated nasal fractures are very common. They vary in the severity of the aesthetic and functional impairment which results. Simple manual or digital reduction of a laterally deviated nasal bone fracture may correct the defect. More complex injuries where severe comminution has occurred, where the nasal airway is compromised or where a significant degree of impaction or intrusion of the nasal capsule has resulted from the injury require definitive correction.
   Late presenting injuries may require interval rhinoplasty.

5. Vascularity. The vascularity of the maxilla and associated bones is maintained well by periosteally derived vessels. Unless much degloving has occurred or injudicious surgery using excess mucoperiosteal stripping is performed, the fractures can be expected to heal well.

6. Teeth. Associated tooth loss may occur, and it is important to ensure that intrathoracic displacement or inhalation of dental fragments has not occurred. Chest X-ray is essential where tooth loss has occurred.

7. Soft tissues. If overlying skin or mucosa is lacerated, early repair ensures that underlying fractures, compound by definition, are not subjected to prolonged environmental exposure. If definitive surgery is to be delayed, immediate closure of soft tissue injuries under local anaesthetic is advised. Delayed primary suture at about 5 days after injury is an option in badly contused or contaminated soft tissue wounds.

Immediate management

1. First aid. Attention to the airway is essential. The upper airway may be compromised by downward and inward displacement of the fractured middle third segment. Immediate reduction manually will avert this problem.

2. IV access is essential. Shock is uncommon in isolated facial injuries. Associated injuries may be present and of greater significance in the early phase.

3. Analgesia. This is an important aspect of early treatment, as patient cooperation is improved and the essential initial phases including X-ray or CT scanning can be completed. If there is an associated head injury, opiates will interfere with pupil reactivity and monitoring of conscious level. Codeine phosphate is therefore the preferred analgesic under these circumstances.

Fracture management

1. Reduction. Closed reduction of major midface segments ensures the security of the upper airway. In badly comminuted injuries, many small fragments may require open reduction and piecing together of a difficult 'jigsaw'.

2. Internal fixation requires wide surgical exposure, location and repositioning of the bone fragments and reconstruction of the facial form with miniplates. Where severe comminution has occurred, it is essential to reconstruct accurately the major bone buttresses and prominences including the orbital rims, orbital walls and lateral facial buttresses. It is important to establish intercanthal distance, dental occlusion and a good range of mandibular opening. Very tiny bone fragments may be removed, particularly if their vitality is in doubt due to loss of periosteal attachments.

3. External fixation. There are many techniques for external fixation in middle third facial injuries. Dental splints or IMF are often required in association with a box frame or universal frame. The vertical dimension of a badly comminuted midface injury may be established using craniomaxillary fixation or by sandwiching the fractured maxilla between an intact or repaired mandible using craniomandibular fixation.

Associated injuries

(a) *Palate splits*: palate fractures are relatively uncommon. Accurate reduction into good dental occlusion with fixation of the fragments will be effective. Direct fixation is rarely required.

(b) *Nasal complex*: disimpaction, reduction and fixation over a nasal pack is required.

(c) *Zygomas and orbital floors*: these injuries may be present as part of a more severe midface injury. They are managed in the same way as isolated zygomatic complex injuries.

Complications

(a) *Malposition* results in poor facial aesthetics.

(b) *Nasal function* and airway volume may be compromised. Rhinoplasty or septorhinoplasty may be required as part of the initial surgery or as a secondary operation.

(c) *Dental occlusion* may be deranged. Immediate postoperative elastic traction aids minor occlusal corrections. Formal orthodontics or orthognathic surgery may be required if major occlusal dysharmony persists.

(d) *Ocular.* Hypertelorism may occur. Enophthalmos and persistent diplopia require orbital reconstruction and the specialist help of an ophthalmologist, respectively.

(e) *Nasolacrimal flow.* Persistent epiphora may occur and dacrorhinocystotomy may be required.

(f) *Postoperative enophthalmos.* A late complication of midface injury and sometimes of the corrective surgery performed for these injuries, it may be very difficult or nearly impossible to correct adequately. Orbital floor grafts using autologous or synthetic materials may be used.

FRACTURES OF THE ZYGOMATIC COMPLEX

Zygomatic complex (ZC) fractures are the commonest pattern of facial injury in most communities. They are typically civilian, urban dwellers' injuries and a frequent outcome of interpersonal violence. Some are associated with simple depressions of the zygomatic arch, other injuries exhibit displacement of the whole ZC and yet others are associated, in addition, with injuries to the orbital floor.

Aetiology

1. Assault. Direct blows with fists or feet or use of weapons to inflict blunt trauma to the midface is often sufficient to fracture the ZC.

2. Sports. Accidental contact with rackets, clubs or fast moving balls may produce ZC injury.

3. Planned osteotomy. During malar osteotomy, lateral orbitotomy and middle cranial fossa access surgery, planned section of the zygomatic arch is performed. Correction of high level midfacial deformity at the LeFort II or III levels requires planned orbital wall osteotomy.

Mechanism of injury

1. Laterally directed trauma will inflict inward collapse of the zygomatic arch, and weapon-induced injury may lead to a sharply indented 'V' pattern fracture of the arch. Severe lateral trauma can produce orbital fractures very similar in type to the classical orbital 'blowout'.

2. Frontally directed trauma will frequently lead to soft tissue contusion alone but if severe enough may lead to comminution of the midfacial skeleton and inward displacement of fracture fragments of the orbital floor into the antrum.

3. Multiple or multi-directional blows lead to a complex pattern of injury, with intrusion and downward displacement of the ZC, arch fracture and comminution of the orbital rim, floor and antral walls.

4. Orbital blowout classically results from a single occluding injury to the orbital rim such that intra-ocular pressure increases suddenly and with sufficient force to fracture the paper-thin skeleton of the inferior and medial orbital walls. The precise mechanism in these uncommon injuries is in reality not so well defined. Orbital injuries indistinguishable from classical blowout fractures do occur in the absence of a consistent history or with a history of a lateral directed blow or from non-occluding injuries rather than frontal trauma. It is suggested that the pattern of force dissipation and fracture propagation in the midface may be different from the simple mechanism of the orbital floor 'burst' pattern fracture due to the sudden increase in intra-orbital hydrosatic pressure from an occluding injury. The precise mechanism of 'orbital blowout' remains unclear therefore.

5. Associations with midface and naso-ethmoid injury. In more complex midface fractures where a ZC injury is part of the clinical picture, the operative sequence often requires reduction of any ZC depression before elevation of the more central portions of the fractured bones are reduced and fixed.

6. Other maxillofacial injuries. Nasal capsule injuries and fractured mandibles occur with similar incidence and may be associated with a midface or ZC injury. As a general principle, reduction of the mandibular fracture before the middle third facial injuries is preferred, as the dental occlusion is more readily established and the profile more easily restored once the mandibular arch form is established.

7. Penetrating facial injuries. Although these injuries are most commonly confined to the soft tissues, military injuries can present complex patterns of fractures and soft tissue damage. Early fracture fixation and soft tissue closure should be the surgical goal. In severely comminuted compound injuries or where the wound is very old or grossly contaminated, delayed soft tissue closure should be employed. Internal fracture fixation should be avoided in principle although in the face, the failure rate of these methods due to infection are lower than in other parts of the body.

Diagnosis

1. Clinical history. A history consistent with trauma of the patterns known to induce ZC injuries is often obtained. Of all those patients, those who actually sustain fractures in addition to the very common midfacial contusions are estimated to be about 4% of the total.

2. Clinical findings. Signs of ZC fracture include soft tissue contusions, midfacial depression, flattening of the malar eminence, step deformity of the orbital rim or lateral rim, tenderness of the malar buttress on compression testing and over fractures on bony palpation, unilateral epistaxis, infra-orbital distribution, sensory disturbance, displacement of the palpebral ligaments, and coronoid entrapment and interference with mandibular excursion.

3. Ophthalmological. If there is orbital floor damage, enophthalmos, diplopia gaze limitation or palsy and ocular damage may all occur. Visual acuity and pupil responses must be assessed and recorded.

4. Radiographic appearances. Occipitomental, submentovertex and PA views will permit diagnosis of most fractures and also allow surgical planning. In complex injuries, comminuted fractures or detailed assessment of orbital floor injuries, CT scanning is preferable. Signs include obvious bony steps or displacement, antral volume reduction, orbital asymmetry and arch contour disruption.

Treatments

1. Expectant. Where symptoms of bony displacement are minimal or where the patient refuses surgery, conservative management is adopted. Follow-up is required to ensure that ocular disturbance does not occur.

2. Closed reduction. Not readily performed with ZC fractures.

3. Simple indirect open reduction. Gilles temporal approach and the sub-buttress use of a Poswillo hook are well-described and straightforward techniques.

Intra-oral elevation is possible but applicable to fewer injuries and therefore less universally useful than the commoner Gilles incision.

4. Open reduction and exploration. Access to the orbital rim is obtained via brow line or skin crease incisions. Orbital floor fractures are approached via one of several incisions including suborbital skin crease, subciliary, blepharoplasty or subconjunctival approaches. With more complex midface injuries, preauricular or bicoronal flaps may be required for direct access to the fractures and to permit accurate reduction and placement of miniplate internal fixation.

5. Fixation. There are many ZC fractures which, once reduced, are stable without use of extra fixation. Bone end interdigitation provides some degree of fixation, and muscle balance is not usually unfavourable as it is with many mandible fractures. However, there are several fixation methods described.

(a) *Wires*: perosseous wires may be inserted at the zygomatico-frontal suture, infra-orbital margin or across arch fractures. This is an uncommon method of fixation in modern practice.

(b) *Miniplates and screws*: low profile and miniaturized titanium internal fixation is available for reconstruction of the orbital rims.

(c) *Transfacial 'K' wire*: using the uninjured contralateral maxilla to suture the fracture segment, a Kirschner wire is driven from the healthy midface across the antral and nasal floors into the reduced and repositioned fracture. Good stability may be achieved. In severely injured patients where a short anaesthetic is required, the facial injury can be corrected satisfactorily by this technique.

(d) *Orbital floor prostheses and grafts*: there is no perfect material for reconstruction of the orbital floor. The choices available include autogenous bone from the antral wall, calvarium or iliac crest, cartilage from the pinna, xenografts including lyophilized dura mater or prosthetic materials such as Silastic. Titanium mesh plates may be screwed *in situ* as reconstruction.

Outcomes

1. Ocular. There should be good visual acuity and no diplopia, the pupillary level should not be canted, there should be no enophthalmos, and full ocular movement in all directions of gaze should be demonstrable and pain free.

2. Cosmetic. Incision placement and closure, particularly with treatment of orbital floor fractures, should be designed to permit all scars to heal with minimal cosmetic disturbance

3. Oral function. Mouth opening should be unimpeded and pain free; coronoid entrapment should no longer be apparent.

4. Sensation. Infra-orbital nerve and its pre-cutaneous branches to the antrum and upper teeth are commonly injured. Sensation returns at a variable rate. No treatment can be guaranteed to improve this. Incisions should do no further damage to the infra-orbital nerve however.

5. Naso-antral. Early treatment of the involved antrum may prevent chronic sinusitis and stuffiness. Mucolytics and decongestants aid clot and mucus resorption and drainage. Nasal fractures associated with the injury should be corrected.

FREE FLAPS

The anatomical origins of such flaps available for use in head and neck surgery include the lower limb, the upper limb and girdle, the chest wall both anterior and posterior, the abdominal wall, the scalp and forehead and sections of the gastrointestinal tract. The most commonly used free flap in head and neck surgery is the radial free forearm flap.

Flaps derived from lower limb tissues include superficial groin flaps based on superficial circumflex iliac artery, deep circumflex iliac groin flaps and dorsalis pedis flaps. Each has their uses and exponents. Upper limb and girdle flaps include latissimus dorsi, scapula and radial forearm flaps. Intestinal tract tissue can be used in pharyngeal surgery particularly and free jejunal, gastric mucosal and omental grafts are all described. Scalp and forehead flaps are also widely used by some. In addition to microvascular surgery, neuro-anastomoses are sometimes undertaken particularly in the field of free muscle and free neuromuscular transplantation in cases of facial palsy and facial paralysis.

Radial free forearm flaps

These flaps are the commonest pattern of free flap currently used in maxillofacial reconstruction. They were first described in China in Shin Yang military hospital in Shanghai and were used extensively to reconstruct burn injured facial tissues. Since then very wide use has been made of radial tissues pedicled on radial artery and cephalic vein. The radial artery is readily anastomosed to the linguo–facial trunk or superior thyroid artery and venous anastomoses to the superficial cutaneous veins or venae comitantes are used. Allen testing and Doppler flow studies demonstrate patency of the collateral ulnar arterial circulation and the adequacy of ulnar supply to the palmar vascular arcade. Bone radiographs demonstrate freedom from disease if radial bone is to be harvested.

This flap is very soft, pliable and ideal for intra-oral reconstruction; a site where a pectoralis major flap produces a bulky and rather stiff flap. Radial bone can be included in this flap to provide revascularized bone at the recipient site. Harvested radial bone can be osteotomized to provide the necessary curvature to reconstruct the mandible where required. The main problems with the radial free flap include the relatively poor quality of bone available, the risk of radial fracture postoperatively and difficulties with the donor defect. The donor defect may be closed primarily or with a full thickness abdominal skin graft. Postoperative splinting, physiotherapy and hand exercises are important. Radial fracture may complicate composite flap harvest and open reduction and fixation may be necessary. Other uses of this flap include facial augmentation and facial reanimation surgery after facial nerve palsy.

Superficial groin flap

The superficial groin region has two separate arterial systems which have a common collateral circulation; the superficial circumflex iliac artery and the superficial epigastric artery. The flap is based with an axis running approximately parallel to the inguinal ligament and a very large outline of skin, fascia and muscle can be harvested using these vessels. The pedicle is a relatively short one however and the nutrient vessels are fine making the dissection difficult. The major advantage of this flap is the very large quantity of tissue which can be harvested and very easy donor site closure without significant scarring or morbidity. Where extensive soft tissue defects are present in the head or neck particularly in burns or badly scarred patients, the groin flap should be considered. Its use in the oral cavity is limited by its bulkiness and very short vascular pedicle. These factors often make the free forearm flap a better choice.

Deep groin flap

The DCIA flap is a useful flap for provision of combined soft tissue and bone for head and neck reconstruction particularly where mandibular reconstruction is required. Iliac crestal bone, with or without a musculocutaneous free flap can be transferred based on the deep circumflex vessels. Where a large quantity of readily harvestable vascularized bone is required, this flap constitutes a good option.

For mandibular reconstruction the ipsilateral iliac crest is chosen. Little recontouring is required and the anterior superior iliac crest can usually provide a well-shaped replacement for a resected mandibular angle. Particular indications for the DCIA flap are a potentially hostile recipient bed usually due to a previous failed flap or infection, large or complex bony defects, requirement for a composite flap involving bone, mucosa and skin, or where no soft tissue replacement is required but vascularized bone alone.

The main disadvantages of the DCIA flap are its soft tissue bulkiness which in small oral defects makes the flap difficult to manage. Patients who have had previous groin surgery such as hernia repair or femoral surgery or those who have had previous iliac crest bone harvest are usually considered to be poor candidates for this flap. Where future restoration of the dentition using osseo integrated implants is planned, the fixtures can be placed in the iliac crest a few months prior to flap transfer surgery if this is an option. The fixtures are then transferred en bloc with the vascularized bone graft; in cancer surgery however, this is rarely an option.

Latissimus dorsi flaps

The free latissimus dorsi flap is a variation on the axial flap and is raised using the same pedicle vessels. The axial flap was initially described early this century as a rotational flap for restoration of the defect after mastectomy and to correct post-mastectomy lymphoedema. In head and neck surgery, uses of the free flap include reconstruction where extensive tissue loss from the scalp has occurred and this, rather than frequent or comprehensive use in maxillofacial surgery, is the case. If it is to be used in head and neck cancer surgery where previous irradiation has occurred it is usually preferrable that microsurgical transfer of contralateral latissimus dorsi is used with or without use of contralateral vein graft. This flap is excellent at producing large quantities of flat malleable tissue. The main contraindications to its use include previous axilliary dissection.

Scapula flaps

This flap provides a large relatively hairless cutaneous flap with a small amount of subcutaneous tissue relatively uniformly distributed. Primary closure of the donor site is almost always possible and the tissue is widely applicable in head and neck reconstruction. The flap is based in the circumflex scapular artery and both cortical and cancellous bone from the scapula can be harvested and transferred en block. Previous axilliary surgery or irradiation constitutes a relative contraindication to the use of this flap.

Inferior rectus abdominus flaps

This flap is useful for providing moderate tissue bulk with a very long vascular pedicle and therefore scalp excisions, skull base or para-nasal sinus lesions, radical tonsillectomy, wide pharyngeal excisions or full thickness maxillary defects can all be reconstructed using this flap. There are no absolute contraindications to its use although patients who have had pelvic surgery which is likely to have resulted in ligation of the deep inferior epiglastic vessels are not good candidates.

Lateral cutaneous thigh flaps

This flap was described in the early 1980s and the skin of the lateral thigh is harvested based on the femoral arterial system. It provides a cutaneous flap of moderate size with relatively thin and pliable tissue; in most patients it is hairless. The vascular pedicle is very long and the vessels are of quite large calibre. An important feature is the cutaneous innervation which can be harvested in conjunction with vessels. Where distal limb reconstruction is contemplated, it can be of great assistance in rehabilitation but in head and neck reconstruction it has as yet found little use. There are no contraindications to use of this flap but bone is not usually harvested and where it is required this flap is not ideal.

Free jejunal grafts

Free jejunal grafts are well proven in reconstruction of the head and neck particularly as a conduit after laryngopharyngectomy and partial oesophagectomy. It provides a good means of reconstructing large mucosal defects after radical head and neck excisions, and it may be used as intact tube or as a patch graft. The principal problems are the postoperative secretion which arises from the graft and the extensive pulmonary care which is required in the early phase to prevent hypersecretion and pooling of secretions in the chest. Tracheostomy is almost routinely required to allow aspiration and suction. Progressive regimes to combat such hypersecretions have been advocated including high volume low pressure cuffs to the tracheostomy tubes with hourly suction and daily bronchoscopy to allow both direct visualization of the graft and intensive suction to be performed. Speech rehabilitation after total laryngectomy and laryngopharyngectomy is a problem whatever reconstructive method is used. The incidence of postoperative dysphagia is reportedly slightly greater with these grafts than with gastric and colonic pull up procedures.

Gastric mucosal and omental grafts

These grafts are based on gastro epiploic vessels. They have been used to close pharyngo cutaneous fistulae and are used during reconstruction of oropharyngeal defects. They are appropriate in previously irradiated tissue which would not be otherwise available to free grafting. The principle advantages of these flaps include the provision of moist, non-hairy tissue which is soft and pliable and easily tailored to fit complex defects. The vascular pedicle consists of fine vessels which are usually low in atheromatous disease even in arteriopathic patients. Omental tissue is richly vascularized and is capable of providing an increased blood flow to otherwise poorly vascularized tissue. The flap is relatively resistant to postoperative infection.

Microsurgical scalp grafts

These are based on superficial, temporal and occipital vessels. The scalp is well vascularized and is good donor tissue for restoration of facial defects. Four classical types of flap designs are described: temporo occipital, occipito temporal, extended temporo occipital, and simple occipital.

Scalp expansion using tissue expanders may be required if very large amounts of skin are required. The classical use of vascularized scalp flaps is in restoration of the anterior hairline in alopecia. This may occur either due to male pattern baldness or after irradiation or burns.

Related topics of interest

Microvascular surgery (p. 256)
Reconstruction – some principles (p. 323)

Revision point

Anatomy of the vascular tree

FUNCTIONAL ENDOSCOPIC SINUS SURGERY (FESS)

Rigid endoscopic examination of the paranasal sinuses is becoming increasingly useful in the management of a range of sinus pathology. The advent of endoscopes with angled viewing ports and the development of appropriate endoscopic surgical instruments have permitted a range of surgical procedures to be evolved which can be performed under endoscopic vision. Inferior meatal puncture and 'Caldwell Luc' pattern punctures afford access for antral assessment and surgery. Access to the higher level sinuses may require a middle meatal puncture. The maxillary sinus can be examined endoscopically in the surgery under local anaesthesia but, where nasal septal deviations are present or disease is suspected higher in the sinus system, general anaesthesia is required. Access is poor until septal deviations are corrected and fronto-ethmoidal surgery is kinder under full general anaesthetic.

Indications

Assessment before and follow-up after open antral surgery
As part of the preoperative planning for open antral surgery, FESS examination may add useful data to that obtained by radiography in defining the extent of mucosal disease. Where lesions have been removed or chronic mucosal inflammation has been treated by surgery, postoperative follow-up by FESS examination is possible.

Pathological examination
Antral tumours, polyps, antroliths and granulomatous lesions can all be investigated and often treated endoscopically. The technique can also be used for removal of foreign bodies.

Ongoing treatment of chronic sinusitis
A diagnosis of chronic hyperplastic sinusitis is not always an automatic indication for surgery, since not all these lesions need surgical treatment. Symptoms of sinusitis include anterior nasal discharge, post-nasal drip, catarrh and nasal obstruction. Septal deviation may cause nasal obstruction. The associated hypertrophy of the inferior turbinates and the mucosal thickening contribute to the condition. Pain, pressure symptoms and anosmia are more typical of acute rather than chronic sinusitis.

A history of ear disease such as variable hearing loss, crackling and itching in the ears, is often related to

Eustachian tube dysfunction. Pulmonary symptoms as well as diseases of the teeth and jaws, allergic symptoms and inflammatory disease of the joints are all important in the diagnosis of chronic sinus disease. Orbital infections, chronic pharyngitis with pain and dryness in the throat, globus sensations and hoarseness are often due to discharge from a chronic sinusitis flowing down the pharynx.

Recurrent acute infection of the sinuses

Although rarely required during an acute episode, samples of muco-purulent fluid for culture and cytology may be obtained. Formal antral washout is no longer considered a useful therapeutic option however. Recurrent acute episodes may be investigated during a quiescent phase to exclude polyposis or hyperplastic mucosal disease as an underlying cause.

Trauma

The role of endoscopy in management of facial trauma is a new use for this technique. In the assessment of the extent of midface injury where sinus walls are damaged it is proving a useful method.

Preoperative assessment

Nasal endoscopy

Inspection of the nose by anterior and posterior rhinoscopy and fibre-optic nasendoscopy are important. The lateral nasal wall, in particular the hiatus semilunaris and the inferior turbinate should be assessed. Pathological features including plugs of mucus lying in the ostium of the antrum or nasal polyps are recorded. Polyps can be associated with ethmoiditis, and small granulations or large polyps may be found protruding from under the middle turbinate or lying in the superior meatus in the region of the posterior ethmoids. Isolated nasal polyposis without sinusitis is unusual. The pedicle of a choanal polyp often arises in the antral cavity, but can originate from the posterior ethmoid. Nasal mucosa that appears normal does not exclude chronic sinusitis. Inflammation or lichenification of the nasal vestibule and the external skin at the nasal introitus should be noted.

Ultrasound scan

Although ultrasound can prove useful in identifying an empyema or an isolated antral cyst and in post-surgical follow-up, it has proved unreliable for the assessment of maxillo-ethmoidal polyposis.

Radiography

Precise information about the type and extent of chronic sinusitis is usually obtained from radiography. The occipitomental (OM) view is useful for demonstrating mucosal swellings of the antral and frontal sinuses. Imaging of the sphenoid cavity is difficult and of the ethmoid is unreliable by OM. Plain films in other planes can be used to delineate these regions. Postero-anterior sagittal views and tilted axial views with highlighting of the ethmoid can be helpful, and lateral views of the frontal sinus are useful. Mucosal hyperplasia, cysts or polyps may all be diagnosed by these means.

Tomography and CT

1. Precision polycyclical tomography. Using 5 mm sections from the root of the nose to the sphenoid sinus, this technique provides excellent images of all three dimensions and is very reliable for the assessment of disease of the sphenoid and ethmoids. It is also suitable for assessment of fractures of the naso-ethmoid region. Tumours of the facial skeleton and the anterior base of the skull can be delineated by intermediate cuts.

2. Computerized tomography provides clearer information with relatively low radiation exposure, particularly using coronal reconstructed sections. These reconstructions allow comparison between normal and affected sides in unilateral lesions. Axial sections with suitable aperture settings permit imaging of the bony walls and assessment of the thickness of the mucosa. The axial CT projection is also suitable for demonstrating localized ethmoid disease. Coronal sections are essential for assessment of the anterior skull base and the ostia. The maxillo-ethmoidal outflow tract into the ethmoid infundibulum is less well shown in axial than in coronal cuts.

Spiral CT scans are not yet widely used in FESS planning.

Magnetic resonance imaging (MRI)

This technique is not yet widely used in preoperative assessment of paranasal sinus disease. Nevertheless, its ability accurately to demonstrate soft tissue disease suggests that it will be increasingly useful in assessment of mucosal disease and tumours. CT is still likely to retain a place in diagnostic work for patients with malignancy due to its superior ability to demonstrate bone involvement in pathology.

Functional tests

Anterior rhinomanometry is a valuable method for assessing the patency of each side of the nose and nasal airway. The pressure difference between the nasal introitus and the choana can be measured, but it does not give any detailed information about the ventilation of individual parts of the nasal cavity and the paranasal sinuses.

Pre- and postoperative olfactometry is sometimes useful for assessing disorders of function of the olfactory mucosa and the results of ethmoid operations.

Other investigations

Allergy testing of patients with chronic hyperplastic sinusitis is a useful clinical step, even if the benefits of desensitization in appropriate cases is relatively low. The demonstration and elimination of allergens can be a useful supplement to surgery. If the skin tests, intranasal provocation and *in vitro* investigations identify the allergen, the patient should be treated conservatively by avoidance of the allergen, topical steroids, systemic medication or desensitization. For patients with polyposis of the sinus mucosa combined with asthma and sensitivity to analgesics, treatment is often disappointing. In these cases, surgery is often the treatment of choice, and allergic management is used as an adjunct.

Dental examination

This measure should not be omitted in chronic maxillary sinusitis. An OPG of the upper jaw is a useful screening test. Dental causes account for 10–20% of cases of sinusitis.

Pulmonary function

These tests can be valuable in asthmatics or patients with bronchitis. As a pre-anaesthetic measure they are useful but as a test for non-specific bronchial hyperreactivity they also help the surgeon to identify patients with a sub-clinical asthma. About 25% of asthmatics suffer chronic hyperplastic sinusitis, this proportion rises to 40% of those who also have analgesic sensitivity. Patients sensitive to analgesics have a worse prognosis and do less well after surgery. Review by a paediatrician is important in children with sinusitis, because of the association with cystic fibrosis.

Complications of FESS

These include haemorrhage, sepsis, damage to olfactory apparatus, optic nerve injury if a middle meatal puncture is performed and recurrent or persistent disease.

Endoscopic diagnosis compared with other diagnostic methods

As a diagnostic tool, FESS permits direct visualization of the paranasal sinus system and access to tissue for biopsy and secretions for culture and cytology. Whether this type of technique proves to be more accurate than CT or MRI scan images in assessment of the extent of disease remains unproven. It is likely that it will prove a useful adjunct to diagnosis. As a therapeutic tool it has already proved effective in a wide range of mucosal conditions.

Further reading

Operative techniques for functional endoscopic sinus surgery
Nasal anatomy
Paranasal sinus anatomy

Related topics of interest

Maxillary sinus (p. 246)
Obstructive sleep apnoea (p. 279)

GENERAL ANAESTHESIA AND SEDATION

The advent of chloroform-induced general anaesthesia in surgery was pioneered in the USA and UK in the mid-nineteenth century. Since then, techniques and drugs have been developed to take into account the specific demands of advances in the different surgical specialties. There are several problems for the anaesthetist that are unique to maxillofacial and head and neck surgery.

Maxillofacial surgery: specific anaesthetic problems

- Shared airway nasal endotracheal tube for oral and dento-alveolar surgery. Armoured oral ETT may be an option.
- Muscle relaxation: widely used but not for parotid surgery.
- Dry: anti-sialogogue at premed or at induction may be used.
- IMF and throat pack: the throat pack should be remembered and the larynx examined before placement of the wire ligatures.
- Sepsis: perioral sepsis and swelling is likely to cause difficulties with intubation.
- Neck arthropathy: neck extension and nasal ETT insertion are often difficult.
- Conscious or bronchoscopic intubation: with large tumours of the posterior tongue or upper airway, as loss of airway control after induction is a hazard. Tracheostomy under LA is an option.
- Hypotensive GA: useful in parotid, orthognathic and extensive neck surgery.
- Vagal reflexes: oculocardiac stimulation and neck dissection associated with manipulation of pericarotid tissues may induce significant bradycardia.
- Neck spaces: once opened surgically, there is an increased risk of surgical emphysema, spread of sepsis and accidental impaction of foreign bodies.
- NG intubation: nasogastral intubation in midfacial trauma is associated with a risk of NG tube passage into the anterior cranial fossa.
- Tracheostomy or surgical airway preparation: required as part of some head and neck operations, particularly tumour surgery and occasionally in trauma.
- Intra-operative turning of patients: posterior, superior iliac crestal (PSIS) bone harvest and elevation of regional flaps, such as latissimus dorsi, require armoured ETT tubes and higher ventilation pressure when lying prone.
- Free flaps: careful selection of limb for anaesthetic use. The position of peripheral vascular access and siting of central venous catheters to avoid the limb and vessels planned for harvest during surgery is essential.
- Chest and rib cage: rib graft and costochondral graft harvest carries a risk of pneumothorax.
- Prolonged anaesthesia: fluid and electrolyte balance, blood glucose and acid base maintenance are important. In oncological surgery, blood loss, autologous transfusion of previously collected blood, clotting studies to prevent dilutional and

DIC-related intra-operative bleeding may be required. Temperature and urine output are essential indicators of adequacy of intravenous volume replacement.
- Surgical adjuncts: antibiotics, anti-thrombotic prophylaxis, steroids, analgesia, haematocrit and clotting status estimations may all be required.

Some specific techniques

Patient-controlled analgesia (PCA)

PCA uses an opiate IV infusion by pump. The dosage is demand fed, with an adjustable lockout to prevent overdosage. This is a useful technique and has wide applications in head and neck surgery, postoperative in cancer surgery and a significant role in palliative and terminal care. Extensive use of PCA is found in other disciplines and in the Intensive Care Unit (ITU) setting.

Patient-controlled sedation (PCS)

PCS uses propofol by IV infusion pump. It is a safe technque as the half-life of the drug is very short. An overdose lockout is available.

Relative analgesia (RA)

No longer as widely used as previously. Nitrous oxide and oxygen are given by continuous or demand-fed inhalation. The technique uses the amnesic and mild analgesic effects of nitrous oxide. The gas mixture is commercially available as 'Entonox' and uses a 50%:50% mix of nitrous oxide and oxygen.

IV sedation

IV sedation involves the use of benzodiazepines and modern analogues given by IV bolus injection. The previously described technique of intermittent IV barbiturates by bolus is outmoded and unnecessarily hazardous, with threat of respiratory depression. Aftercare of patients is important, as a large apparent volume of distribution and redistribution phenomena exhibited by the kinetics of most sedative drugs used is apparent in the hours after the surgical procedure. It can constitute an important hazard for patients unless they are warned appropriately. Reversal agents and pulse oximetry for monitoring should be available.

Day case surgery

Uses and indications

- Short procedures, usually less than 30 min duration.
- Simple operations or investigations are usually considered appropriate uses.
- Frequently performed operations may not necessarily constitute ideal procedures for performance under day case arrangements.
- An uncomplicated postoperative course should be anticipated.
- Analgesia requires meticulous attention as discharge in the early postoperative period allows no opportunity for revision of prescribed drugs.
- Travelling distances must be short and transport arrangements straightforward.
- Access to immediate follow-up must be available if required.
- Social circumstances must be adequate to permit discharge and a suitable escort must be available.
- Recruitment of experienced surgical and anaesthetic staff is important.

Use of IV sedation and LA

Many patients demand GA, as fear and anxiety about surgery makes LA an unpopular choice. Good patient–clinician rapport will alleviate the anxiety for many patients.

Oral premedication or IV sedation techniques may offer an alternative to GA. But they are no substitute if GA is in reality required. The contraindications to GA apply fully to the use of IV sedation techniques and the risks are as great.

The patient needs monitoring, and full postoperative recovery facilities are required. Reversal agents and full resuscitation facilities should be available. The 'Poswillo' report sets down the detailed statutory requirement for use of sedation techniques outside the hospital service in the UK.

Revision points

Anaesthetic agents and their pharmacology.
Care of the unconscious patient.
Emergencies and complications.
Preparation and fitness for GA.

GENIOPLASTY

The surgical alteration of the chin form can be performed as an isolated procedure or as part of a more complex orthognathic operation. Planning requires careful consideration of the hard and soft tissue profile as well as frontal views, both radiographic and clinical. Genioplasty can be designed to augment or reduce chin size, to straighten an asymmetric face or lengthen a short face.

Augmentation genioplasty

1. Augmentation of the chin can be required in antero-posterior, vertical and transverse dimensions. The problem of short face syndrome requires particular care in planning to achieve the necessary increase in length at the chin segment. A lengthening genioplasty is possible if the more major parts of the surgical procedure are insufficient to correct the lack of anterior face height. In particular, where ramus or occasional body osteotomies have been performed, a genioplasty may be required in addition to achieve the necessary increase in vertical face height, antero-posterior mandibular length and chin projection.

2. Sliding augmentation genioplasty is performed for brachiocephalic or normocephalic faces where the lower face height will tolerate an increase in conjunction with increased prominence of the chin. It is performed via a lower vestibule degloving incision, and care is paid to tension or traction on the mental neurovascular bundle. A digastric myotomy may be combined with this operation. This usually requires an external approach. A single cut osteotomy or multiple, stepped osteotomies are possible, depending on the degree of correction required. The angulation of the bone cuts can also be varied if desired. Fixation is achieved with plates, but wires remain an option if necessary.

3. Alloplastic or autogenous augmentation is an option for genioplasty when an increase in lower face height is less advantageous but a transverse diameter increase is desired. It is not a very reliable method and is dependent for success on the material chosen and on operator experience with the chosen material. Chin prominence increases in all dimensions. The operative procedure usually requires an external incision, and a subperiosteal envelope is prepared for the implant or graft. The new tissue is secured with sutures or fine stainless steel wires.

Reduction genioplasty

1. Vertical dimension reduction. This is the commonest indication for chin reduction.

2. Macrogenia may be osseous, and soft tissue form and lip habits are important. The correlation between cephalometry and clinical appearance should be assessed as what appears to be a gross skeletal macrogenia may not be too bad from the point of view of facial aesthetics, and vice versa. Osseous macrogenia can occur along several growth vectors, giving rise to excessive growth in anterior or vertical planes. Some patients exhibit a combination of these patterns.

3. Surgery for reduction of the bony chin can be performed via a full symphysis degloving approach, but soft tissue compensation occurs and the aesthetic result is often disappointing. This can be improved by minimizing the extent of mucoperiosteal stripping on the portion of chin to be retained. Soft tissue apposition to the chin in its new position is therefore undisturbed.

Derotating genioplasty

In patients undergoing major corrective surgery for facial asymmetry, the element of chin asymmetry is often corrected incompletely and a derotating procedure is required as part of the main operation. A horizontal genial osteotomy via a minimal degloving incision is the commonest and best proven technique. Care in achieving harmony of the facial and dental midlines is important.

GRANULOMATOUS CONDITIONS

Lesions labelled as granulomas may be true granulomas or may represent proliferation of granulation tissue. The histology typical of many granulomatous lesions is well illustrated by the non-caseating lesions of sarcoidosis.

Sarcoidosis

Of unknown aetiology, although a transmissable agent is postulated. Widely disseminated lesions are common; lungs, lymph nodes, skin, eyes, skeletal tissues and nervous system involvement are all described. Various immunological disturbances are described, but their contribution to the clinical course is unclear. Orofacial sarcoid is not very common. Cutaneous sarcoid affecting the face is more so. Labial biopsy may demonstrate granulomas. Kveim testing may provoke their formation and serum acetylcholinesterase (ACE) levels, although not very specific, may aid diagnosis. Corticosteroids may be inhibitory, particularly for lung disease and in uveoparotid fever. Intra-lesional steroid injections of triamcinolone are used with benefit.

Tuberculosis (TB)

Human TB is caused by mycobacterium tuberculosis infection, producing caseating granuloma formation in tissues. Typically, the lungs are affected although other organs may become diseased. Kidneys, skin, brain, bowel and disseminated disease may all occur. Oral manifestations of TB are quite uncommon. Tuberculous ulceration affecting the tongue, buccal mucosae and palate are described. Oral mucosal lesions usually present as linear ulcers with undermined edges. Commisural lesions are occasionally noted. Tuberculous lesions are painful, often severely so. Serological testing and vaccination is widely available. Treatment with a combination of specific anti-tuberculous drugs is curative. Tuberculous cervical lymphadenitis (scrofula) is occasionally seen amongst non-immunized Asian immigrants in the UK. Discharging abscesses, cervical masses and deep scars if the condition is chronic are typical. Occasionally, surgical drainage may be required but care is required as chronic fistula formation is a risk.

Leprosy

This is caused by *Mycobacterium leprae*. It is characterized by slow but progressive tissue destruction and granuloma formation. Leprosy exists in both lepromatous and tuberculoid forms. Oral manifestations include lepromatous tumour masses, ulcerated lesions and gingival hypertrophy. Twenty percent of patients have lingual lesions, and perivermillion cicatrix formation results in a scarred microstomic patient. Alveolar bone destruction is associated with gingival hypertrophy. Treatment with Dapsone and Clofazimine is the current preferred regimen, although recommendations change quite frequently as the incidence of bacterial drug resistance is increasing. Reconstructive surgery is possible in biochemically cured or disease-free patients.

Sexually transmitted diseases

Syphillis, yaws and granuloma inguinal (Donovanosis) may all present with granuloma formation.

Crohn's disease

Crohn's disease is principally a disease of the GI tract, although extra-intestinal manifestations are common. It is of unknown aetiology. In the gut, transmural inflammation, fissural ulcers, lymphoid aggregations and non-caseating granulomata formation are pathognomonic. Oral manifestations include corium lesions with normal or ulcerated overlying mucosae. Oral aphthous pattern ulcers, cobblestone lesions and facial swelling are characteristic. Evidence of Crohn's lesions in other systems should be sought. Local or systemic salazopyrin is effective, and severe exacerbations of GI disease may require steroids.

Melkerson Rosenthal syndrome

An uncommon triad of tongue fissuring, unilateral facial palsy and facial swelling comprise this condition. Cheilitis granulomatosa occurs when lip swelling occurs in the absence of other features, but the histology is typical of the full syndrome. Histologically, lesions are similar to Crohn's oral lesions.

Mycoses

Lesions due to tissue invasion with fungi or yeasts are commonly granulomatous. Tissue reaction to fungal antigens may provoke the condition but the organisms may also provoke a foreign body pattern reaction in some instances. Some examples include blastomycosis, histomycosis, aspergillosis, phycomycosis and actinomycosis.

Wegener's granulomatosis   This condition is a systemic granulomatous vasculitis. It affects nasal mucosa, skin, gut, lungs and kidneys. Joint and neurological disease is also described. It presents as a bloody discharge typically from affected mucosal surfaces, but organ failure results if kidneys are affected. Oral involvement occurs in about 50% of patients, with the gingivae, tongue and palate being the commonest tissues affected.

Lethal midline granulomas   Chronic progressive destruction of the midline structures of the nose and maxilla occurs. These conditions rarely affect lungs or kidneys and are thus distinguished from Wegener's granulomatosis although histologically they are similar. Steroids, radiotherapy and anti-neoplastic drugs have all been tried. Prognosis is poor.

Histiocytoses   *1. Eosinophilic granuloma.* This is the commonest form in adults. Lytic lesions in the skeleton occur and pulmonary involvement is typical. This form has a moderate prognosis.

2. Letterer Siwe disease. This form is usually fatal in early childhood. There are widely disseminated granulomatous lesions which respond poorly to chemotherapy. There is little effective treatment.

3. Hans Schuller Christian's disease. Bone granulomas, exophthalmos and diabetes insipidus characterize this condition. Pulmonary lesions also occur, and sarcoid-like hilar lymphadenopathy is typical. Some resolve spontaneously, and steroids and cyclophosphamide may be beneficial.

GUN SHOT WOUNDS

Gun shot wounds of the head and face are not common in UK civilian practice but constitute part of the pattern of injury in 30% of all battle casualties. In the USA, they are far more frequent as outcomes of street violence. In the UK, their frequency is reportedly increasing. Deliberate self-harm and attempted suicide are common causes currently in the UK, and the most frequent choice of weapon is a shotgun. Handguns are less common, and high velocity weapons are almost never used in self-inflicted injuries.

The projectile

The important characteristics of the weapon used in the injury are;

- the number of shells or fragments involved
- the velocity or energy transfer of the fragments
- the range from the muzzle to the patient at discharge.

Shotgun wounds inflicted from any distance are rarely deeply penetrating as the cartridge is designed to give a large number of low-velocity pellets effective over a short range. Farming or hunt accidents are commonly of this type. Point blank shotgun discharge can produce multiple deeply penetrating fragments and leave the patient with pellets and wadding lodged in surgically inaccesible sites. They are foci of potential sepsis, and the decision to remove such fragments from inside the cranial cavity or close to major cervical blood vessels is determined by the need to prevent abscess formation.

Military issue semi-automatic weapons fire shells which are designed for maximum anti-personnel effect and with very high muzzle velocity or energy transfer. The injuries which result are different from low-velocity injuries. Their characteristics include the production of small entry ports, extensive tissue damage in the track of the projectile which is exacerbated by generation of a vacuum within the tissue in the wake of the missile. Cavitation and massive environmental contamination result and are associated with wide loss of viability in adjacent tissues.

Other forms of projectile injury include fragmentation pattern injury ('shrapnel wounds') and injuries from specialist projectiles such as soft-tipped or explosive-tipped bullets. Shrapnel injuries were one pattern of military wound sustained from a cannon shell designed to fragment in flight and to produce maximum damage to enemy personnel numbers. As a description it is inaccurate, but it is used widely to describe wounds due to fragments of environmental debris immediately following an explosion. Glass is one common such example. Such fragments can be quite high velocity and induce the high energy transfer pattern of wounding.

Initial management

1. Active resuscitation. Airway security, blood volume replacement, high-dose IV antibiotics and analgesia are essential.

2. Other injuries. Screening for other injuries particularly to the chest, abdomen and limb vascularity is important. Priority setting for the sequence of any necessary surgery is essential.

3. Radiography and CT scanning. This permits assessment of the degree of tissue loss, damage to adjacent vital structures, fractures, soft tissue comminution and the number and position of projectiles or fragments.

4. Surgery. Early operation is planned in all but the most minor shotgun injuries.

Soft tissue management

For low velocity wounds, for instance shotgun pellet wounds, superficial removal with extensive antiseptic washing may be all that is required when minimal penetration has occurred.

High-velocity shells leave a wide contaminated devitalized track which must be opened widely and debrided thoroughly. Primary closure is absolutely contraindicated, and removal of all shell fragments and wadding is essential. Meticulous nursing is required to prevent contamination during dressing changes and for turning to prevent pressure damage to healthy skin.

Where extensive soft tissue loss has occurred, salvage of all vital tissue is helpful, and delayed closure is performed either by primary suture or by local flaps of free grafts once the recipient bed is clinically clear of infection; a problem universal in all projectile injuries.

Specific head and neck sites

1. Intracranial. Shot pellets may be left *in situ* or removed, depending on the neurosurgical assessment of the risk of abscess formation against the risks of surgery. Antibiotics and anticonvulsant therapy may be required.

2. Ocular. Intra-ocular foreign bodies should be removed. More severe disruption may require enucleation of the globe. Orbital reconstruction may be required. Bone grafts, titanium mesh reconstruction and osseointegrated implant-retained prostheses may all be useful in this clinical setting.

3. Neck. Exploration is often advisable to prevent gross sepsis later in the clinical course and to repair vascular damage if necessary.

4. Gross soft tissue loss. Thorough debridement and achievement of maximum skin cover are the surgical aims. Where possible, skin cover should be obtained early in the post-injury phase. Reconstruction is planned as an interval procedure once initial healing has occurred and the site is infection free.

Fracture and bone loss

Fractures are all compound and infected by definition. Extensive bone fragmentation may occur, and debridement including necrotic adjacent muscle is required. Neurovascular repair is essential where damage has occurred. External fixation and delayed closure or bone grafting is often necessary. In head and neck wounds, the orthopaedic strictures against internal fixation are less stringent.

Psychosocial

In deliberate self-harm, a thorough psychiatric assessment is required with the intention of preventing a repeat of the episode in survivors. Battle casualties have specific psychiatric needs which can be provided for by specialist clinicians. Post-traumatic stress disorder may manifest weeks or months after the initial injury. Any major facial injury carries in its wake the bereavement due to loss of normality, the need to adjust to a new appearance and often less than perfect orofacial functioning and the requirement to adjust to the reactions of family, colleagues and friends. If functional loss is marked, the psychological aspect of this cannot be overlooked.

Long-term rehabilitation

1. Functional rehabilitation. Swallowing, speech, chewing and facial expression may all need specialist help.

2. Surgical reconstruction. Alloplastic tissues such as titanium mesh, autogenous bone grafting either with non-vital or vascularized bone and combinations of these techniques offer useful reconstructive options to restore bony facial contours. Palate reconstruction using bone or titanium palate reconstructon is possible. Soft tissues can be restored using local flaps, axial flaps or free tissue transfer. Fine features of facial form pose particular difficulties. Vermillion lip margins, nasal architecture, maxillary or malar prominence and pinna form may all require specific attention.

3. Camouflage makeup. This is available in some units if surgery is not an option or if it has not been successful in scar revision and removal.

4. Maxillofacial prosthetics. There are many options, including osseointegrated implant placement.

5. Long-term feeding may be required if oral function is inadequate in spite of careful surgery and aftercare.

HEAD AND NECK ONCOLOGY – BIOLOGICAL ASPECTS

Eight percent of all human malignancies occur in the head and neck; 90–95% of all head and neck malignancy is squamous cell carcinoma. The larynx is the commonest affected site in the head and neck. Lymphomas, salivary gland tumours, neurogenous lesions and other lesions of connective tissue origin also occur. The highly specialized tissue of the orofacial region gives rise to uncommon and unique patterns of neoplastic disease; for example the odontogenic tumours.

Tissues of origin of head and neck tumours

Primary lesion	Commonest site	Commonest lesion	Relative frequency (%)	Lymph node metastases at time of presentation (%)
Lip	Lower lip	scc	15	5
Oral cavity	Tongue	scc	20	40
Oropharynx	Tonsillar fossa	scc	10	40–80
Hypopharynx	Pyriform sinus	scc	5	80
Larynx	Vocal cords	scc	25	5–35
Nasopharynx	Roof	scc	3	80
Sino-nasal tissues	Maxillary antrum	scc	4	15
Salivary glands	Parotid	psa	15	25
Other lesions	–	–	3	–

scc, squamous cell carcinoma; psa, pleomorphic salivary adenoma.

Squamous cell carcinoma

Aetiology

1. *Tobacco.* Implicated forms of tobacco preparation include smoked, particularly as cigarettes, chewed, as 'Skoal bandits', or snuff.

2. *Alcohol.* Ethanol or methanol both exhibit a synergistic effect with tobacco in the genesis of some tumours. This effect is most noticeable in oral, hypopharyngeal and oesophageal lesions.

3. Urban dwelling. City dwellers are affected more often than rural. The effect is likely to be multi-factorial, with urban pollution, occupational stress, domestic overcrowding and dietary differences featuring in the causation of tumours. It is not a very marked effect however.

4. Male sex. Head and neck malignancy is variously estimated to be five to nine times more common in males than in females, although the incidence in women in the UK is increasing.

5. Age. Although older patients are commonly affected, recent biphasic incidence curves have been demonstrated with increased rates of tumours amongst patients in the second and third decades.

6. Site-specific carcinogens.
(a) Nasopharynx

- hardwood dust
- Epstein–Barr virus (EBV) in Chinese
- HPV 6 and HPV 11.

(b) Buccal mucosa

- paan
- araca nut or betel nut
- tobacco.

(c) Malignant melanoma

- UV exposure.

7. Diet. This is a less clear effect than with stomach and colon tumours for instance. Vitamin A and C deficiencies have been suggested as aetiological factors. No very clear link has yet been demonstrated however.

8. Radiation exposure. The importance of ionizing radiation in causation of head and neck cancers is well demonstrated. Therapeutic use of radiotherapy is implicated in some second head and neck primary malignancies.

9. *Pre-malignancy.* Patterson–Brown–Kelly syndrome is implicated in some hypopharyngeal carcinomas. The syndrome comprises iron deficiency anaemia associated with post-cricoid web formation and dysphagia.

Epithelial dysplasias and dyskeratoses. The leukoplakias and erythroleukoplakias arguably exhibit premalignant potential. At the very least they often share a common aetiological pattern and require careful monitoring and occasional biopsy for exclusion of associated frank malignancy.

Immunology

Immune surveillance against tumour growth is dependent upon intact cell-mediated immunity. Expression of tumour cell antigens is important in immune recognition of tumours and may provide diagnostic and prognostic indicators as future developments have their effect on clinical medicine.

Secretory IgA present in saliva and nasopharyngeal secretions may be protective to mucosal surfaces. Its role in protection against mucosal malignancy is not yet fully elucidated.

Anti-EBV immunoglobulin may be protective against nasopharyngeal carcinoma, and serum IgA elevation is occasionally detected.

Lymphoid infiltration suggests a well-differentiated lesion and a good prognosis. Lymphocyte infiltration is common in squamous lesions but the cell toxicity of the infiltrating cells appears attenuated. The mechanism of this moderation of the immune cell response is not known. Interleukin 2 may reverse this down-regulation effect.

CD4 (H) titres are commonly reduced, and the T(H):T(S) ratio is similarly affected. If the helper:suppressor ratio is significantly reduced this may be an indicator of a poorer prognostic significance in patients with squamous tumours. Radiotherapy (DXT) selectively impairs T(H) number and functionality. T(S) cell responses to DXT are inverse to the response of T(H) cells.

The importance of humoral mediators in the immune response is of interest. γ-Interferon, interleukins and prostaglandins modulate the effectiveness of immune responses. Prostaglandin production mutes the overall response.

Genetics

RNA virus genomes have been demonstrated to bear a close genetic relationship to human oncogenes. The demonstration of proto-oncogenes, cell transformation in cell culture and the identification of oncoproteins and tumour regulator proteins is the stuff of current research.

Mutation of tumour suppressors or anti-oncogenes such as p53 are demonstrably linked with high rates of squamous malignancy *in vitro* and in animal models. The link with human disease is less clearly defined. A series of other genes has been documented. For instance, cytokeratins are of relevance in squamous cell carcinomas but whether they will be useful as markers for disease progression remains to be demonstrated.

DNA repair enzymes and failure of expression of cellular stability genes may be responsible for oncogenesis and increased rates of metastases seen in some patients.

There remains as yet no single cohesive genetic explanation for tumour genesis, and it is still considered that multiple error-inducing events occurring sequentially are required for malignant disease to occur.

Growth factors and markers

Epidermal growth factor (EGF) and receptor proteins are present in normal tissue. Reduced sensitivity or reduced requirement for induction of cell division is suggested as the hallmark of tumour cells. The expression of EGF receptors in head and neck malignancies may result in an amplification effect in receptor status.

Other growth factors include transforming growth factor-α, fetal EGF, platelet-derived growth factor, fibroblast growth factor, insulin-like growth factor and nerve growth factor. The precise relationship of the different factors to biology of specific tumours remains unclear.

Clinically useful markers such as carcinoembryonic antigen, ferritin and circulating immune complexes have all been studied, but few reliable markers for head and neck cancer have as yet been indentified.

Prognostic indicators

In squamous cell carcinomas of the head and neck, survival rates are related to age, sex, T stage and general medical state.

The effect of age is apparently important, but is much less marked when corrected for untreated malignancy, second tumours and intercurrent disease.

Women in general do less well even with treatment of their disease than age-matched male counterparts.

General health status does influence prognosis. In terms of tumour progression and spread, and in response to treatment, intercurrent disease correlates well with a poorer outcome than in age- and sex-matched but medically fitter patients.

The influence of pathological grading is relatively non-significant, except where extracapsular lymph node spread is demonstrated on postoperative histology.

In late or end stage disease, the Karnovsky status, clinical response to chemotherapy and cellular ploidy are important in determining prognosis.

Recent studies suggest that of all possible prognostic factors considered, the most significant ones are tumour stage, surgical margin clearance, the number of pathologically positive neck lymph nodes and blood transfusion. The latter factor appears to correlate with long-term outloook. Use of blood transfusion has been demonstrated to impair the outcome of surgery for large bowel malignancies, and this effect is also apparent in patients with head and neck tumours, albeit to a lesser degree. It may be related to immune suppressant effects of repeated antigen loading as a result of blood transfusion.

Second primaries

A second primary cancer in head and neck squamous lesions is a common event. Estimates suggest that at diagnosis, 5% of patients have second lesions and up to 20% of all patients eventually manifest synchronous or metachronous disease. This effect is most marked with tongue and palate lesions. The concept of field change is well documented and is particularly associated with tobacco- and alcohol-related lesions.

Lymph node disease

The pattern of lymph node spread in head and neck disease is important. The principal mode of spread is via local growth and invasion and by lymphatic dissemination. The pattern of nodal spread is largely predictable once the primary site is known. The anatomy and drainage patterns of the head and neck lymphatics are well described. Lymphatic spread occurs by permeation and seeding. Nodal metastases in the neck occur in a stepwise fashion, with the first echelon nodes becoming involved before the vertical perijugular chain of nodes. Skip lesions in nodal disease are almost unknown in metastases from a head and neck squamous cell carcinoma.

Pathologically, the most important factor is extracapsular nodal spread of tumour cells. Where the first echelon nodes are involved in tumour spread but no extracapsular breach has occurred, the prognosis is only a little worse than for N0 disease.

Distant metastases

Distant metastases are relatively uncommon in head and neck squamous lesions. Bone, lung and nervous sytem may all be affected nevertheless. Paraneoplastic syndromes do occur, but only occasionally.

The occult primary

The problem of advanced disease of the cervical lymph nodes without evidence of obvious primary tumour occurs in the head and neck. Supraclavicular primary disease will sometimes produce nodal secondaries and present with a nodal mass as the sole presenting feature in some patients. This suggests that the primary lesion is pharyngeal; 60% of such lesions will be nasopharyngeal, 20% oropharyngeal and 10% arise in the pyriform fossa. Thoraco-abdominal disease will account for many of the remainder.

HEAD AND NECK ONCOLOGY – PRINCIPLES OF PATIENT MANAGEMENT

Diagnosis

History and examination

1. Presenting features and complaints. The important details include the presence of non-healing ulcers, swellings or lumps around the mouth, face or neck, a change in pigmentation and bleeding. Pain, neurological deficits, functional deficits including speech, swallowing and saliva production are all noted. Changes in sense of smell, taste and systemic symptoms of anorexia, insomnia and weight loss are documented.

2. Past medical history. Major concomitant illnesses, a history of previous malignancy, previous cancer surgery, radiotherapy or chemotherapy are all important. Current drug therapy and details of allergies should be noted.

3. Social history. Ethanol or other alcohol abuse and tobacco use as smoked, chewed or as snuff are all central to diagnosis of head and neck cancer. Other lifestyle habits including paan or araca nut chewing and drugs or substance abuse are important.

4. Dental and oral conditions. Restorative or prosthodontic states are documented. The decision regarding the need for an immediate or temporary obturator is made and early dental impressions taken. Discussions regarding osseointegrated implants and jaw reconstruction are valuable in the surgical planning phase.

5. Clinical examination. A full examination is performed. Some salient features include details of the condition of the mouth, teeth and restorations, face and scalp, and the neck for masses and lymphadenopathy.

6. Pre-malignancy. Note the presence, chronicity, progress and past treatment of any oral lesions suspected of pre-malignant potential. Leukoplakia, erythroplakia, speckled erythroleukoplakia, erosive lichen planus, oral submucous fibrosis, sideopaenic dysphagia and Patterson–Brown–Kelly syndrome and early melanomata may all be detected or have been previously documented.

7. Functional assessments of swallow, speech and thyroid status are useful. Examination of the chest and abdomen in a search for metastatic disease and of the CNS, particularly the cranial nerves, aids in determining the stage of the disease. Limbs are examined, and an Allen test performed if surgery is planned to include reconstruction using radial free flap harvest.

Investigations

1. Imaging
(a) *OPG*: to delineate bone invasion by oral cancers. The most accurate and clinically useful method to determine the presence of bony invasion, and therefore the need to resect the jaw during surgery, remains debatable. Plain X-rays, axial tomography, isotope scintiscanning and clinical examination at operation are all options.
(b) *Chest X-ray*: important as a pre-anaesthetic check in patients with known pulmonary or airways disease and to demonstrate tumour metastasis to lungs or hilar lymph nodes, ribs or vertebral.
(c) *Scans*: CT axial tomograms of the primary site and suspected sites of distant metastases, and MRI scans of the neck to delineate the extent of cervical node metastases are essential.
(d) *Barium or 'Gastrograffin' contrast studies*: to demonstrate causes of dysphagia and to outline the extent of ulceration and fistula formation in the upper aerodigestive tract.
(e) *Doppler duplex flow studies*: in planning radial free forearm flaps, the clinical findings of the Allen test can be confirmed using these imaging techniques.
(f) *Angiography*: in planning lower limb free flaps, the adequacy of distal tibial vessel 'run off' and the likely length of the microvascular pedicle can be

estimated from angiograms. Fibula free flaps require such investigation during surgical planning.

(g) *Endoscopy*: flexible fibre-optic nasendoscopy, rigid pan-endoscopy under GA during examination under anaesthesia and gastroscopy for PEG insertion may all be required.

2. *Cytology.*

(a) *Fine needle aspiration cytology (FNAC)* of a mass in the head and neck is a useful routine procedure. FNAC is of particular usefulness in the diagnosis of salivary gland and cervical lymph node disease. The usefulness of FNAC in making the decision to embark on neck dissection is in some doubt. Whether the presence of a palpable lymph node should of itself determine the need for neck dissection irrespective of FNAC findings or whether a 'reactive' FNAC sample in such a patient should lead to deferral of surgery remains an arguable matter.

(b) *Endoscopic brushings or washings:* not as commonly used in head and neck surgery as in upper GI tract and thoracic surgery. In patients with pharyngeal lesions, endoscopic examination often permits formal biopsy rather than cytology.

(c) *Imprint cytology:* for accessible oral lesions, glass slide imprints allow surface cells of the tumour to be sampled. Cytological examination may give a tissue diagnosis.

3. *Biopsy.*

(a) *Frozen sections* of tissue harvested intraoperatively aids in surgical decision making. Determination of the presence of tumour cells in an excised lymph node may help in 'fine tuning' the plan for neck dissection. If a low level cervical node is involved with the tumour, the need for radical neck dissection is established whereas reactive nodal tissue from such a sample may permit less radical surgery to be performed. The limitations of frozen section biopsy include poor demonstration of extracapsular spread of tumour and increased uncertainty in histological interpretation. With this in mind, reliance on frozen section diagnoses is considered inappropriate by some surgeons in the UK.

Determination of marginal clearance by use of frozen section is arguably of more help. The final clearance of the primary tumour if complete is associated with enhanced survival and low local recurrence rates. Radiotherapy to deal with incomplete marginal excision is an option, but surgical clearance is the goal in curative surgery.

(b) *Paraffin sections* of incision or excision biopsies or of postoperative resection tissue remains the final method of definitive histological diagnosis.

(c) *Other sampling methods:* fine needle biopsy differs from FNAC by sampling tissue with preservation of cell relations and tissue architecture. Punch and 'TruCut' biopsies are less commonly used in head and neck surgery but punch biopsy of thick oral mucosal lesions is sometimes useful.

4. Microbiological. Microscopy, Gram staining, culture and antibiotic sensitivity determination are important in the analysis of samples of fluids, pus and some cellular samples.

Preparations for surgery and for GA

Patients planned for cancer surgery often require extensive preparation.

Venous blood for assessment of baseline haematology and biochemistry should be sampled. Blood for cross-matching and venesection for autologous transfusion may be necessary. *Autologous blood transfusion* has several advantages. It reduce risks of transfusion, transfusion reactions, cross-infection and the suggested increased risk of developing a second malignancy.

Intensive pre-operative feeding may be required and insertion of a PEG is often necessary.

Liaison with the anaesthetist regarding siting of central and peripheral vascular access points is essential if free flap harvest is planned and use of limb vessels for microvascular transfer is to be performed.

It is important to consider clotting status, DVT prophylaxis, perioperative antibiotics and concurrent medication.

It may be wise to plan a preoperative visit to ITU.

Principles of treatment

1. *Surgery.*
   (a) *Ablative or tumour resection* with good margin of non-involved adjacent tissue. Most surgeons regard a 1 cm margin as adequate. *Resection* must account for tumour biology and for any mucosal field change.

   The extent of margins remains a balance between tumour clearance and reconstructability with good postoperative function.
   (b) *En bloc excision:* primary tumour resection in conjunction with the entire field of lymphatic drainage and all intervening tissues comprises classical radical cancer surgery. Preservation of vital structures results in modified *en bloc* excision or functional surgery. The benefits of radical surgery versus functional or conservative operations are still a matter of debate particularly in head and neck cancer patients.

2. *Reconstruction.* There are many methods of reconstruction after resection of cancers of the head and neck. They include primary closure of mucosa or skin, allowing surfaces to granulate or to heal by secondary intention, use of grafts, local or regional axial flaps, or harvest and placement of free flaps to replace excised bone, muscle, mucosa or skin.

3. *Rehabilitation.* After major resections, restoration of function is important and often time consuming. Attention is required to speech, swallowing, facial appearance, with prostheses or camouflage in some cases. It may be necessary to plan long-term feeding via PEG or an in-dwelling central venous line where oral feeding is not possible. Where limbs are stiff and joint posture is sub-optimal after free flap harvest, intensive physiotherapy may be required.

4. *Non-surgical treatments.*
   (a) *Radiotherapy.* (DXT) may be given pre or postoperatively. The important aspects may include:

- Planning and mask construction.
- Enrolment in international or multicentre trials.
- Curative or palliative radiation dose: a decision made in liaison with the surgeon.
- Administered on inpatient or outpatient basis.
- Complications and their treatment; mucositis, and xerostomia and osteoradionecrosis are common after head and neck radiotherapy.
- Pre DXT dental treatment, hyperbaric oxygen, pilocarpine and artificial saliva may help with these problems.

(b) *Chemotherapy.* Not as widely used in head and neck malignancy as in treatment of other cancers. Some regimens may benefit late stage or disseminated disease in squamous head and neck primary lesions.

(c) *Modern adjuncts.* Many are still experimental and some are little better than speculative. They include immune modulation, use of bacterial toxins, interferon or bacille Calmette–Guerin (BCG) vaccines.

Prognosis   Accurate staging of the patient's disease allows some degree of precision with prognosis determination. Discussions with the patient and their family are essential, and the best estimate of likely prognosis should be given. However, overemphatic or too certain an estimate of the outcome for an individual patient is likely to be unhelpful.

Related topics of interest

Head and neck oncology – biological aspects (p. 178)
Tissue sampling techniques (p. 400)

Revision point

Principles of clinical examination

HEADACHE AND FACIAL PAIN

A common complaint. History and clinical examination is directed towards exclusion of serious intracranial disease and there are rarely any positive physical signs.

Causes of headache

Psychogenic tension headache
A constant band-like or poorly-localized superficial pain experienced deeply over vertex, occiput or behind the eyes. Associated with occupational stress, lifestyle factors and mild depression. Anxiety about circumstances, hypochondria and fear of underlying brain tumour are reported by some patients. Simple analgesia relieves once reassurance and appropriate simple psychotherapy are instituted.

Post concussion pain
The pain is similar in type to simple tension headache but associated with a variety of other symptoms including dizziness and tinnitus. Personality change, poor concentration and litigation awareness may aggravate the headache.

Raised intracranial pressure
Intracranial space occupying lesions such as tumour, haematoma or abscess may cause headache. Pain is worse on rising in the morning, on lying down, associated with vomiting and exacerbated by sneeze, cough or straining at defaecation. Papilloedema may occur but visual disturbance is less common. Alcoholic binge produces a hangover headache of similar character.

Focal disease and headache
Subarachnoid haemorrhage ('the worst headache I've ever had'), meningeal irritation, and extracranial disease including, dental sepsis, sinus disease and cervical lesions all cause headache in some patients. Orbital lesions are associated with headache only late in their course.

Systemic hypertension
This condition rarely if ever causes headache. Malignant hypertension may be causative however.

Migraine
There are several types. Classical, complex and variant types are all described. Classical migraine occurs in young patients typically. It may be associated with the

onset of multiple sclerosis (MS) but usually occurs without antecedent or underlying illness. There are clinical associations with female sex, oral contraceptive pill use, emotion, stress and various foods. There may be a family history or unexplained childhood abdominal pain. There is typically a prodromal aura of widely varied visual, auditory or other sensory or perceptive disorders. The headache is often severe and the post-headache phase is associated with drowsiness and a diuresis. A vascular or vasospastic phenomenon, the headache is usually unilateral and has a pulsatile quality. Complicated migraine is associated with a variety of transient neurological focal signs including in some patients hemiparesis and facial weakness. It is responsive to analgesics in combination with ergotamine, methysergide or pizotifen. Antiemetics may also be required.

Management of headache

Investigations are planned to exclude major underlying disease. Baseline haematology and ESR will exclude connective tissue disease in particular arteritis. Chest X-ray will exclude bronchial carcinoma and skull imaging to exclude stigmata of raised intra-cranial pressure may be required. Clinical follow up will permit detection of progressive symptoms or evidence of underlying disease including psychiatric illness. Only occasionally will CT scanning or angiography be required. Treatment is for diagnosed underlying illness and analgesia and reassurance are usually required.

Causes of unilateral facial pain

Migraine

The headache of migraine is typically unilateral and in some patients is experienced in the whole of one side of the face. The other clinical features of migraine aid in establishing the diagnosis. Treatment for migraine will alleviate the facial pain.

Migrainous neuralgia or cluster headaches

Typically a severe episodic unilateral periorbital and frontal pain. Episodes occur in clusters, six or eight attacks often occurring at night for 2–3 weeks. The patient remains pain free thereafter for prolonged periods of months before another cluster occurs. Eye symptoms are common during a cluster and local treatment may be required. This sort of pain requires differentiating from trigeminal neuralgia and is responsive to migraine therapy.

Trigeminal neuralgia

Always presents as a very severe, lancinating pain occurring in the distribution of a branch of the trigeminal nerve. Most commonly affects the lower divisions of the trigeminal nerve. This condition is a disease of the elderly and is more frequent in females. In young patients with classical symptoms, demyelination should be suspected. Trigger zones, afterpain and fear of the lancinating pain are typical. Suicides are reported due to the severity of the pain. Carbamezepine is effective. Other anticonvulsants may be useful and local anaesthetic injections into the trigger zone may aid diagnosis. If symptomatic relief is obtained, percutaneous phenol neurolysis or surgical ablation with cryotherapy, diathermy or nerve excision may be required.

Glossopharyngeal neuralgia

The pain is very similar to that described for trigeminal neuralgia. Glossopharyngeal neuralgia is much rarer. The pain is usually provoked by swallowing. Carbamezepine is effective.

Post-herpetic neuralgia

A history of previous facial or mucocutaneous herpetic infection with vesiculation and crusting is usually available. Ramsey–Hunt syndrome with geniculate herpes is sometime associated. The onset of neuralgia is often delayed by many weeks and is typically severe. Carbamezepine, strong analgesia and tricyclic antidepressant treatment in combination may be effective. Antiherpetic treatment is ineffective after the onset of the neuralgia.

Temporal arteritis

Giant cell temporal arteritis is a local arteritis which may be part of a more widespread connective tissue disorder. It may be very localized or may mimic TMJ pain. TMJ pattern dysfunctional symptoms presenting in an elderly patient should arouse suspicion. Overlying scalp tissues may be inflamed and tender. Masticatory claudication or sudden unilateral blindness may result from extending arteritis. Temporal artery biopsy is diagnostic and high dose corticosteroids rapidly control the condition.

Atypical facial pain

A poorly localized usually unilateral midface pain. It typically affects young or middle aged women and is strongly associated with an underlying mild psychiatric disturbance; usually depression. There are usually no abnormal physical findings and all investigations if performed are normal. Reassurance, psychotherapy and antidepressant treatment is effective in some patients.

TMJ related pain

Arthritides, post-trauma and post-dislocation pain are all described. There are a variety of internal joint derangements described including meniscal and condylar head movement dysharmony with consequent disc damage and early arthritic change. The largest group of patients have essentially normal joints with dysfunctional symptoms. Simple physical therapy, bite adjusting appliances, occlusal therapy if appropriate and analgesia may all be effective. Dysfunctional symptoms are often prolonged but ultimately self limiting. Surgery and arthroscopic investigation are available for very prolonged or intractable joint disease.

Referred facial pain

Any disease process arising at a distance from the face may present as unilateral facial pain. These sites include, cervical spine, ear, eye and orbit, pharynx, tongue, dental tissues and myocardium.

HIGH LEVEL MAXILLARY OSTEOTOMIES

Le Fort II osteotomy

This osteotomy is the principle surgical treatment for patients with nasomaxillary hypoplasia, mild deficiency of the infra-orbital margin and pseudo-proptosis. The Küffner modification of the Le Fort III osteotomy avoids alteration of the nasal architecture and is preferred where nasal surgery is not required. The operation offers a more limited range of movements and is therefore less versatile than the Le Fort I osteotomy. Downward rotation and forward translation of the maxilla is possible, but impaction or upward movement is not. It is not possible to combine a Le Fort I level osteotomy with this procedure.

It is classified into three types.

Anterior Le Fort II osteotomy (Converse)	A naso-orbital maxillary osteotomy that combines an intra-oral pre-maxillary osteotomy, but which does not include the posterior maxilla or infra-orbital rims. The nasal capsule and medial orbital skeleton only are mobilized. Palatal osteotomy similar to a Wunderer pattern osteotomy may be required for completion. This operation is unsuitable for cleft patients.
Pyramidal Le Fort II osteotomy	A midface osteotomy similar to the Le Fort II fracture pattern, the principle indication being nasomaxillary hypoplasia. It is the commonest pattern of Le Fort II osteotomy and there are several established modifications. These include dento-alveolar segment inclusion or exclusion and modifications in cleft palate cases.
Quadrangular Le Fort II osteotomy; (Küffner-modified Le Fort III)	First described by Küffner (1971) and subsequently modified by several others. The indications are significant maxillary deficiency that extends to the infra-orbital rims and zygomas but with normal nasal projection. This operation leaves the nasal capsule unaltered and mobilizes the maxillae and zygomas *en bloc*. The orbital osteotomies and sagittal splitting of the zygomas require incisions similar to those for subcranial Le Fort III osteotomies. Keller and Sather described a wholly intra-oral approach to the quadrangular Le Fort II osteotomy .
Laterally extended Le Fort II osteotomy	A further Küffner-like modification which becomes almost indistinguishable from a subcranial Le Fort III

osteotomy. Lateral orbital walls may be included in the maxilla-malar movements.

Combination osteotomies Combined midface and separate malar ostetomies are described.

Techniques *1. Preparations.* Tarsorrhaphies, submucous septal resection and tracheostomy should be considered.

2. Incisions. Access to the medial orbital floor is made via subciliary, blepharoplasty or medial skin crease incisions bilaterally. A central supranasal incision over the nasal bridge or glabella region is required. Intraorally, buccal sulcus incisions either in the horseshoe pattern similar to that for Le Fort I osteotomy or bilateral buccal incisions from first molar to canine regions. Adequate degloving and protection of infraorbital nerves, lacrimal tissues and medial canthal ligaments is required.

3. Osteotomies. Bilateral orbital rim cuts are performed passing antero-posteriorly between the infraorbital nerve and nasolacrimal duct, passing medially behind the lacrimal sac on to the medial orbital wall. The midline glabellar level cut is made and joined to each medial orbital osteotomy. A nasal septal section is made in the infero-posterior direction. Le Fort I level maxillary buccal cuts are made and pterygoid disjunction is performed.

4. Mobilization. Performed in the downward and forward direction.

5. Bone grafting. Cancellous bone from the iliac crest is harvested and fixed into osteotomy sites. Rib grafting for augmentation of malar prominences may be used.

6. Fixation. Requires miniplate fixation, craniomandibular fixation and IMF if bimaxillary procedure has been performed. Craniomaxillary fixation with frontal or superciliary, pinned external fixators and universal joints is possible. Suspensory wires may be required. There are several available systems of external fixation, including Mount Vernon and Levant frames.

The Le Fort III osteotomy

The first total midface osteotomy at Le Fort III level was reported by Gillies and Harrison. However, extensive pioneering work by Tessier in 1960 established the feasibility of routinely performing the Le Fort III osteotomy to correct severe midfacial congenital deformities found typically in the craniofacial dysostoses such as Aperts, Crouzon and Pfeiffer syndromes.

The Küffner modification of the Le Fort III osteotomy is usually reserved for the treatment of severe infra-orbital recession with normal nasal profile and central projection. It is useful in malar-maxillary advancement.

The subcranial approach is similar in design to that described for Le Fort II osteotomies.

In craniofacial syndromes, the technique often requires a transcranial approach in conjunction with the neurosurgeon. Orbital depth and volume may be altered. In syndromic patients, the Le Fort III osteotomy is usually performed at an early age, often at 7 or 8 years of age. A Le Fort I osteotomy may subsequently be required after cessation of growth. Le Fort III osteotomies are quite stable procedures. When undertaken in young, growing children, relapses may occur and are related to continued mandibular growth rather than midface relapse. Interpositional bone grafts play an important role in stability.

Techniques

1. Incisions. These are similar to those described for the Le Fort II procedures.

2. Osteotomies. The bone cuts are made across the orbital floor, laterally through the base of the lateral orbital margin and vertically downwards through the zygomatic bone, half way or two-thirds of the distance from the orbital margin, which creates inverted L-shaped separation.

The osteotomy crosses the medial orbital wall on each side. The frontal process of the zygomatic bone is split in the sagittal plane. The lateral wall of the orbit is therefore split and the cut is continued inferiorly to complete division of the zygoma. The osteotomies are joined through the fronto-nasal area. Pterygoid disjunction and septal separation are then completed. The central facial block is mobilized.

3. Bone grafting. Iliac crest bone grafting is usually required after mobilization.

4. Occlusion. Dental relationships are established using an inter-maxilliary wafer.

5. Fixation. Craniomaxilliary fixation is often required, but intra-operative IMF can usually be removed.

6. Adjunctive procedures. Transposition of orbital fat and fascia through an inferior incision, repositioning of muscle attachments and tongue reduction may be required in selected cases.

Malar osteotomies

Indications

Congenital malar hypoplasia, post-traumatic zygomatic depression and craniofacial syndrome-associated lateral facial disharmony are indications for isolated malar surgery.

Techniques

Incisions. Access using the subcranial approach described for Le Fort III osteotomies is used. In craniofacial surgery, a bicoronal flap is commonly used for access to the fronto-naso-orbital region and excellent access to the zygoma can by achieved in conjunction.

Osteotomies. Bone cuts are similar to the lateral wing of a Küffner-modified Le Fort III osteotomy. Independent mobilization and correction of each malar can be performed.

Adjunctive procedures. May include separate midfacial osteotomy or malar augmentation with bone or alloplastic materials. Lower level dento-alveolar osteotomies or cleft deformities may also be required.

Related topics of interest

Cephalometric analysis (p. 58)
Osteotomies (p. 297)

Revision point

Post natal facial growth

HIV DISEASE – OROFACIAL ASPECTS

AIDS may be defined as a persistent defect in cell-mediated immunity with no other known cause other than demonstrable infection with Human Immunodeficiency Virus (HIV).

Epidemiology

1. At risk groups. Homosexuals (72%), IV drug abusers (15%), haemophiliacs and blood transfusion recipients (2%). Children and heterosexual partners of affected patients are at risk.

2. Indicator diseases may permit a preliminary diagnosis of AIDS before definitive laboratory results are available. They include oesophageal or pulmonary candidiasis, disseminated cytomegalovirus (CMV) infection, and cryptosporidial diarrhoea or mucocutaneous herpes simplex ulceration lasting more than 1 month. Kaposi's sarcoma or primary cerebral lymphoma in patients under the age of 60 or interstitial lymphoid pneumonia in young children are suggestive of HIV infection.

Immunology

The triad of decreased T4 (CD4) count, polyclonal IgG hypergammaglobulinaemia and impaired delayed or attenuated delayed hypersensitivity response characterise laboratory findings. Absolute lymphopaenia, reduced cytotoxic responsiveness of CD8 and NK cells, impaired monocyte function and circulating immune complexes are typical findings. Impaired cell-mediated immunity follows. The antibody response or seroconversion occurs between 6 and 18 weeks from infection. In some a 'flu like' seroconversion illness occurs. A small number of infected and infectious patients never seroconvert. Virus isolation and antigen detection are capable of establishing the diagnosis in affected patients. ELISA tests for HIV antigen detection are now available. These permit earlier detection than dependence on antibody testing alone and if measured levels are persistently raised it is associated with a poor prognosis.

Virology

The infectious agents are RNA reverse transcriptase producing retroviruses. Mutations are common. The agent is now known as HIV but already HIV2 is well characterized. Demonstration of the virus may be obtained using electron microscopy, cellular assays to demonstrate cytopathic effect or antigen expression, reverse transcriptase detection in supernatants, and nucleic acid genetic probes for detection of viral nuclear material. Pharmacological inhibition of the RNA reverse transcriptase enzyme with zidovidene is a possible therapeutic step. There are newer analogues under trial currently. Clinical benefit is variable.

Infections

1. *Opportunistic infections.* Protozoal infections causing pneumocystis pneumonia or cryptosporidium diarrhoea, disseminated or extensive candidiasis, viral (CMV) colitis or encephalitis.

2. *Other infections.* Tuberculosis, salmonella septicaemia, HIV encephalitis and lymphoid interstitial pneumonia in childhood AIDS are all noted as closely associated features of HIV infection.

Tumours

Kaposi's sarcoma, B-cell non-Hodgkin's lymphomas and increased risk of other cancers are documented.

Clinical aspects

Classifications. CDC classification. There are four subgroups. In sequence they are acute HIV infection, asymptomatic infection, persistent generalized lymphadenopathy (PGL) and full AIDS. There are other more complex staging classifications available (such as the Walter–Reed system) but the CDC is simple and workable.

Phases and progression

1. *Acute seroconversion illness.* Characterized by fever, macular rash, disseminated lymphadenopathy and pharyngitis.

2. *Persistent generalized lymphadenopathy.* Widespread enlarged lymph nodes. If prolonged over 3 months in an at risk patient PGL is very likely to be due to AIDS.

3. *AIDS related complex (ARC).* A systemic illness without recurrent major episodes of opportunistic infection.

Orofacial disease

Occurs very commonly, particularly in later stage patients.

1. Thrush. Oral candidiasis is very common owing to the disease itself and to extensive antibiotic use often required in AIDS patients. Oesophageal, tracheobronchial and pulmonary candidiasis are common in AIDS patients but rare in non-HIV infected patients.

2. Leukoplakia. Hyperkeratinisation and Epstein Barr virus (EBV) infection all contribute. Hairy leukoplakia is rare amongst non-immunocompromised patients but frequent in AIDS.

3. Gingivostomatitis. Poor mouth care and hepetic stomatitis are additive in their deleterious effects.

4. Recurrent oral ulceration. Viral and non-infective aphthous pattern ulcers occur more commonly than among non-AIDS patients.

5. Sinusitis, otitis media and otitis externa are commonly seen.

6. Parodontal sepsis and neck space infections occur and require aggressive antibiotic treatment. Quinsy is more common than in non-affected patients. Surgery for abscess drainage is required in association with high dose antibiotics.

7. Facial skin conditions. Folliculitis, shingles, molluscum contagiosum, seborrhoeic dermatitis, papilloma viral warts, both intra-oral and facial, and dermatophyte infections are all described. Increased rates of malignant melanomas and basal cell carcinoma (BCC) are a problem in AIDS patients.

8. *Kaposi's sarcoma* can affect skin or mucosa. Treatment by excision, radiotherapy or intra-lesional chemotherapy may be effective.

Further reading

Farthing *et al.* AIDS, Wolfe Atlas.

HYPERBARIC OXYGEN

The combination of increasing both the fractional concentration of oxygen in the inspired gas mixture (FiO_2) and its ambient pressure is known as hyperbaric oxygen. Hyperbaric oxygen (HBO) therapy finds several uses in maxillofacial surgery.

Indications for HBO

- Radiation necrosis of bone and soft tissues
- Healing of wounds
- Compromised skin grafts and flaps
- Chronic refractory osteomyelitis
- Crush injuries and traumatic ischaemia
- Gas gangrene
- Diabetic ulcers
- Carbon monoxide and cyanide poisoning
- Acute smoke inhalation
- Decompression sickness
- Gas embolism.

The major use of HBO therapy in head and neck surgery is for management of non-healing wounds after tumour excisions and as treatment for osteoradionecrosis. The biological problems in wounds that fail to heal include sepsis, failing vascularity, fracture site mobility, residual or recurrent tumour and nutritional deficiencies. These damaging biological effects are due to free radical generation, and the failure of their absorption and neutralization is well described.

Free radical-related disease *Failure of free radical generation* in chronic granulomatous disease results in neutrophil dysfunction and severely impaired intracellular killing of microorganisms.

Phagocytosis and superoxide radical generation fail and frequent episodes of staphylococcal skin infections occur and may be complicated by hepatorenal damage and osteomyelitis.

Free radical scavenging failure: typically an endarteritis is associated. It may be that the poor vascularity that underlies the failure of wound healing is related initially to free radical arteritis.

Induction or promotion of neoplasia may follow from nuclear or chromosomal damage related to free radical activity.

Clinical problems

Non-healing of wounds	• poor vascularity • oxygen demand exceeds supply • impaired local nutrition • mobility of fractures • foreign bodies
Pain	• ischaemia • sepsis • inflammation • neurogenic; if residual tumour is present
Debility	• chronic disease • cachexia • malnutrition • anaemia
Associated medical problems	• diabetes mellitus • poor peripheral vascular status • immunocompromise • drugs

Delivery of HBO therapy

Delivery requires a specialized chamber and gas supply. There are two patterns.

The chamber delivers pure oxygen (FiO_2 = 100%) at increased pressure.
The chamber is air filled and the pressure is increased and the patient breaths 100% oxygen from a mask.

The protocols followed mirror those used in management of diving accidents. Each session is referred to as a 'dive'.

The duration of each dive is determined according to tables similar to those used in the management of decompression illness in divers. One typical protocol developed by Marx for treatment of osteoradionecrosis is detailed.

Stage 1:   30 dives.
            If improvement; further 30 dives completed (60 total).
            If no improvement; go to stage 2.

Stage 2:   Transoral sequestrectomy and primary closure, then complete 60 dives.

            Failure; wound dehiscence, fistula persistence or pathological fracture.
            If failure or progression occurs go to stage 3 or 3R.

Stage 3:   Mandibular resection, then complete 60 dives.
Stage 3R: 20 dives followed by reconstruction followed by 20 dives.

The dive counts may be exceeded if clinical improvement is continuing after the protocol is completed.

Contraindications to use of HBO include:

- intercurrent or new malignancy
- optic neuritis
- relative contraindications include age and physical infirmity such that use of the chamber is impractical.

Osteoradionecrosis   *1. Prevention.* It is wise to complete all dental treatment prior to DXT. It is essential to cover dental surgery with oral hygiene optimization, antiseptic mouthwashes and antibiotics. Consider pre-surgical HBO.

2. Initial conservative treatment. Antibiotics, mouthwashes and debridement are options.

3. HBO. If healing is not achieved, the patient enters the protocol at a point appropriate to the clinical presentation. If persistent fistula or pathological fracture is already present stage 2 is appropriate. Surgery is therefore required in addition to HBO.

4. Other methods for overcoming reduced local tissue vascularity may include pedicle flaps and free tissue transfer. If the problems of the recipient bed remain unaddressed, ischaemia and sepsis are likely to lead to flap failure.

5. Combination therapy with high frequency ultrasound and antibiotics has been shown to be effective.

Further reading

Wood GA, Liggins S. Does hyperbaric oxygen have a role in management of osteoradionecrosis? *British Journal of Oral and Maxillofacial Surgery,* 1996; **34:** 424–7.

IMAGING

There are many clinical uses of imaging techniques in maxillofacial surgery.

Plain radiographs

In oral and facial surgery a wide variety of plain films are commonly requested.

1. Intra-orals. Useful for diagnosis of dental lesions. Bitewings and periapicals are the principle films used in diagnosis of dental caries and periapical disease. Standard occlusal projections permit localization of ectopic, unerupted teeth if used in conjunction with a periapical film using a parallax technique.

2. OPG. Orthopantomographs are very widely used projections. OPG is an example of axial tomography which gives good images of the body and ramus of the mandible, the maxillary alveolus and moderate views of the antra. The images of the anterior alveolar tissues are less good unless on standard OPG films. More modern equipment allows adjustment of the centre of rotation and an elliptical path to be traced by the film cartridge rather than the circular pattern used by older equipment. The changes in the path travelled about the axis result in improvement in the focus and detail available. Magnification of 10–15% results from most OPG machines and localization is possible if used in conjunction with an intra-oral projection. These films are used in assessment of intra-alveolar lesions, in trauma and in orthognathic surgery.

3. PA face or PA jaws. Postero–anterior views allow good visualization of transverse relationships of the mandibular angles with respect to the body in mandible fractures. Commonly 'winging' of the posterior fracture segments occurs due to unfavourable muscle action. Assessment of the condylar neck and head in fractures and fracture dislocations is possible with this view. Mid third facial bone positions can be assessed and this projection has some use in orthognathic surgical planning.

4. *Lateral cephalometric views.* Assessment of skeletal jaw relationships and follow up of orthognathic patients undergoing presurgical orthodontics. Facial growth and skeletal maturation can be followed by serial films. These views are essential for orthognathic plotting and surgical planning.

5. *Occipitomental views.* Taken at various angulations from 10° to 30° these projections are useful as sinus views and in assessment of zygomatic complex and orbital floor injuries.

6. *Submentovertex.* Used in assessment of zygomatic arch fractures.

7. *TMJ views.* There are several available views. Transorbitals, transpharyngeals or reverse Townes views in open and closed positions allow assessment of static joint positions and delineation of gross joint disease.

8. *Cervical spine.* Laterals and AP views are required showing the full length down from atlas to the lower border of C7 to exclude fractures. An open mouthed odontoid peg view is essential in major trauma. Oblique views may also be useful.

9. *Chest and thoracic inlet.* PA chest films may be required for pre-anaesthetic assessment in patients whose medical history suggests the necessity. Thoracic inlet views are occasionally required in preparation for thyroid excision if retrosternal extension of goitre is present.

10. *Skull films.* In trauma when cranial bone fracture or intra-cranial foreign bodies are suspected. Assessment of head injury may require such views.

11. *Limbs or abdomen.* In the preoperative stage for patients with head and neck malignancy in whom free tissue transfer during surgery is planned.

12. Soft tissue films. Impacted foreign bodies and in laryngeal trauma, soft tissue penetration films may aid localisation and assessment.

Fluoroscopy

Screening of a sequence of X-ray exposures allows assessment of swallow in dysphagia, bulbar palsy and obstructive sleep apnoea. Endoscopy has largely superseded this technique in practice.

Ultrasound scans

Fluid filled swellings can be delineated by ultrasound scans. It is a useful technique for diagnosis in cysts, salivary gland lesions, and cystic tumours. Diagnosis of obstruction of salivary glands due to calculi and duct strictures is a frequent use. Intra-luminal ultrasound probes placed in the oesophagus permit assessment of mediastinal masses and duplex scans are useful in blood flow studies for neck disease and in limb vessels prior to free tissue transfer.

CT scanning

Computerised tomograms are widely indicated in trauma, FESS planning, assessment of extent of primary oro-facial malignancy and neck node involvement and in detailing cleft deformities in adults. 3D computerized reconstruction allows planning of surgery in complex syndromes and in conjunction with jig cut models from reconstructed scans accurate model surgery is possible.

MRI scanning

Magnetic resonance scans are good at producing soft tissue images. They are based on the spin resonance properties of water molecules in a magnetic field rather than relying on X-rays. Useful in delineating meniscal displacement and synovial disease in TMJ syndromes, they are thought nevertheless to exhibit a high rate of false positive diagnoses for meniscal displacement. The diagnostic significance of TMJ images is often uncertain therefore. In facial pain assessment and diagnosis of lymph nodes in neck disease secondary to intra-oral malignancy MRI images are useful.

Contrast techniques

Barium or Gastrograffin swallow X-ray sequences are used in assessment of dysphagia. Sialography is performed by cannulation of salivary gland ducts and is used in duct obstruction and assessment of salivary gland disease. Angiography in free flap planning may be used although Doppler scans are less invasive and more commonly employed. Digital substraction angiography (DSA) is used in diagnosis of CVA and angiography may be useful in management of trauma and in planning of haemangioma embolisation. Contrast enhancement of CT scans is possible and gadolinium salts will enhance the images produced on MRI scans.

Nuclear medicine

Isotope scans are useful in assessment of bone and thyroid disease. Vitality of vascularized bone grafts and functionality in thyroid lesions may be determined. Bone scintiscanning in determining the activity of growth centre in craniofacial asymmetry and in syndromic patients may be used.

Other techniques

Cine radiography and xeroradiography are described. Bone densitometry may be applied to bone reconstructions in the postoperative period. Soft tissue planning and assessment prior to complex orthognathic surgery can be aided by laser digitized imaging. Localization techniques including needle guidance to pathological foci may be used aided by ultrasound or CT scanning. Photography, digitized imaging and orthognathic plotting and predictive algorhythms extend the usefulness of the radiographic methods in planning facial surgery.

Overlap with endoscopy

The choice of investigations for an individual patient is determined by the availability of specialist equipment and local expertise in most cases. The correlation of endoscopic and radiological appearances enhances the usefulness of both techniques.

Interventional radiology

The application of Seldinger techniques for catheter insertion permits endoluminal surgery in vascular and urological surgery. Research into endovascular techniques in major vascular reconstructions continues and may find application in head and neck surgery in the future. As yet there is relatively little application in extracranial maxillofacial surgery.

IMPLANTS

In maxillofacial surgery, the need for techniques to replace or reconstruct tissues lost in trauma, by disease or after surgical excision is common. Implants are one useful method of providing firm support for prosthetic tissue replacement and for retention of surgical devices such as hearing aids. Proprietary intra-oral and extra-oral implant systems are available.

Types of implant

Diodontic

Single dental unit replacements have been the subject of much interest, and alternately extolled and condemned. The advent of osseointegrated implant techniques has improved the options for this pattern of implant. Removal of the apical portion of a dental root will permit placement of a combined implant–endodontic post-pattern fixture. The implant part of the fixture is allowed to osseointegrate with the apical bone and the endodontic part is in firm contact with the dentinal surface of the root canal. This part of the fixture requires luting.

Subperiosteal

Cast non-ferrous alloy frameworks are made to a bone surface impression taken during the first stage surgery. A second operation is required for placement of the implant. The submucosal framework is completely covered with alveolar mucosa, and the transmucosal posts, integral to the cast structure, are uncovered at placement. The failure rate as determined by mucosal dehiscence is significant. Bone grafting or osseointegrated implant techniques have superseded this technique.

Transmandibular

For extensively atrophic mandibles, a combined intra- and extra-oral approach permits insertion of transosseous implants secured with lower border baseplates and an alveolar superstructure. This is a very 'operator-sensitive' technique that remains of largely unproven long-term benefit.

Osseointegrated

Many proprietary systems are available. The Branemark system is rapidly becoming the standard. A staged technique with strict adherence to prescribed technique is required to achieve the high published success rates. Titanium oxide is the basis of the implant coating and is associated with bone growth and biological integration.

Uses

Dental arch reconstruction

Intra-oral osseointegrated implants can be used to replace single teeth or to support a denture or full arch prosthetic appliance. The use of this technique in reconstruction of the atrophic, edentulous mandible in conjunction with bone grafting is becoming more common. The ability of titanium oxide-coated fixtures to retain the volume of bone grafts is well documented. In advanced periodontal bone loss, a combined approach involving implant placement, alloplastic bone replacement and guided tissue regeneration techniques with membrane placement are described. In the maxilla, antral floor augmentation with bone grafts after 'sinus lifting' approaches is often successful.

Post-tumour excision and reconstruction

The intra-oral aspect of postoperative reconstruction for cancer patients has been much improved with the advent of osseointegrated implants. Where mandibular alveolus has been excised, implant-retained dentures offer a stable reconstruction where previously an unsatisfactory, bulky and unstable denture was the only real option. Extra-oral fixtures pemit orbital and facial prostheses to be firmly retained. Poor tissue healing and osteoradionecrosis are contraindications.

Post-traumatic tissue loss

Like cancer patients, major trauma may lead to patients presenting with similar needs for complex prosthetic restoration of orofacial tissues. The techniques used in post-oncological reconstruction are often appropriate.

Extra-oral techniques

These may include provision of support prosthetic eyes, ears and nasal superstructure.

Bone-anchored hearing aids (BAHA)

Extra-oral fixtures provide a very firm foundation for these devices.

Surgery of the extremities

Digital implants may permit finger reconstruction after amputation.

Future uses	Major joint replacement such as hip or knee may eventually replace cemented prostheses. The future for osseointegrated TMJ prostheses remains far from clear however.

Aspects of the technique

Staged reconstruction	Fixture placement must be performed 6–9 months before second stage surgery. This will allow osseointegration to occur before any surgery to establish the transmucosal phase of healing is done.
Intra-oral placement	For intra-oral placement, submucoperiosteal flaps are raised. Bone sites are prepared using high flow water cooling and slow bone preparation to prevent necrosis, infection and subsequent implant failure. Fixtures are inserted under slow, well-cooled rotational action. Complete mucosal cover is achieved. After allowing 6–9 months for osseointegration to occur, a second procedure to uncover the fixtures, attach transmucosal abutments and to place healing caps is required. Once a sound epithelial cuff has formed around the implant and osseointegration is sound, prosthetic work can begin.

Failure of osseointegration will occur if cooling is inadequate, if infection supervenes, if premature loading is permitted or tumour recurrence in adjacent tissue occurs. External beam radiotherapy-related osteoradionecrosis, if untreated, will result in failure of the implant, but the use of hyperbaric oxygen may reduce the failure rate in such patients. In most cases, previous DXT constitutes a contraindication to the use of osseointegrated implants. Clinical signs of failure include mobility, persistent sepsis or inflammation and sinus formation. Removal and resiting of the fixture is usually required.

Extra-oral implant placement	A transcutaneous incision and bone surface exposure are required for extra-oral placement. The clinical steps are essentially similar to those for intra-oral placement.
Bone augmentation	Osseointegrated implants have the effect of stimulating bone deposition. In-grafting autologous bone at the time of implant placement further enhances this effect. Sinus

lifts, via a Caldwell Luc approach but external to the antral mucosa, allow bone grafting and provision of a greater depth of bone into which simultaneous maxillary implant placement can be performed. Prior insertion of implants into the donor bone site, such as the iliac crest, will permit harvest of a combined graft–implant block and insertion of an already osseointegrated fixture into the recipient site. The use of bone morphogenetic protein remains unproven in this treatment but may emerge as a useful adjunct.

Tissue–implant interface

Soft tissue factors, both epithelial and fibrous, are important in long-term retention of osseointegrated implants. Meticulous surgery and care with surgical soft tissue flap design and apposition on completion of operative procedures is essential. A true gingival crevice cannot in reality be formed but a sound, infection-free peri-implant epithelial cuff can be. Whether combined use of guided tissue regeneration techniques may aid this aspect of the technique remains under investigation. The local flora is altered due to the non-physiological anatomy.

Prosthetic aspects

Placement of single or multiple dental units, Dolder-type bars for denture support, effective restoration of occlusal vertical dimension and facial contouring are all possible. Retention with custom precision-type attachments and magnets is used. For extra-oral sites, site-specific retention devices are available.

INCISIONS AND ACCESS TO THE FACIAL SKELETON

Surgical exposure of the facial skeleton and access to deeper structures is becoming a specialty related art. New approaches must significantly enhance access and ease of performing the desired surgery, be relatively swift to execute and simple to reconstruct without cosmetic deficit.

Intraoral incisions

1.   Gingival. Either gingival margin subperiosteal incisions or buccal envelope type incisions allow ready access to the alveolar segments and routine dentoalveolar surgery may be performed using these techniques.

2.   Intraoral degloving. Extended buccal incisions are used during orthognathic surgery of mandible and maxilla. They allow excellent access and easy sound wound closure.

3.   Palatal. Palatal access is best achieved via a flap incised at the gingival margins. Only rarely need palatal mucosa be transected; typically during segmental osteotomy or during flap design in cleft palate repair.

4.   Supraperiosteal. If a safe approach around the cutaneous nerves of the face is required or if periosteum is to be excised with a biopsy specimen, these techniques are used. In nerve sparing approaches, the incision is deepened through the periosteum once the nerve trunk has been identified and preserved.

Extraoral approaches

1.   Periorbital. Access to the orbital skeleton can be achieved via suborbital incisions, lateral orbitotomy, malar osteotomy, supraciliary incisions and pericranial flaps. Transantral and pernasal middle meatal approaches are described but not widely used in facial surgery.

The relatively common isolated orbital floor injury can be approached via infraorbital skin crease, subciliary, transconjunctival or blepharoplasty incisions.

2. Frontocranial and occipital. The hemicranial or bicoronal flap is the 'workhorse' incision for cranial vault surgery, as access for galeal–pericranial flaps and osteoplastic flaps for use in facial reconstruction and for neurosurgical access. Temporoparietal and occipital flaps are widely used in neurosurgery.

3. Pituitary. Trans-sphenoidal, transantral or subfrontal approaches are all described. Currently, the pernasal trans-sphenoidal approach is widely in favour.

4. Nasoethmoid. There are several eponymous subtypes of surgical approaches to the medial orbital wall. Bicoronal flap elevation may be required if extensive dissection is required.

5. Perinasal. Rhinoplasty techniques create the need for intranasal and peralar incisions. Open or lateral rhinotomy gives good access to the external nasal skeleton, midfacial bones and inferior orbital rim.

6. Lateral midface. Gillies' temporal approach to zygomatic arch fractures is a common approach for relatively minor trauma. Preauricular, temporal and suborbital approaches are all described.

7. Midface degloving. Weber Ferguson and Altemir incisions allow excellent access to the midface in extended maxillary surgery or maxillectomy. Upper lip splitting and combined intraoral buccal mucosal incisions are required to permit development of the midface soft tissue flap.

8. Pre-auricular and TMJ. For parotid surgery and access to the temporomandibular joint for elective and post-trauma surgery the preauricular skin crease incision is common. This incision may be extended into the mastoid and submandibular region in parotid surgery and into the temporal region for joint surgery. Transaural and post-auricular approaches to the TMJ are described. Temporal extension of this incision allows ready harvesting of tempralis fascia in myringoplasty and closure of OAF. This incision is modified for use in rhytidectomy and requires post-auricular extension into the skin above the hairline, the edges being bevelled to minimize damage to the hair follicles.

9. Mandibular ramus. External and intraoral approaches may be used. For low level access an extended third molar buccal mucosal incision may be used, particularly in fractures in the region of the angle. For orthognathic surgery, this incision needs to be augmented by elevation of a lingual subperiosteal flap or by submandibular external incision. For higher ramus surgery a preauricular incision is often preferable. Access to the coronoid is possible via an upward extension of the buccal incision described.

10. Tonsillar fossa and posterior tongue. Direct tonsillar fossa approach with suitable neck extension and mouth prop allows tonsillectomy, biopsy or quinsy drainage to be performed without difficulty. For extensive dissection in malignant disease or for posterior dissection, lower lip splitting and mandibular osteotomy allow much better access to this region. Reconstruction is straightforward and usually complication free. Some surgeons advocate segmental mandibulectomy to prevent compression of vascular pedicles where local or free flaps have been used to reconstruct a large intra-oral defect.

11. Neck incisions. Submandibular incisions are designed to preserve the marginal mandibular branch of the facial nerve and to allow access to the submandibular gland and the suprahyoid triangles, both submandibular and submental, during neck dissection.

- *McFee.* Upper and lower parallel neck incisions allow access to the neck for purposes of neck dissection and tunnelled access for transmission of pectoralis and latissimus dorsi pedicled flaps. This incision is reportedly associated with fewer wound dehiscences in previously irradiated tissues.

- *Crile and variations*. Either Y, T or H patterns are widely used to give a triangular three flap pattern and good access to all regions of the neck.
- *L pattern*. The vertical limb is made over sternomastoid and the horizontal limb passing forwards over the anterior neck to the midline. This allows access for thyroid, laryngeal and oesophageal surgery combined with neck dissection.
- *Supraclavicular*. Transverse to allow sampling of the lymph nodes in this region.
- *Thyroid*. For benign thyroid disease a transverse skin crease incision is used. For extensive or malignant disease a more extensive incision is preferable. One of the incisions used for neck dissection is often a better choice.
- *Vertical*. Uncommon in the neck but hemilaryngectomy may be performed via such an approach. Midline vertical incisions may be used in tracheostomy to preserve lateral tissues for inclusion in flap elevation during reconstruction if the stoma is part of a major ablative operation in malignant disease.
- *Posterior*. Scalp incisions for removal of soft tissue tumours or flaps for infratentorial neurosurgical access are all described. Posterior or occipital and mastoid triangle dissection may be required in nodal metastases from posterior scalp malignancies.

Osteotomy techniques

Mandible splitting, Le Fort I osteotomies and malar osteotomies are all used to gain access to different parts of the head and neck. Posterior tongue and pharynx can be approached with a midline or parasagittal mandibulotomy, Le Fort I osteotomy gives excellent access to the upper cervical spine and nasopharynx as well as to the cranial base. Lateral cranial base surgery and posterior orbital approaches are all enhanced by zygomatic osteotomy. Palate splitting may be an adjunctive procedure in maxillary osteotomy as access to midline cranial base in excision of large tumours.

LE FORT I OSTEOTOMY

This is an extremely versatile operation and can be adapted for many uses.

Indications

1. *Maxillary–mandibular disproportion.* Jaw disproportion and malocclusion at the dento-alveolar level may be corrected in conjunction with pre-surgical orthodontics and possibly with combined mandibular surgery. This is the commonest indication for low level maxillary surgery.

2. *Late cleft surgery.* In the post-adolescent phase, hypoplasia of the middle third of the facial skeleton may be extreme. This is particularly true if early or extensive surgery has been required for closure of palatal clefts. Le Fort I level maxillary advance often requires prior or simultaneous bone grafting to repair residual alveolar clefts and to close oro-nasal fistulae.

3. *Combined with high level advance.* Le Fort III osteotomy for major craniofacial deformity can be combined where necessary with a dento-alveolar advance.

4. *Cranial base access.* Access to the nasopharynx, upper cervical spinal and cranial base is greatly facilitated by use of this osteotomy.

5. *Post-traumatic.* Correction of a late presentation of an old fracture is possible.

6. *Obstructive sleep apnoea (OSA).* Maxillary advance is sometimes advocated as part of the treatment of OSA.

7. *Down's syndrome.* The relative macroglossia and associated drooling of saliva can occasionally be improved by osteotomy.

Planning

1. *The maxillary dento-alveolar component,* once mobilized, can be moved almost in any direction.

Backward or upward movements (impactions) are more difficult to perform than forward or downward ones. As part of a bimaxillary procedure in combination with a sagittal split mandibular osteotomy, very large alterations in facial form can be achieved.

2. Segmental maxillary osteotomies may allow additional modification to the Le Fort I technique; however, the limitations of unmodified segmental osteotomies will still apply.

3. Soft tissue form. Lip length and resultant dento-alveolar visibility may present problems. With Le Fort I techniques, soft tissue adaptation to the new skeletal position is usually excellent, nevertheless a degree of overcorrection should be built into the surgical plan to allow for a degree of relapse due to the limitations imposed by the soft tissue envelope.

4. Psychological aspects and patient motivation are essential aspects in determining suitability for orthognathic surgery. Poor compliance with preoperative orthodontics or unresolved or untreated psychiatric illness constitute relative contraindications to such elective surgery.

Preparations

- Clinical examination.
- Full records including photographs.
- Trimmed and articulated study models.
- Radiographic assessment to determine dental status, presence of unerupted or supplemental teeth and presence of alveolar pathology is essential.
- Cephalometric radiographs and tracings are required for detailed skeletal analysis and osteotomy planning.
- Soft tissue form and function and any parafunctional habits are documented. High relapse rates can be expected in patients with uncorrected habits such as digit sucking. Endogenous tongue thrusts and bruxism are relative contraindications to surgery.
- Prediction of soft tissue form postoperatively is difficult and the subject of ongoing research.

- Pre-osteotomy surgery; removal of third molars and unerupted teeth is essential in the months prior to osteotomy. Nasal airway surgery can be considered preoperatively if symptomatic or if a large degree of mandibular intrusion is planned.
- Pre-surgical orthodontics is usually essential.

Technique

1. Incision. Extended buccally from the distal aspect of the first molar tooth on one side to the same point on the opposite side leaving a generous skirt of unattached mucosa to facilitate suturing later. Distal extension beyond the first molar may compromise the vascularity of the osteotomized segment and is not necessary. The muco-periostial flap is raised. Distal subperiostial reflection from the end of the incision line to the posterior aspect of the tuberosity is made on both sides, and curved retractors are placed in the pterygoid buttress posterior to the maxilla on both sides, Infra-orbital tissues are exposed and the neurovascular bundle protected. The mucosa in the floor of the nose is reflected.

2. Osteotomy cuts.
(a) From the lateral wall of the nose at the pyriform fossa at approximately the level of the soft tissue incision in the buccal aspect of both sides of the maxilla. Distal extension of the osteotomy cuts into the pterygomaxilliary fissure behind the posterior aspect of the maxilla on both sides permits disarticulation with the pterygoid osteotome.
(b) The horizontal buccal maxilliary cut often has to be angled around a prominent zygomatic buttress.
(c) At the nasal floor, the septum needs separating from the maxilla, the lateral nasal walls are osteotomized and the inferior turbinates may need trimming.

Once completed, these cuts should allow down fracture of the maxilla.

3. Jaw movements.
(a) *Maxillary intrusion or maxillary set up*: careful trimming of septum, inferior turbinates and the margins of the buccal cuts is required in order to

remove sufficient bone to permit repositioning of the dento-alveolar fragment.

(b) Maxillary set down: interpositional bone grafting may be required.

(c) Interpositional acrylic wafers are essential for most operations. Two wafers are required if a bimaxillary osteotomy is performed.

4. *Modifications.*

(a) Midline palate split in maxillary setback will facilitate the achievement of satisfactory buccal occlusion.

(b) Wedge tuberosity reduction may also be necessary.

(c) *Alloplastic material or bone chip placement* to augment the maxillary prominence may improve final aesthetics.

(d) *Segmental osteotomies or corticotomies* may occasionally be helpful where pre-surgical orthodontics has not been possible.

5. *Fixation.* Rigid fixation with titanium plates and screws is usual in modern orthognathic surgery. Postoperative IMF is rarely required, but light elastic traction may aid final positioning in some patients.

Temporary intra-operative IMF secured on to orthodontic brackets or preformed arch bars and is used in conjunction with intra-operative acrylic wafers to establish the occlusion. The antero-posterior and lateral position of the maxilla is determined in relation to the mandibular occlusion, but final orientation in all dimensions is difficult to establish with complete accuracy. Research continues to determine new techniques which will permit accurate maxilla positioning.

Complications

1. *Intra-operative.*

(a) *Unfavourable osteotomy*: most occur at the pterygoid and palatine regions.

(b) *Haemorrhage:* primary bleeding may occur from the maxillary artery, pterygoid veins and greater palatine vessels.

(c) *Difficult positioning and fixation:* inadequate mobilization, bone reduction in impaction osteotomies or insufficient bone contact after movements will make esablishing the new maxilla position difficult.

(d) *Nasal and airway problems:* septal reduction and turbinate trimming is often required and, if inadequate, makes the postoperative nasal airway inadequate.

(e) *Damage to teeth:* direct damage during segmental surgery or inadvertant apicectomies are described complications.

2. *Postoperative.*

(a) *Haemorrhage:* reactionary haemorrhage in the hours immediately after surgery may occur from the maxillary vessels and the pterygoid venous plexus. IV resuscitation, nasal packing (anterior or posterior) and re-operation may be required. Embolization of bleeding vessels under angiographic control or external carotid artery ligation are described options. Late haemorrhage usually results from sepsis, and high dose antibiotics are required. It is uncommon.

(b) *Sepsis:* local infection may occur but is not commonly troublesome. Bony sequestra or sinusitis may occur in some patients.

(c) *Plate failure:* screw loosening and mucosal dehiscence may require plate removal.

(d) *Relapse:* planning issues include selection of patients for correct operations, good pre-surgical orthodontics, bone grafting if required and slight overcorrection in planned jaw movements. Predisposition to relapse is due to continued facial growth, inadequate fixation and wrong choice of operation. Bimaxillary procedures tend to be more stable than single jaw operations, maxillary impactions are more stable than downward movements and cleft osteotomies are more likely to be unstable than surgery in non-cleft patients.

(e) *Neurological dysfunction:* damage to the infra-orbital nerve may occur.

(f) *Dental problems:* vitality is lost if apical damage has occurred, and loss of sensitivity may result from transection of the posterior superior alveolar nerves in the antral walls.

(g) *Aesthetics:* soft tissue factors including the length of the upper lip, the appearance of the nose and the amount of gingival tissue visible on smiling are all potential sources of patient dissatisfaction.

(h) *Velopharyngeal incompetence:* has been described after large forward movements of the maxilla.

(i) *Iatrogenic oro-nasal fistula:* this may occur if rapid maxillary expansion has been performed preoperatively.

Postoperative requirements

1. Liquid or semi-solid diet. This is important if miniplate fixation has been used and is all that is possible if the patient is in IMF.

2. Analgesia. Individual analgesia demands vary widely. Opiates by PCA pump are useful for the first 24–48 hours, but thereafter NSAID analgesia should be adequate for most patients. Persistent or increasing analgesia demands should arouse suspicion of sepsis or local complications.

3. Antibiotics. Most surgeons give antibiotics if internal fixation has been placed. Three or four postoperative doses are as effective as a prolonged oral course.

4. Occlusion. Intermaxillary elastics may be required.

Follow-up

- *Orthodontic:* postoperative finishing orthodontics is commonly required.
- *Surgical:* normally only required in the immediate postoperative weeks.
- *Combined orthodontic and surgical follow-up:* usually recommended for record keeping and monitoring for 5 postoperative years.
- *Audit* of results is required.

LIP SURGERY

Surgical anatomy

The important features of the lips for surgical planning include the following.

- *Vermillion borders*: non-keratinized, translucent and without skin adnexae.
- *White line*: immediately to the cutaneous side of the mucocutaneous junction. Important in lip repair after trauma and in cleft lip closure.
- *Orbicularis oris*: provides sphincter function to the mouth and contributes to lip competence. The depth from the skin surface is only 2 mm, therefore mucocutaneous malignancies fix skin to deep structures early in the disease course.
- *Vascular supply*: facial, submental and inferior and superior labial arteries.
- *Lymphatic drainage*: dual supply travelling in both the submucosal and subcutaneous planes. Lower lip medial lymphatics pass to the submental nodes and lateral ones to submandibular nodes. The upper lip lymphatics drain to the pre-auricular, pre-parotid and submandibular nodes.
- *Philtrum and Cupid's bow*: the midline structure of the upper lip is important in reconstruction, particularly in cleft lip patients.
- *Commissures*: excisional surgery should attempt to preserve this region as reconstruction is particularly difficult.

Surgical pathology

Benign lesions

1. Benign mucosal lesions. These include fibroepithelial polyps, fibromata, neuromata and salivary mucoceles.

2. Benign cutaneous lesions. These include pyogenic granulomas, common in pregnancy, benign naevi and keratoacanthoma.

3. Granulomatous disease. Sarcoidosis, Crohn's lesions and syphilitic chancres may occur.

Cheilitis

1. Angular cheilitis. Maceration and infection of the mucocutaneous tissues occurs in patients with a combination of oral *Candida,* reduced occlusal vertical dimension and iron deficiency anaemia. Painful commissural splits and poorly healing tissues are pathognomonic.

2. *Granulomatous cheilitis.* This occurs in Crohn's disease, sarcoidosis and Melkersson Rosenthal syndrome.

Clefts

Upper lip clefts occur as isolated lesions and as part of various head and neck syndromes. Rare Tessier clefts affecting the midface and very rarely the lower lip and chin are described.

Neoplasia

1. *Melanoma.* Both cutaneous and mucosal melanomas occur.

2. *Carcinoma.* Ninety seven percent of all lip tumours are squamous carcinomas. There are three types: verrucous, exophytic and ulcerative. Verrucous lesions of the lip are uncommon, and exophytic or mixed ulcero-exophytic patterns are the commonest. Lymph node metastases are present in only 12% of patients with lip cancer unless the commissures are affected. Of these patients, about 20% will have nodal disease at presentation.

Lip surgery

Cosmetic

1. *Augmentation and reduction* in the amount of vermillion visible is sometimes performed. Vermillion advancement is advocated by some surgeons. Collagen or dermal fat injections are also used.

2. *Dento-alveolar and orthognathic procedures.* Associated with such procedures, alteration in the form and prominence of the upper lip in particular can be anticipated.

Excisions

1. *Lip shave.* Excision of the vermillion border is effective treatment for dysplastic or dyskeratotic lesions.

2. *Wedge excision.* A wedge-shaped full thickness excision may be used to excise carcinoma of the lip. Closure with accurate approximation of the mucosal and muscle layer gives a good cosmetic and functional result.

Reconstruction

3. Combination. A combined shave and wedge excision will deal with carcinoma and associated dysplastic field change in the vermillion tissues.

1. Primary closure. Good apposition is possible after excision in which one-third of the width of the lip is involved. Greater tissue loss than one-third dictates formal lip reconstruction.

2. Vermillion advance. Used to reconstruct and replace vermillion tissue after lip shave. It is of no use when full thickness tissue loss or loss of width has resulted from excisional surgery.

3. Abbe rotation or switch flap. After excision of lower lip carcinoma, a similar width of the opposing upper lip is raised as a full thickness flap pedicled on the labial artery. The medial limb of the flap stops short of the white roll and vermillion border, and the flap is rotated permitting apposition of the excisional wound margins. This is a variation on the Abbe rotation used in correction of the short, tight upper lip after closure of primary clefts of the lip. In the post-cancer reconstruction, the commissure is excluded by the first stage Abbe operation and a second procedure is required, a double Z plasty, in order to restore commissural continuity with the rest of the lip.

4. Bernard–Fries. This is not commonly performed. If very large amounts of lower lip tissue are excised, advancement of the margins is possible by bilateral removal of triangles of tissue immediately lateral to the two commissures. Inward rotation permits marginal apposition.

5. Burrows flap. After excision of malignancies of the central upper lip, subalar full thickness ellipses are excised and the excised areas are joined by a subnasal incision. The excision margins may then be approximated.

6. Karapandzic flaps. This is the most functional repair of excised or amputated lip tissue. Skin and muscular layers are dissected free in the lateral nasolabial regions bilaterally. The flaps so raised are rotated inwards and the flap margins once approximated permit function to be restored as the muscle layer is reconstructed. The aesthetics of this flap are acceptable, but subsequent vermillion advancement is possible.

7. *Estlander flap.* After excision of commissural lesions, a flap pedicled on the superior labial artery and prepared parallel to the nasolabial groove allows reconstruction. Subsequent revision of the commissure may be required.

8. *Upper lip reconstruction.* This is difficult if full-length excision is performed. Bilobed forehead flaps or inverse Karapanzic flaps are required.

9. *Commissure reconstruction.* Most immediate restorations after tumour excision or after traumatic lip amputation result in a rounded commissure. Correction of this is achieved using a double Z plasty technique.

Upper lip lesions account for 5–8% of all lip cancers. They pose difficult management problems. Reconstruction requires extensive flaps to be raised, and if nodal metastases are present the wide dissemination of lymphatic drainage makes such tumours essentially inoperable.

Prophylactic bilateral supra-omohyoid neck dissections in large lower lip tumours remains controversial. Radical neck dissection will be required if nodal metastases are found in surgical specimens.

Radiotherapy in lip cancer patients results commonly in lip muscle atrophy and lip stiffness. Increased risk of malignant change in residual tissue, particularly on sun exposure, is noted. Subsequent excision of irradiated tissue may be required.

Related topics of interest

Cleft lip and palate (p. 69)
Cleft lip deformity (p. 75)

LOCAL ANALGESIA

Local anaesthetic agents can be given parenterally, topically as creams, ointments, or as a eutectic mixture of local anaesthetic (EMLA), or to the airway mucosa by inhaled or nebulized aerosol. They can be mixed with steroids for intra-articular injection or with analgesic or general anaesthetic agents.

Locoregional analgesia

This provides a field of anaesthesia over the extent of the anatomical distribution of the nerve subjected to blockade. Most dento-alveolar surgery can be performed by this means. Other procedures which are suitable include excision biopsy and minor soft tissue surgery, insertion of osseointegrated implants, removal of rigid fixation, upper airways endoscopy and pernasal antral puncture.

Regional anaesthetic techniques

1. *Perioral* blockade of inferior or superior alveolar nerves usually for surgical removal of teeth and mental nerve blockade for surgery on anterior mandibular teeth or on the soft tissues of the chin.

2. *Percutaneous* access for establishing anaesthesia in the distributions of maxillary, mandibular, anterior ethmoidal, zygomaticotemporal and zygomaticofrontal nerves are all described.

3. *Infra-orbital nerve* injections allow an extensive area of numbness to be produced on the anterior facial skin, upper anterior teeth and adjacent gingivae as well as the sinus mucosa to a variable degree. It is a useful technique in management of trigeminal neuralgia and for removal of maxillary plates and screws.

Topical techniques

- *EMLA cream*: prior to insertion of IV canullae.
- *Lignocaine paste*: for mucosal application prior to infiltration techniques.
- *Eye ointment or drops.*
- *Benzydamine mouth* rinse for treatment of painful oral mucosal lesions.
- *Nebulized lignocaine* prior to endoscopy, intubation or tracheostomy.

hypopharyngectomy and gastric 'pull up' for hypopharyngeal carcinoma, a thoracic epidural infusion is useful.

Guidelines for procedures appropriate for LA

- The planned operation should be short (i.e. less than 30 min).
- The surgical site should permit easy access. The posterior pharynx, post-nasal space and soft palate therefore constitute difficult access problems which in most patients demand GA even for relatively simple procedures such as biopsy.
- The patient should be capable of willing cooperation.

Advantages of LA
- Avoidance of the necessarily inherent risks of GA.
- Operation on a non-starved patient who is conscious and therefore capable of ongoing implied consent throughout the procedure.
- There is usually no conflict of interest with maintenance of the airway as the gag reflex is maintained and the pharynx remains under conscious control of the patient.

Contraindications to LA
- Pus or active local infection where LA agents are ineffective.
- Sepsis adjacent to perinasal anterior facial soft tissues as the risk of spread of infection is significant.

Revision points

Anatomy of trigeminal nerve and branches for regional blockade.
Basic sciences of pharmacology of different groups of LA drugs.

MALIGNANT NECK DISEASE

The diagnosis and treatment of malignant cervical lymph nodes is central to the management of head and neck cancer.

Location of cervical lymph nodes

- Level I.   Submental and submandibular triangles.
- Level II.   Upper jugular group including nodes adjacent to the accessory nerve and carotid bulb up to the skull base.
- Level III. Middle jugular group comprising nodes from carotid bifurcation to cricothyroid notch.
- Level IV.   Lower jugular group extending from cricothyroid notch to clavicle.
- Level V.   Posterior triangle including supraclavicular nodes.
- Level VI.   Anterior group comprising visceral nodes from hyoid down to supra sternal notch.

There are several clinical scenarios with regard to cervical nodal metastases which require consideration.

Clinically negative neck
In primary head and neck cancers with no palpable lymph nodes (N0 disease) the decision about management of the neck is often difficult. MRI scanning may reveal enlarged lymph nodes which are impalpable on clinical examination. Enlarged cervical nodes even close to an intra-oral primary lesion may prove inflammatory or reactive on histological examination.

1. The 'no treatment' option. This may be preferred by the patient. Regular follow up is required if this option is adopted.

2. Prophylactic neck dissection. Where scanning fails to demonstrate evidence of nodal disease a decision regarding prophylactic neck dissection is required. It is common practice to offer neck dissection to patients about to undergo surgical excision of the primary lesion where the tumour is large, advanced, cytologically or histolocically high grade or in a site known to be frequently associated with nodal metastases. These sites include base of tongue, posterior floor of mouth, pyriform fossa and supraglottic larynx.

3. *Supraomohyoid clearance.* Squamous lesions of the head and neck usually metastasize to cervical nodes in a relatively orderly fashion. In oral lesions it is unlikely therefore that if the first echelon nodes are clear of tumour more distant ones in the jugular chain are involved. Supraomohyoid clearance as a node sampling procedure in association with intra-operative frozen section is an attractive option under such circumstances.

4. *Functional neck dissection.* In the absence of frozen section facilities or where the primary lesion is considered to present a significant likelihood of micrometastaic disease, function sparing neck dissection may be performed.

5. *Radical neck dissection* cannot usually be justified as a prophylactic measure.

6. *Survival benefit* for prophylactic neck dissection remains to be demonstrated.

Clinically positive neck in presence of diagnosed primary lesion

1. *The single palpable lymph node (N1 disease).* Most of these nodes are likely to be reactive. FNAC will demonstrate high lymphocyte counts under these circumstances. If malignant cells are found on FNAC in the first echelon nodes, either radiotherapy or functional neck dissection is usually required. Extracapsular spread is uncommon in N1 disease and radical neck surgery is not usually necessary but is advocated by some.

2. *Larger or multiple unilateral nodes (N2 or N3 disease).* The risk of extracapsular spread is much greater with N2 disease and radical neck dissection or radical cervical radiotherapy is required. Recurrence of neck disease appears to be reduced by addition of radiotherapy after surgery.

3. *Bilateral or contralateral nodes (N2c disease).* Only 5–10% of patients present initially with bilateral or contralateral cervical nodes. The prognosis is however more closely related to the presence of extracapsular spread than to laterality related to the side of the

primary lesion. The morbidity of bilateral neck dissection is considerable and at least one internal jugular vein should be preserved. Interval bilateral radical neck dissections may be performed if necessary and it is considered that sacrifice of both internal jugular veins is required.

Late presenting neck nodes after treatment of head and neck primary

Where no treatment to the neck was given with that of primary lesion, radical neck dissection or radiotherapy is required. Recurrence of tumour on the previously treated side of the neck requires consideration of radiotherapy if none was originally given in a patient who underwent neck dissection. Radical surgery in a previously un-operated but irradiated neck is possible. Second look surgery is less preferable but conversion to a radical pattern neck dissection can be considered if limited operation was performed previously. Contralateral disease in a previously treated neck may occur. Late contralateral radical neck dissection is possible and is associated with an approximate 30% 5-year survival.

Clinically positive neck with an occult primary

Cytology or histology of the node metastasis may reveal the likely primary site. The decision to search for the primary and decisions about management of the neck disease are dealt with in a separate chapter.

Massive or advanced neck disease

Constitutes N3 disease. Less than 5% of head and neck cancer patients present with massive nodal metastases. Decisions regarding operability are important. Invasion of the internal jugular vein, carotid arterial system, or base of skull are makers of probable inoperability. Palliative radiotharepy and tracheostomy may be required.

Lymphoma, adenocarcinomas, infra-clavicular pulmonary lesions and occasionally sarcoma, may present with malignant cervical lymph nodes.

MANDIBULAR RAMUS OSTEOTOMIES

There are a number of patterns of mandibular ramus osteotomy. The sagittal split mandibular osteotomy is commonly performed in the UK and is described in detail in a separate chapter. The vertical subsigmoid, horizontal or oblique and inverted L or C pattern osteotomies are the other major types.

Vertical subsigmoid osteotomy

A versatile and a relatively straightforward procedure, the vertical subsigmoid (VSS) osteotomy can be carried out via an intra-oral or extra-oral approach. The intra-oral osteotomy is slightly more complex technically and often requires a right-angled oscillating saw.

1. Indications include correction of the narrow or atrophic mandible. It is more useful for small mandibular setbacks rather than lengthening procedures. It is useful in the edentulous patient where a small osteotomized correction is required prior to implant placement or in pre-prosthetic surgery where setback rather than lengthening is required.

2. The extra-oral approach via a skin crease incision below the angle of the mandible. Structures at risk include the cervical and marginal mandibular branches of the seventh cranial nerve. The flap is raised, dividing skin, subcutaneous fascia, platysma, and deep fascia. The flap is developed taking the branches of the facial nerve in the upper aspect. Muscle and periostium are stripped upwards towards the sigmoid notch on the outer aspect of the ramus of the mandible and the appropiate channel retractors are placed. The antilingula is a useful landmark so that a vertical cut from the sigmoid notch down towards the anterior aspect of the angle of the mandible should avoid section of the inferior dental neurovascular tissues. The osteotomy is completed with an osteotome. The contralateral osteotomy is performed, planned movements completed and fixation is placed. The wound is closed over a vacuum drain and routine post-osteotomy instructions are instituted.

3. The intra-oral approach is similar to that required for a sagittal split osteotomy. An extended buccally placed triangular incision is made as a flap developed subperiosteally. The lateral surface of the ramus of the mandible is exposed widely, and the osteotomy is performed as described previously.

4. Medial ramus approach. The flap development is essentially the same as for a sagittal split technique except for minimal buccal stripping . A forked coronoid retractor and ramus channel retractors are inserted above the level of the lingula. Having established good medial access, an oblique cut passing upwards and forwards from the angle to the sigmoid notch is made. The osteotomy is completed with an osteotome.

Subcondylar osteotomy

This operation is performed via a similar approach to an intra-oral VSS osteotomy. It permits a range of corrective movements of the mandibular dentition using a relatively quick and simply performed osteotomy. The cuts run from the sigmoid notch in an infero-posterior direction to the posterior border of the ramus.

Horizontal or oblique ramus osteotomy

This operation is a variation of the VSS procedure where the osteotomy cut is placed at a much less vertical angle. The direction of subsequent mandibular movement is determined by the angulation of the osteotomy cuts, but the extent of such a movement is limited. The procedure can be performed from a medial or buccal approach and is usually done from an intra-oral incision similar to that described for a VSS operation.

Inverted L and C or arcing osteotomy

1. Indications. These osteotomies are valuable when an increase in the height and length of the ramus is required in conjunction with a change in the length of the mandibular body. In congenital or post-traumatic mandibular hypoplasia, or post-fractured condyle and occasionally when previous surgery has disturbed the bony or periosteal anatomy, these operations may be useful.

2. Procedure. Similar to a sagittal split procedure, it usually requires a bone graft to make up the deficiency left after the advancement of the tooth-bearing fragment of the mandible. The technique is similar to that of an extra-oral subcondylar osteotomy, with the exception that there is a horizontal cut placed from the anterior border of the ascending ramus passing distally behind the lingula and joining the vertical downward angled cut towards the lower border of the mandible adjacent to the angle. The bone cut is close to the antegonial notch and may be designed as an L, inverted L or C shape. The latter pattern is used where rotational movement or arcing is required.

Interpositional intra-operative wafers can be used to stabilize the mandible in the new position whilst bone grafting and final fixation are placed. Bone for grafting is obtained from the iliac crest or rib and fixed with rigid bone plating. This procedure may be performed in isolation or in conjunction with maxillary osteotomy, in which case the upper jaw surgery should be performed and completed first. The wound is closed in layers over vacuum drainage.

Body osteotomies

These operations are not commonly used in orthognathic surgery. They are usually performed in the pre-molar or first molar region and most are vertical in design, although stepped or oblique osteotomies are described. The mandibular canal is always at risk in these procedures. They are most commonly performed as part of access to the floor of the mouth or lateral border of the tongue during oncological surgery.

Related topics of interest

Osteotomies (p. 297)
Mandibular surgery (p. 238)

MANDIBULAR SURGERY

The range of procedures and indications for surgery on the mandible is extensive. Some operations are designed to deal with conditions affecting the temporomandibular joint. These conditions may be dysfunctional, or organic with ankylosis, sepsis, degenerative arthropathy and tumours such as villonoduar synovitis featuring in the differential diagnosis. Other procedures are pure orthgnathic operations performed to correct jaw disproportion, mandibular asymmetry or abnormalities of the dental occlusion. Pathology of mandibular bone may be primary or secondary. Sepsis, primary bone tumours or alveolar atrophy after dental extraction may be present and spread of local malignancy to affect the mandible is quite common. Metastases from distant malignancy occurs classically from lung, breast, colon, kidney and prostate primary tumours.

Excisions

1. Local curettage. Approached via an intra-oral incision, this pattern of mandibular excision is appropriate for infected or cystic lesions with localised osteitis and for some benign odontogenic tumours. Wide curettage is appropriate in the first line treatment of ameloblastoma but more extensive resection is often required if the tumour recurs.

2. Block excision. Removal of a block of mandible may be necessary for aggressive odontogenic tumours such as ameloblastoma, for very extensive excision of malignancies of the oral floor and for recalcitrant osteomyelitis or osteoradionecrosis. It is avoided where possible as the discontinuity is difficult to rehabilitate without reconstruction.

3. Alveolar excision or rim resection. Where removal of mandibular bone invaded by spread from an adjacent malignancy is necessary, alveolar bone alone may be removed preserving the lower mandibular border intact. This preserves facial contour and is easier to rehabilitate subsequently.

4. Partial or hemimandibulectomy. An extended pattern of block resection which may involve removal of the angle, the ramus or even in some cases the condylar head. Even in 'full' hemimandibulectomy, excision of the TMJ is not commonly required but in patients previously treated with full dose radical radiotherapy where surgery is for salvage purposes or for management of recalcitrant osteoradio-necrosis, joint disarticulation is sometimes performed. Removal of the anterior part of the mandible across the symphyseal region without preservation of the lower border produces the very disfiguring, so called 'Andy Gump' deformity.

Coronoidectomy

1. Indications. Idiopathic coronoid enlargement, impingement syndromes, and for access to the condylar neck during intra-oral condylar neck surgery and after impaction Le Fort I osteotomy.

2. Approach. Intra-oral external obliqe line incision followed by temporalis tendon stripping and subperiosteal exposure of the medial and lateral faces of the ramus. Bone cuts are made with an oscillating saw and the coronoid process is removed. Surgery may be required bilaterally.

Condyle surgery

Condylectomy

1. Indications. Joint ankylosis, inflammatory or degenerative arthropathies, tumours for example osteochondroma or villonodular synovitis, idiopathic condylar hyperplasia, mandibular asymmetry including hemifacial microsomia and unilateral mandibular hypertrophy or elongation are all accepted indications for surgery. Persistent or recurrent intractible TMJ dysfunction or internal joint derangement may constitute a requirement for surgery if conservative measures have failed.

2. Cephalometric measurements. May be used to determine the amount of condylar head to be excised and calculate the change in height of condyle in the PA plane by measuring from gonion to intermastoid line.

3. Surgical technique. A pre-auricular incision with temporal extension for improved access is usually used. Horizontal osteotomy through the neck of the condyle at the predetermined level is made and the deepest portion of medial bone is sectioned with an osteotome. The lateral pterygoid muscle and joint capsule is stripped and the condyle fragment is mobilised and removed. The joint capsule is closed primarily and a vacuum drain is placed. Firm pressure bandaging is no longer considered necessary. Fixation is not usually required but training elastics or a short period in IMF may be required

Condylotomy or subcondylar osteotomy

Indications

- Correction of mild mandibular prognathism.
- Occasionally used to treat TMJ internal derangement.
- Horizontal, oblique and low subcondylar variants are described.

Principles

The condylar head should remain in the glenoid fossa and the neck fragment should overlap the ramus of the mandible on its lateral aspect. Variations of the condylar or subcondylar osteotomy have been suggested to facilitate condylar placement. Use of IMF is debatable. A period of 4–6 weeks has been used but joint stiffness and mobility is impaired if long periods of non-use are imposed. Early mobilization with good analgesia are preferred. Rigid fixation of fragments is possible and offers a good alternative.

Approaches

1. Extra oral

- *Incisions*; retromandibular, submandibular or pre-auricular.
- *Osteotomy*; condylar neck is sectioned obliquely and mandible is repositioned posteriorly.
- *Fixation*; Simple overlap of condylar neck is all that is required for union. Microplating systems are available.

2. Intra-oral (most common approach)

- *Incisions*; buccal flap based on external oblique ridge in the subperiosteal plane.

- *Osteotomy*; condylar neck is sectioned obliquely and mandible is repositioned posteriorly. Difficult access is improved with special retractors for use in condylar region.

3. *Closed condylotomy*

- Described first by Kostecka in 1931.
- Later reviewers included Ward (1961) and Banks and MacKenzie (1975).
- Uses a blind percutanaeous approach.
- Gigli saw blade is passed around condylar neck.
- Significant risk of damage to facial nerve and mandibular nerve.
- Unpredictable haemorrhage from maxillary artery may occur.

Post-condylar grafts

First described by Trauner (1954) and modified technique described by Banks and Ardouin (1980). Not commonly performed in modern practice.

Indications
- Used as an initial step in the management of severe mandibular retrusion.
- To minimize the degree of advancement of mandibular osteotomies that are required subsequently.

Surgical technique
- The condyle, capsule and meniscus are all advanced onto the articular eminence.
- A block of cartilage graft is attached to articular fossa.
- IMF applied for 1 week.
- The cartilage graft calcifies therefore a permanent advancement of condyle is obtained.
- In postoperative months a new articular fossa forms interior to the graft site and the eminence appears to migrate forwards.

Complications
- graft infection;
- facial nerve damage;
- temporomandibular pain and dysfunction;
- damage to external acoustic meatus.

Other condylar neck operations

Although not strictly performed as part of orthognathic surgical procedures, there are other operations principally designed as part of surgical management of TMJ disease or dysfunction. Surgical access is similar to that described for orthognathic operations on the condyle and the risks to the facial nerve and local branches of the external carotid artery are similar. A combined pre-auricular and Risden incision may be used or an extended approach similar to that used for parotidectomy may be appropriate. The operations include high condylar shave, articular eminence surgery, meniscal surgery and insertion of TMJ prostheses.

The atrophic mandible

The problem

Loss of teeth results in loss of physiological loading of the alveolus and consequent resorption of alveolar bone. Preservation of dental tissues is therefore of importance in order to prevent the increasing numbers of elderly in the population from presenting with the late effects of alveolar resorption. Increased risk of fracture, poor nutrition and severe difficulties with dentures are common in this age group.

Trauma

Minimal periosteal stripping during surgery for fracture fixation is essential in order to maintain vascularity. Use of existing full dentures or prefashioned acrylic bases as Gunning pattern splints is possible but requires insertion of IMF.

The elderly patient is likely to tolerate this poorly. TMJ arthritis, and joint stiffness may follow after immobilization. Osteoporosis is a risk. Internal fixation is possible with modern screw and plate systems. Senile osteosclerosis makes the procedure more difficult than in younger patients. Insertion of 'K' wires or external fixation particularly for compound injuries is possible. Non-union occurs occasionally. The causes include, sepsis, excessive periosteal loss and reduced vascularity, local bone pathology and metabolic disturbance.

Management

Diagnosis. A history of chronic dissatisfaction and difficulty with lower full denture retention is always elicited and impact pain due to pressure on mental nerve trunks or muscle attachments may be present. Radiographs reveal poor density of bone and severe reduction in mandibular height from lower border to alveolar crest. Bone densitometry may be available and reveal osteoporosis in some patients although atrophy does not require the presence of osteoporosis for the diagnosis.

Treatment. Muscle attachment reduction and genial tubercle reduction; mental nerve repositioning and musosal modifications including vestibular flap elevation and repositioning may be offered. Tissue conditioner or periodontal dressing allows healing under the fitted basoplate to occur. Epithelial grafting and inlay techniques provide increased soft tissue area and sound base for future denture construction. Edlan technique and Russell–Hopkins vestibuloplasty are options.

Cast submucosal onlays. Two stage surgical technique. Cast chromium alloy framework made to impression taken of bone surface during first surgical stage. Transmucosal abutments are integral to the cast structure and are inserted at a second stage operation. This technique has a high complication rate, principally failure of the implant due to sepsis, and is not commonly performed.

Osseointegrated implants. Insertion of mandibular implants requires a minimum depth of basal bone. Once *in situ*, implants permit physiological axial loading and retention of bone. Bone grafting simultaneously with implant insertion is possible and pretransplant implant placement in the bone donor site is described. For example, the anterior superior iliac crest is capable of receiving implants months before transplantation of the bone–implant block to the oral site.

Osteotomies. Ramus osteotomies are possible but rarely overcome severe alveolar atrophy. Alveolar height may be restored by Wisor sagittal osteotomy. Sandwich osteotomy is a good option for increasing the alveolar height. Segmental osteotomy may restore localized deficiencies in bone depth but is not so widely advocated.

Transmandibular implants. A combined intra- and extra-oral approach permits insertion of base and alveolar surface bone plates secured and united by transosseous screw implants. Simultaneous bone grafting and muscle attachment repositioning is possible.

Cartilage and bone grafting. Costal and costochondral grafting is possible but long-term bone stability is rarely achieved.

Biotechnology. Titanium alloy trays and Dacron mesh trays in conjunction with bone grafting may permit reconstruction of severely atrophic mandibles but remain the subject of ongoing research.

Mandibular reconstruction

Indications for reconstruction

- Late presenting trauma;
- fracture non-union;
- ablative tumour surgery;
- hemifacial microsomia;
- gunshot wounds;
- condylar hypoplasia;
- pathological fracture;
- atrophic mandible;
- failed prior surgery.

Prerequisites

- *Infection.* The recipient site for bone or soft tissue grafting should be infection free.
- *Concomitant medical conditions.* Good preoperative control is essential.
- *Rehabilitation.* Ideally the patient should be a likely candidate for subsequent occlusal rehabilitation.

Aspects of surgery

- *Bone harvest.* The iliac crest is a good source of bone. Vascularized bone may be harvested from the radius, fibula, scapula or iliac crest if required. In treatment of mandibular growth disorders, costochondral grafts provide donor bone with a degree of growth potential. Split rib grafting for mandibular augmentation resorbs rapidly and is a relatively poor choice for this reason.

- *Biotechnology.* Titanium mesh trays are available and can be custom made to an impression. Cortical bone chips are compacted into the tray and once bony union has occurred, osseointegrated implants may be inserted.

Related subjects

TMJ disease and diagnoses
TMJ surgery
TMJ arthroscopy

Related topics of interest

Implants (p. 210)
Mandibular ramus osteotomies (p. 235)
Osteotomies (p. 297)
Segmental osteotomies (p. 346)

MAXILLARY SINUS

The maxillary sinus is the most inferior of the paranasal sinus system: it is a system of intrabony cavities whose ostea all converge on the lateral wall of the nose. Pyramidal in shape with a volume of about 15–30 ml, the maxillary sinus osteum opens into the middle meatus. Blood supply is derived from facial, maxillary, infra-orbital and greater palatine arteries, and lymphatic drainage is to submandibular and deep cervical nodes. Intra-uterine development commences at 3 months of gestation as an outpouch of the middle meatus. At birth it is tubular and reaches 60% of adult size by 9 years; by 12 years its floor parallels that of the nose and it achieves full adult dimensions by about 18 years of age.

Surgical anatomy

The important relationships of the maxillary antrum are:

- superiorly: orbital contents
- inferiorly: infra-orbital vessels and nerve roots of upper cheek teeth
- posteriorly: pterygopalatine fossa and maxillary artery
- medially: lateral nasal wall and nasolacrimal duct
- anteriorly: bucco-alveolar sulcus.

These relationships make the sinus a common site of involvement in midfacial trauma and one possible route of surgical access to the orbital floor in fracture, and to the middle portion of the maxillary artery in control of troublesome epistaxis. Its anterior and medial relationships are sites of elective surgical access in Caldwell Luc antrostomy and functional endoscopic surgery respectively.

Physiology

Air circulation
The antra are ventilated mostly during expiration (assuming nasal respiration) with many respiratory cycles required for full exchange of contained air.

Mucous secretion
Mucociliary transport has been studied using Indian ink, charcoal fragments and radioisotopes, and all studies demonstrate a complex spiral pattern of movement in the mucous layer which converges on the osteum.

This movement is readily impaired by pathology and by surgical breach of the antral walls and, even after intra-nasal antrostomy, almost all mucous drainage still occurs via the natural osteum.

Ventilation

This can be much improved by surgically created ostea. The role of air circulation in taste and olfaction is poorly understood.

Radiology

The X-ray views of choice include occipitomental and submento vertex projections. These views allow visualization of the sinus lumen and the bony margins. If oro-dental disease is suspected, OPG is helpful, or if complex fractures are present or surgery for malignancy is being planned, CT scanning is required.

Maxillary sinus disease

Sinusitis

1. Infective sinusitis. Acute sinusitis may present as a toxic patient with pain in his midface causing changes of head posture. It may be associated with a viral URTI or with secondary infection in the immuno-compromised. Ten percent of acute sinusitis episodes are dental or periapical in origin, and a handful are related to facial fractures. Treatment with antibiotics, analgesics and mucolytics is usually effective. Chronic sinusitis may be associated with low-grade persistent infection but is more commonly sterile and unresponsive to anti-infective therapy. The possibility of immunodepression and cystic fibrosis should be considered in these patients. Iatrogenic lesions after dental extraction and the presence of a persistent oro-antral fistula require appropriate treatment before the sinusitis will settle.

2. Non-infective sinusitis. Perennial rhinitis of allergic or vasomotor varieties is associated with florid nasal mucosa and hypertrophied inferior turbinates. Polypoid nasal and sinus mucosa most frequently affect the ethmoid lining but also the maxillary antral mucosa in some. It is a common association and of greater incidence in aspirin-sensitive patients. Decompression injuries in divers (sinus barotrauma) are well described as an antecedent to chronic sinusitis. Untreated deviations of the nasal septum predispose.

3. Complications of sinusitis. Contiguous spread to other sinuses producing a pansinusitis, otitis media and cavernous sinus thrombosis are all described but are uncommon due to the wide use of antibiotics early in the course of the illness.

Paediatric sinus problems

1. Acute sinus disease. Measles, chicken pox and other childhood exanthemata may produce a florid maxillary sinusitis. Childhood sinusitis is more likely to be associated with distant spread than is the adult condition. Intra-cerebral abscess, especially in diabetics, frontal osteitis and orbital cellulitis are occasionally seen in affected children.

2. Upper airway obstruction. The clinical picture of chronic nasal obstruction in a child who is an obligate mouth breather is common. It is associated with adenoidal enlargement in many and with tonsillar hypertrophy in some. The development and maturation of the midfacial skeleton is associated with improvement in nasopharyngeal patency and hence in symptoms. Adenotonsillectomy is often required in the childhood years before the adolescent growth spurt achieves this. An associated chronic sinusitis may be present in these patients.

3. Atopy. The common diagnosis of childhood asthma in such patients often masks the relationship between coincident atopic sinus mucosal hypertrophy and asthma. There is an uncommon association with chronic catarrhal inflammation of the naso-sinus mucosal system, chronic laryngitis and pulmonary sepsis in the susceptible.

4. Foreign body. Nasal foreign bodies, if missed or untreated, can produce chronic mucosal inflammation.

5. Syndromes. Cystic fibrosis and Kartagener's syndrome are characterized in part by increased susceptibility to pansinus disease due to abnormalities in mucous secretion and mucociliary function respectively.

Clinical notes	*1. Cheek swelling* is rarely due to maxillary sinusitis alone and is most commonly of dental origin. It may imply antral carcinoma where the dentition is healthy.
	2. Proptosis. Frontal or pansinusitis in children should be suspected and the possibility of malignancy in adults should be excluded.
Tumours	The maxillary sinus can be the seat of primary malignancy, can become involved in destructive processes affecting the lateral nasal wall and can hide less destructive lesions arising in any of its closely adjacent structures for a significant time without producing symptoms. Incidental discovery on facial radiographs of sinus opacities is a relatively frequent clinical event. Antral polyps, osteomas, antroliths as well as antral carcinomas can present late or in this coincidental manner. Ringertz tumours, Wegeners granulomatosis and lethal midline granuloma can all destroy the medial antral wall. Intra-luminal tumours of odontogenic origin can occur. Benign odontogenic tumours such as ameloblastoma, odontogenic fibroma and cementomas have all been described as involving the antrum. Malignant odontogenic lesions such as ameloblastic sarcoma have also been noted.

Fractures involving the maxillary sinus

In patients with zygomatic complex fractures, it is common to find either comminution of the antral wall, reduction in its radiographic volume or reactive mucosal oedema and fluid levels. There are, in addition, specific instances when clinical presentation of sinus breach requires early recognition and prompt surgical attention. The most important of these is orbital floor fracture with entrapment of the orbital fat or fascial sheath. It is now recognized that most symptomatic orbital floor fractures result from herniation of orbital fat and entrapment of fibrous septae in the fatty tissue rather than true muscle entrapment. Entrapment of the orbital contents results in limitation of globe movement and acute diplopia. Infra-orbital nerve paraesthesia including the maxillary teeth is common in damage to the anterior wall, and comminution of the bony skeleton of the sinus results in epistaxis quite frequently. In more major injuries involving the middle third of the facial skeleton, sinus involvement is almost inevitable. All such fractures are compound by definition and require antibiotic treatment.

Maxillary sinus surgery

Antral washouts
Diagnostic in cases of chronic mucopurulent sinusitis, washouts can be performed under local or general anaesthesia. They are of little therapeutic value.

Intra-nasal antrostomy
This acts as an aid both to ventilation and to mucous drainage. Ventilation is the major therapeutic benefit. Access during endoscopic procedures is possible via a middle meatal antrostomy, but the standard approach for lateral nasal wall puncture is an inferior meatal one. Submucous resection of septal cartilage is often required to permit access to the lateral nasal wall and thence into the antrum.

Caldwell Luc antrostomy
This is performed via the canine fossa via an intra-oral incision, the anterior wall of the antrum is windowed. Inspection under direct vision is possible via this approach. Good access to intra-luminal pathology is achieved. Some surgeons advocate covering intra-nasal antrostomy. The procedure is occasionally complicated by permanent fistula formation, infra-orbital anaesthesia and damaged teeth apices.

Endoscopic surgery
Access to the paranasal sinus system is gained via the osteomeatal complex. Instrumentation of the sinus system is possible via this approach, and good visualization of the orbital floor as well as access to the ethmoid air cells is achieved. Preoperative coronal reconstructed CT scans are required before attempting access to the periorbital sinuses. Accidental or inadvertent breach of the lamina papyracea can result in optic nerve damage and blindness.

Oro-antral fistula

An oro-antral fistula is an epithelial lined track between the mouth and antrum. The commonest cause is iatrogenic. Dental extraction of maxillary posterior teeth, especially those with chronic periapical, or periodontal infection, can result in this complication. Tuberosity fracture during extraction, clot destruction, dry socket formation and chronic odontogenic antral infection all predispose. Antral malignancy can produce fistula. The history differentiates easily between the principle causes of oro-antral fistula. Initial symptoms include passage of drink via the fistula down the ipsilateral nostril, passage of air into the mouth, alteration of voice, unilateral epistaxis or unilateral nasal obstruction. If untreated, it can include persistent sinusitis, unilateral nasal discharge, intra-oral antral polyp, cacogausia and facial pain.

Treatment   Ideally, close the fistula immediately. Where this is not possible, conservative treatment with a dressing plate or modified upper denture can be considered. An antral regime of antibiotics, ephedrine nasal drops, mucolytic inhalations and analgesia should be prescribed. Instructions about avoiding nose blowing are important. Many fistulae will close spontaneously but, after 4 or 5 weeks, little further resolution can be expected. In fistulae with diameters greater than 4 mm or depth of surrounding alveolar bone less than 5 mm, spontaneous closure is unlikely.

Surgery   There are several well-recognized techniques for surgical closure. Excision of the fistula lining is important. Advancement of a buccal mucoperiosteal flap can be used in patients where the depth of the buccal vestibule is adequate and there is no risk of impairing later provision of well-fitting dentures. Palatal rotational or island pattern flaps are possible and offer a good source of tissue to close the fistula. Temporalis fascia from a post-auricular incision, bone from a Caldwell Luc operation or collagen implants have all been tried with varying degrees of success.

Related topics of interest

Cleft palate surgery (p. 78)
Functional endoscopic sinus surgery (FESS) (p. 161)

Revision points

Midface embryology
Sinus anatomy

MAXILLOFACIAL PROSTHETICS

The development and advances in maxillofacial prosthetics have mirrored those in reconstructive surgery. Decisions often revolve around the choice of the best treatment option; whether prosthetic or surgical reconstruction. This is particularly true in cancer surgery. Other subdisciplines within maxillofacial surgery may benefit from liaison with the technician.

Clefts

- Initial impressions for plaster model records
- feeding plates
- pre-surgical orthopaedics (an uncommon requirement in modern practice)
- obturators for residual fistulae
- pre-surgical orthodontics if orthognathic surgery is needed during teenage years.

Obturators

The most common reason for construction of an obturator is after hemimaxillectomy for excision of midface malignant disease.

1. Primary obturators.

- Resection plate plus 'bung'.
- Resection plate may be one piece or split.
- Split plates are united by a midline bar or an interlocking slide pin.
- 'Bung' construction uses gutta percha, foam or self-curing silicone fashioned in the operating theatre immediately after resection.
- Retention is secured by peralveolar or suspension wires, or by transalveolar or transpalatal screws.
- The obturator allows retention of facial contours, feeding and oro-nasal continence. 'Palatal' integrity is restored and therefore speech, although nasal in quality, is much improved.
- Modern materials remain relatively clean.
- Skin grafting of maxillectomy cavities is optional; graft retention is aided by a well-fitting bung.
- Primary obturators are removed after about 2 weeks.

2. Permanent obturators

- Impression after first 'bung' change.

- Silicone or gutta percha as impression material.
- Acrylic baseplate acts as a special tray for impression.
- If radiotherapy is required, it is usual to allow cavity healing to progress and any skin graft to take before commencing DXT.
- Obturator construction can proceed but shrinkage and reduction in cavity volume will occur and bung change will be necessary.
- A permanent bung is constructed from acrylic (e.g. Molloplast B).
- Baseplate and bung assembly may be a single unit or in two parts. A two-part system permits independent removal of the plate and bung and revision or renewal of each part separately as required.
- Teeth may be placed on the baseplate in the fashion of an upper acrylic denture.

3. *Other uses of obturators.*

- Acquired clefts
- mature unclosed residual clefts
- oro-nasal fistulae
- traumatic clefts and gun shot wound.

Facial reconstruction

Major or substantial facial tissue loss is a demanding clinical problem. Surgical reconstructive options have advanced rapidly in recent years. Free tissue transfer, vascularized bone transfer and advances in biomaterial grafts have altered the outlook dramatically for patients requiring extensive facial reconstruction. Nevertheless, facial prosthetic reconstruction remains a good option for many patients.

Causes of extensive facial tissue loss
- Congenital deformity
- iatrogenic; planned excision in malignancy
- traumatic
- military injuries
- burns.

Tissues reconstructed
- Ears: soft acrylic pinnae retained with adhesive pads or osseointegrated implants.

- Orbits and eyes: titanium mesh and 'Silastic' for orbital walls. Osseointegated implants for prosthetic globe retention. Hydroxyapatite ocular prostheses.
- Calvarium: titanium plates or acrylic to recontour skull tissue.
- Facial skin: denture retained with or without integral obturator. Spectacle-retained tissue is still in use. Osseointegrated implant fixtures may be placed for retention purposes.

Materials	
	- Titanium
	- silicones
	- soft acrylic
	- high impact acrylic
	- cast alloys
	- magnets.

Trauma

Splints	Hard acrylic splints or soft polymeric 'blow downs' are useful in dento-alveolar trauma and for retention and fixation in maxillofacial fractures.
Arch bars	These may be wrought, pre-formed or constructed as cast cap splints.
Halo frames and universal box frames	Used in fixation of high level middle third facial fractures or complex midface injuries.
Facial reconstruction	If extensive tissue loss has occurred, secondary facial reconstruction may be required.

Orthognathic surgery

Serial study models	These are required for assessment, treatment planning and recording outcomes.
Intra-operative wafers	During orthognathic surgery, once dento-alveolar units or segments are mobilized, pre-planned jaw positions are imposed on osteotomized units by means of temporary IMF and interpositional occlusal wafers. Preoperative plotting from true lateral cephalometric films and articulated model surgery determines the

occlusal positions and form of the intra-operative wafers.

Pre-surgical orthodontics   Functional appliances and fixed appliances have a role in preparation for orthognathicsurgery.

Facial palsy

- Contoured dentures
- prosthetic slings
- eyelid gold weights.

Medical

Dressing plates   Surgery for patients with clotting diatheses may require clear acrylic full coverage plates.
A tamponade effect is suggested to minimize postoperative bleeding.
Local haemostatic measures may also be required.

Dento-alveolar

Oro-antral fistula closure   Dressing plates.
Temporary obturators may be required.
Surgical closure is preferred.

Other roles for the maxillofacial technician

- Distraction osteogenesis
- improved ocular and ear protheses
- hydroxyapatite ocular implants
- bone-anchored hearing aids (BAHA).

MICROVASCULAR SURGERY

Free tissue transfer is used increasingly in head and neck reconstruction after ablative surgery for malignant disease. The use of these techniques is also becoming increasingly applicable to post-traumatic and post-burn reconstruction. Some technical aspects are considered here.

Preoperative medical status Relative contraindications to the use of free flap tissue transfer include; diabetic patients, heavy smokers, collagen degenerative diseases, previously irradiated patients and poorly controlled local sepsis. Donor site factors include the requirement to demonstrate patency of collateral circulation and distal run off in the lower limb where a section of the arterial tree is to be harvested. In the forearm, good ulnar circulation and in the lower limb angiographic evidence of distal run off are necessary.

Operative techniques There should be two surgical teams operating simultaneously if possible. The first team performs the tumour excision and neck dissection, the second prepares the flap. The dissected flap remains in continuity with the donor blood supply until it is required for anastomosis.

Meticuluous perivascular dissection and careful use of diathermy are needed to preserve the vasa vasorum of the vessels to be used in the anastomosis.

Microvascular techniques *1. Optical aids.* Loupes or an operating microscope are required and the assistant will require similar optical aids.

2. Vessel preparation.

- Gentle handling of vessels
- meticulous dissection
- correction of diameter mismatch by dilation, bevelling and spatulation are all possible
- adequate but not excessive removal of adventitia prevents interposition in anastomosis.

3. Suture techniques. Modification of established vascular surgical techniques is required. Sutures traversing the vessel lumen result in almost certain failure of anastomosis. Kinking or twisting of the vessels imposed by the suture position are hazardous. Non-resorbable material on atraumatic needles are used.

4. Position and construction of anastomoses. End to end anastomoses for arteries and end to end or end to side for veins is satisfactory. The pedicle should be positioned to ensure it is protected from severe bending or kinking and so it lies beneath sound tissue where possible. Non-constricting suture ligatures may be placed to secure the pedicle course in the neck. The flap and anastomosis should be tension free. Vessel length is important and, if too short, interpositional vein grafts harvested from local veins or from long saphenous vein can be inserted.

5. Prevention of thrombosis. Endothelial damage initiates thrombus formation. Limited endothelial damage may induce self-limiting thrombus formation and intimal repair begins rapidly. Initial organization and healing is complete at 2 weeks postoperatively, and no evidence remains at 8 weeks. A high degree of accuracy in surgical apposition of the intima is required to minimize thrombus formation. Malalignment, poor contact and edge inversion all result in an increased incidence of anastomotic failure and vessel leakage. Through and through suture placement, oblique orientation to suture lines and incorrect knot tension all contribute to anastomotic failure and thrombosis.

6. Reflow problems. Problems after anastomosis may have a number of other underlying causes:

- capillary leakage
- vasovasorum thrombosis
- microcirculatory sludging due to excess viscosity or low perfusion pressure
- vessel thrombosis
- superoxide free radical formation due to prolonged ischaemia time.

7. Prevention of haematoma and abscess. Careful haemostasis includes ligating all side branches of the donor vessels so that when blood flow is restored, no leakage can occur from the pedicle into the neck.

8. Pharmacology. Use of heparin saline solutions locally during microvascular anastomosis is common. Widespread use of systemic papaverine solutions or anticoagulants other than 5000 IU subcutaneous heparin is not necessary. Dextran solutions have been used to produce intra-operative reduction in coagulability. Theatre temperature (warmed), patient temperature and preoperative or perioperative venesection to reduce haemoglobin to 10 g/dl are all advocated. Aspirin, heparin, low molecular weight dextrans and dypyridamole have all been tried. It is more important to perform technically correct microvascular surgery.

9. Patency testing. Various milking techniques and methods of demonstrating flow across the microanastomosis are described. They are traumatic and best avoided if possible. Performing the arterial anastomosis first will demonstrate flow across the flap vascular bed with obvious venous outflow. Completion of the final venous anastomoses should result in a well-perfused flap with normal capillary return and blanching on gentle pressure. Free bone grafts pose problems in demonstrating viability. Isotope assays are currently used to demonstrate blood flow but are unreliable and difficult to interpret.

Related topic of interest

Reconstruction – some principles (p. 324)

Revision points

Pathophysiology of blood flow
Blood clotting mechanisms

NASAL AND ANTRAL TUMOURS

Tumour types

Benign tumours
- Osteoma
- chondroma
- ossifying fibroma
- fibrous dysplasia
- haemangioma

Intermediate tumours
- Ringertz tumour (inverted papilloma)
- haemangiopericytoma
- basal cell carcinoma
- extracranial meningioma

Malignant tumours
- Squamous carcinoma
- adenocarcinoma
- tumours of minor salivary glands
- malignant melanoma
- osteogenic sarcoma
- malignant histiocytoma
- lymphoreticular tumours, midline reticuloses, non-Hodgkin's lymphoma, multiple myeloma
- olfactory neuroblastoma

Epidemiology

The approximate incidence is 10 new reports per million per year in UK. In Japan, Far East and parts of Africa the incidence is probably nearer 30 cases per million per year. There is a male preponderance and the most frequent age of diagnosis is in the sixth decade of life.

Aetiological factors
- Hard-wood dust in the timber industry (adenocarcinoma)
- nickel refining industry
- leather workers
- isopropyl oils exposure
- snuff usage (Bantu populations)

Incidence of sino-nasal malignancies

Site incidence
- Maxillary antra   50%
- ethmoid sinuses   25%
- nasal carcinoma   24%
- frontal sinus   1%

Rate of metastatic disease
- Cervical nodes   30%
- distant spread   30%
  (squamous cancers)

Ohngren's line

Arbitrarily divides midface cancers into supero–posterior and antero–inferior. Although artificial, this division correlates well with operability and prognosis. Tumours arising above Ohngren's line are more commonly inoperable and have a poorer prognosis than those occurring below.

Incidence of different histological types of midfacial cancers
- Squamous carcinoma   50%
- anaplastic carcinoma   15%
- adenocarcinoma   5%
- salivary gland neoplasms   5%
- reticuloses   10%
- sarcoma   5%
- other tumour types   10%

Surgical pathology

Squamous lesions of antrum

1. Nasal spread. Bone erosion of the lateral nasal wall, nasal stuffiness, facial swelling and pain are characteristic.

2. Orbital spread. Occurs via the infra-orbital fissure, and unilateral proptosis and diplopia results.

3. Ethmoid spread. Midfacial swelling occurs late in the course of the tumour. Unilateral proptosis occurs once the orbit is involved.

4. Oral spread. Typically presenting as a mass in palate, or with complaints of poor denture fit. These lesions may be painful.

5. *Buccal mucosa.* Cheek swelling and redness occur.

Squamous ethmoid carcinoma	Orbital, sphenoidal, antral and nasal spread all may occur. Intracranial spread across the cribriform plate to involve the anterior fossa may also occur.
Adenocarcinomas	These lesions exhibit similar bone erosive properties and a similar potential for cervical node metastastic spread as squamous lesions.
Adenoid cystic carcinoma	Usually arise from minor salivary glands or nasal mucous glands. Perineural spread across peripheral nerve trunks and intracranial invasion via skull base foraminae is possible. Distant metastases are common.
Mucoepidermoid carcinoma	Arise from nasal and antral mucous glands. Very malignant lesions which metastasize early.
Malignant melanoma	These tumours arise more frequently from nasal septal tissue than sinus mucosa. The cutaneous classifications and methods of assessment are not relevant to mucosal melanomas. The biological behaviour of these tumours is unpredictable with some lesions progressing to kill the patient within weeks and other relatively indolent ones permitting survival for years. They comprise 1% of all sino-antral cancers.
Malignant histiocytoma	Associated with previous bone irradiation. Paget's disease and fibrous dysplasia predispose.

Investigations

Radiology	• Plain radiographs including chest X-ray. • *CT scan.* To assess extent and degree of bone erosion. • *MRI scan.* To assess soft tissue oedema and status of cervical nodes.
Tissue diagnosis	• *FNAC* of neck nodes if palpable may be helpful. • *FESS* for biopsy of sinus mucosal lesions.
Laboratory indices	These investigations are important for exclusion of myeloma, for baseline indices and as preoperative screening where appropriate.

Treatment

1. Benign tumours. excision via fronto-ethmoidectomy or lateral rhinotomy for fronto-ethmoidal lesions and Caldwell–Luc approach for antral lesions.

2. Transitional cell and inverted papillomas require limited or partial maxillectomy.

3. Lymphomas are staged and then treated with combined chemotherapy and radiotherapy.

4. Cutaneous lesions may require wide excision and facial reconstruction.

5. Malignant tumours. Fifty to 60% are likely to be incurable by surgery alone. Twenty per cent of these are likely to be considered inoperable due to the extent of tumour. Particular surgical difficulties arise where the following structures are involved.

- *Eye.* Orbital exenteration should be considered if there is evidence of peri-osteal breach or if there is doubt about the likelihood of surgical clearance where eye preservation is planned. Orbital recurrence is likely to be inoperable.
- *Nasopharynx.* Extensive involvement makes surgical resection with adequate reconstruction practically impossible.
- *Intracranial.* Intracranial spread suggests inoperability.
- *Pterygoid region.* Surgical clearance is difficult but as wide a resection as possible should be planned for this region in any maxillectomy operation.
- *Midface contours.* The decision to obturate or reconstruct remains a matter of debate.
- *Salivary glands.* Not commonly involved in squamous disease but may require inclusion in an en bloc resection.
- *Radiotherapy.* Exclusion of the cornea and contralateral eye from the irradiated field is required. Side-effects include mucositis and xerostomia. Occipitoparietal alopecia may occur. Brachytherapy with the isotope included in the

facial mask and intra-cavitary radiation sources have been used.

Revision points

Anatomy of maxillary antrum, pterygoid region and infra-temporal fossa
Anatomy of the midface
Anatomy of the paranasal sinues
Embryology and development of the midfacial paranasal sinuses
Ethmoid sinuses
Lateral nasal wall, nasal floor and nasal cavity
Lymphatic drainage of sinuses
Nasal septum
Orbit

NASO-ETHMOID INJURIES

Naso-ethmoid injuries are relatively uncommon, but when they do occur they are usually serious and carry a significant mortality. The immediate threat to life arises due to concomitant head injury, airway compromise and from associated injuries in a multiple trauma setting.

Mechanisms of injury

Isolated naso-ethmoid injuries arise from assault using a hand weapon such as an axe or similar blade, from industrial injuries whilst using high-speed rotary machinery such as circular or band saws, and from projectile injuries.

Immediate assessment	• airway • conscious level • eye and visual status • other injuries • haemorrhage.
Investigations	• plain X-ray films • CT scans • standard trauma X-ray series.
Immediate medical management	• resuscitation • anaesthetic assessment • head injury monitoring
Associated early problems	*1. CSF leak.* If present, a CSF leak poses a surgical problem. Most will settle without surgery, but admission, close observation particularly with an associated head injury and possible use of antibiotics are essential steps. Neurosurgical closure requires bicoronal flap access, frontal craniotomy and anterior fossa repair with development and introduction into the wound of a dural or pericranial flap to seal the leak. Subcranial injuries can be treated via the same approach at the same operation once the dural repair is completed. Complex midfacial injuries carry an increased risk of sepsis and meningitis. *2. Epilepsy.* After a significant head or craniofacial injury the risk of fits is increased and, during the year

immediately following the injury, close follow-up is required as post-traumatic epilepsy may become persistent.

3. Orbital contents and optic nerve. Direct globe or nerve injury may occur during the incident. Blindness may result but, unless traumatic optic nerve section or avulsion occurs, some degree of recovery can be expected. *Fractures* involving the orbital walls or rims can lead to blood, air or naso-antral mucus being introduced into the orbit, with serious consequences for the eye. Early treatment of orbital injuries is important where globe damage or muscle damage has occurred, and repair to prevent ingress of naso-antral mucus should be undertaken.

Later problems

- enopthalmos
- traumatic telecanthus
- antral mucosal disease
- nasal airway function impaired
- nasolacrimal function; epiphora may result
- facial and cranial skeleton form.

Immediate definitive treatment

(a) Surgical access: there are several approaches including bicoronal flaps and midface incisions.
(b) Fixation: open reduction facilitates miniplate fixation. External fixation and cranial suspension are options.
(c) Nasal capsule: classification of injuries is useful in treatment planning. Three layers are described, the most superficial detailing nasal cartilage injury only and the deepest describing a complex capsule injury.
(d) Orbit: treated as for orbital injuries alone.
(e) Nasolacrimal duct: damage often results in chronic obstruction and may lead to chronic epiphora. Dacrorhinocystotomy may be required.
(f) Sinuses: frontal exenteration, cranialization or obliteration of the ethmoid and frontal sinuses may be required.
(g) Medial cantral ligament reconstruction may be required to prevent traumatic telecanthus.
(h) Cranium: skull contours are important.

Late correction

Osteotomies, dacrorhinocystostomy for epiphora, cranial or craniofacial reconstruction and orbital reconstruction for enophthalmos may each be necessary. Bone grafts and alloplastic materials such as titanium mesh are used.

NECK DISSECTION

Since Crile's description of excision of the interfascial fat and its contained lymphoid tissue in 1906, there have been several seminal modifications of technique and approach.

Indications

Palpable lymphadenopathy   In the presence of oro-facial malignancy, palpable cervical nodes should be considered for neck dissection. Careful orientation of the operative specimen for the histopathologist permits accurate description and location of the nodes containing the tumour and those demonstrating inflammatory reactivity. Decisions regarding the patient's need for postoperative radiotherapy are guided by histological evidence of tumour spread to the nodes and in particular to the extracapsular tissues.

MRI scan   This is a more sensitive method of determining the presence of lymphadenopathy. The reliability in determining the extent of tumour invasion and cervical nodal involvement is dependent on the interpretive skill and experience of the radiologist.

FNAC-positive reports   Where palpable nodes have revealed tumour cells on FNAC sampling, neck dissection is usually required. The problem of management of patients with negative FNAC reports from palpable neck nodes remains debated.

Recurrent disease   Where nodal malignancy in the neck recurs or presents after control of a local primary tumour, if neck dissection was not performed or a limited dissection was used at the initial surgery, the patient should be offered full neck dissection.

Disputed role of 'prophylactic' neck dissection   The issue of neck dissection where there is no clinical, radiological or cytological evidence of cervical nodal disease is contentious. In general, formal neck dissection is delayed until evidence of nodal disease presents. This is not universally true however.

Clinical problems

N0 neck

In patients with no clinically palpable nodes in the neck or without CT or MRI scan evidence of cervical disease, the decision is between continued clinical observation or prophylactic treatment of the neck. The rationale for prophylactic neck dissection is to gain the benefit of reduced likelihood of late presentation of metastatic nodal disease. It is difficult to demonstrate survival advantage. The same problems obtain if radical radiotherapy is the prophylactic regimen of choice. Prophylactic surgery, if undertaken, should be functional rather than radical.

N1 neck

A high percentage of palpable first echelon nodes are likely to be reactive rather than metastatic. FNAC will aid differentiation. A policy of conservative management is employed by some surgeons with a negative FNAC result, but many units are offering functional neck dissection to this group of patients. Where positive evidence of tumour is present in nodal FNAC, radical neck dissection should be considered.

N2 to N3 necks

Due to the increasing risk of tumour metastasis and extracapsular spread when nodal disease is advanced, radical neck dissection is commonly required. Radical radiotherapy may be considered.

Issues

Radical, functional or limited neck dissections

The limited, supra-omohyoid neck dissections should be considered as node-sampling operations. Postoperative radiotherapy is more likely to be required, and recurrence, if present, is likely to occur at the resection or radiotherapy field margins. In N0 necks, functional neck dissection is justified but, where clinical or scan evidence of nodal disease is present and surgery is intended to be curative, a radical pattern of dissection is required.

Tracheostomy

Extensive resections, with excision of posterior floor of the mouth primary lesions or bilateral neck surgery are likely to be associated with significant postoperative oedema, and a planned tracheostomy is wise.

Incision patterns	Crile, Schobinger, 'Y' or half 'H' incisions all give good access but, in previously irradiated necks, a McFee incision often heals better with less flap dehiscence.
Internal jugular vein	Tumour permeation and intimacy of the vertical lymphoid chain make this structure a key one in planning curative surgery. In demonstrable nodal disease, the internal jugular vein must usually be sacrificed in order to achieve nodal clearance. It is preserved in functional neck dissection and may be used as the recipient for microvenous anastomoses in free tissue transfer to reconstruct the defect after radical excision of the primary lesion.
Carotid arterial system	Tumour involvement is uncommon and suggests inoperability. Shunting is possible and late invasion of the arterial wall predisposes to 'blow out'. The branches of the external carotid artery supply donor vessels for microvascular reconstruction of primary defects.
Brachial plexus and phrenic nerve	Dissection should proceed in the plane superficial to the pre-vertebral fascia to protect these vital structures.
Subclavian region	The subclavian vein and lung apex are at risk.

Complications

Immediate	• Haemorrhage and haematoma formation • facial oedema.
Intermediate	• Chyle leak • Horner's syndrome • sepsis.
Late	• Contracture • recurrence of tumour.

Related topic of interest

Malignant neck disease (p. 232)

Revision point

Technical aspects of neck dissection

NECK SPACE INFECTIONS

The neck is anatomically subdivided by fascial boundaries into a series of potential spaces or planes. These spaces may intercommunicate and free access from the neck into the chest and mediastinum exists. Each of these fascial planes forms potential spaces in which collections of mucus, air, blood or pus can collect and in which foreign bodies may lodge.

Causes

- *Odontogenic sepsis.*
- *Tonsillitis* (particularly in children).
- *Salivary gland* disease.
- *Penetrating trauma* and stab wounds (pre-auricular wounds may involve the parotid space).
- *IV drug abuse* with immunocompromize and introduction of unusual organisms increases the risk of spread of sepsis.

Microbiology

1. Mixed oropharyngeal flora

- *Aerobes.* Staphylococci and streptococci are common.
- *Anaerobes.* Periodontal and gastrointestinal organisms such as bacteorides and coliforms are often present.

2. Immunocompromised patients. Fungal infection must be considered.

3. Most cases. No identification of causative organisms is achieved.

Antimicrobial therapy

Broad spectrum penicillin or cephalosporins are used. Metronidazole will treat anaerobic infection and systemic antifungal therapy may occasionally be necessary. The benefit of systemic corticosteroids on toxaemic patients has been demonstrated in other clinical settings but remains to be proven in patients with deep neck space infections.

Clinical problems

- Airway. Inevitably at risk with the oedema associated with severe infection in the neck.
- Toxaemia.
- Drooling and dysphagia.
- Potential emergencies include carotid 'blow-out',

internal jugular vein thrombosis and lateral sinus thrombosis.

Neck spaces

1. Submental. A subdivision of the submandibular space and anatomically located between the anterior bellies of the digastric muscles. Infection arising around the apices of the lower anterior teeth can point in this region. Discharge of pus under the chin is typical. There are lymph nodes which may present as acutely inflamed submental masses.

2. Sublingual. The upper part of the submandibular space is found on the oral aspect of the mylohyoid muscle. It contains the sublingual gland and infections arising in it present as a swelling in the floor of the mouth. Ranulae can become infected and plunging ranulae penetrate the mylohyoid muscle to present as a swelling in the neck below the mandibular lower border. Sublingual gland excision may be required and is performed via an intra-oral approach. Mandibular dental or periapical infections may occasionally discharge into this space. It is an uncommon presentation of dentoalveolar sepsis however.

3. Submandibular. The part of this space below and behind mylohyoid is principally occupied by the submandibular gland. The mandibular cheek teeth if the apices are foci of infection may discharge into this space. This is a common presentation of infection arising in the lower posterior teeth. Ludwig's angina is an acute submandibular space infection; more accurately a spreading cellulitis of this space and adjacent tissues. It constitutes a potentially serious risk to the airway. Treatment with high dose IV antibiotics is essential and early surgical drainage may be required. Infections arising in the submandibular gland will usually require interval operation to remove the chronically infected gland once the acute episode is resolved.

4. Buccal. The tissues deep to buccinator constitute a potential space and permit the spread of pus from discharge arising around the upper or more typically the lower molar teeth. Penetration of the buccinator muscle may occur. Swelling may be diffuse and will often become localized particularly with antibiotic therapy. Removal of the affected teeth with or without abscess drainage is curative.

5. Submasseteric. Deep to the lower attachment of masseter between the muscle and the outer cortex of the mandibular ramus there is a potential space. It is occasionally a focus for pus collection from dental infection or sepsis of mandibular bone origin. Occasionally a missed mandibular fracture or one which presents late may be associated with a submasseteric abscess. It is characteristically very painful and requires urgent surgical drainage.

6. Periparotid. The parotid gland is enveloped in a facial envelope or sheath. Infection of the gland parenchyma or sepsis arising in the parotid lymph nodes may present as a parotid abscess. Immediate treatment with IV antibiotics is required. If surgical drainage is required, a formal parotidectomy incision is required to avoid the risk of damage to the facial nerve. Interval parotidectomy may be required.

7. Mastoid. Mastoiditis is rare in modern practice due to prompt treatment of otitic infections with oral antibiotics. It is an acute complication of progressive otitis media and may result in lateral sinus thrombosis and internal jugular vein thrombosis. Cortical mastoidectomy is usually required.

8. Subgaleal. Scalp infections may arise from skin lesions such as sebaceous cysts or furuncles. Usually infection spreads via superficial cellulitis. Occasionally deep penetration occurs and the subgaleal plane is a preformed anatomical pathway for rapid spread of sepsis. Calvarial osteomyelitis or post-craniotomy sepsis may occur and spread along this route.

9. Parafollicular. Spread of pus from a tonsillitis into the para tonsillar space is a 'quinsy'. The space is medial to superior constrictor muscle. Typically such a collection points into the lateral pharyngeal wall. Treatment with IV antibiotics is preferred rather than immediate drainage. Once systemic toxicity is controlled, drainage may be required and interval tonsillectomy is usual although not mandatory after a single episode.

10. Parapharyngeal. Lateral to the constrictor muscles and bounded laterally by the lateral pterygoid muscle. This space contains the carotid sheath and associated structures. This space is the site of drainage for infection arising in the tonsil, mastoid or third molar region. It is a rare complication in modern practice and requires wide incision along the sternomastoid muscle to establish adequate drainage. Multiple drains are usually required.

11. Retropharyngeal. Lying posterior to the pharynx and anterior to the cervical spine this space contains a few large lymph nodes. These may be become the focus of infection in children secondary to an upper respiratory tract infection. Cervical spine tuberculosis may cause 'cold abscess' formation in adults. IV antibiotics are the treatment in the acute phase and if appropriate, antituberculous therapy. Although this space communicates with the mediastinum, spread of infection is a rare event.

12. Prevertebral. Continuous with the retropharyngeal space, this region if involved in spreading infection may be the site of presentation of spinal tuberculosis. Lateral spread may result in cutaneous fistulae formation and discharge adjacent to sternomastoid. It is possible for spread to continue downwards as far as the coccygeal region from a prevertebral focus.

13. Pretracheal. The principal contents of this space are the thyroid and parathyroid glands. Colloid cysts may rupture or become infected. Pretracheal lymph nodes may become foci of infection. A true pretracheal collection is uncommon.

14. Substernomastoid and carotid sheath. Deep to sternomastoid there is an extensive collection of lymph nodes closely associated with the jugular venous system. These may be the focus of metastatic disease or infection. A collection of pus deep to the muscle may occur. Tracking around the anterior margin is possible but in tuberculous lymphadenitis, a classical 'collar stud' abscess may result from pus penetrating through the muscle belly and forming a cutaneous fistulous track.

15. Supraclavicular. The supraclavicular region has lymph nodes which drain both head and neck viscera as well as thoracic and abdominal organs. A collection of pus is uncommon in this site; malignant lymphadentits is more common.

16. Mediastinum. Subdivided into superior, anterior, middle and posterior compartments. There is free communication between the fascial planes of the neck and the superior and anterior mediastinal spaces. To a lesser degree the middle mediastinum may be affected by downward drainage of infected material from the neck. Tracheal or oesophageal perforation by a foreign body or from iatrogenic perforations during endoscopy may result in both air and subsequently pus being present in the mediastinum.

Principles of management
- Clinical history and examination.
- Ultrasound scan or CT may indicate which space is involved and the amount of fluid present
- IV fluids and high dose antibiotics.
- Surgical drainage of any pus collections.
- Definitive surgery once acute phase has resolved.

Related topic of interest

Neck dissection (p. 267)

Revision points

Anatomy of the fascial planes of the neck
Anatomy of the mediastinum

NEUROLOGY OF THE HEAD AND NECK

The cranial nerves serve the major somatic and visceral functions of the head and neck.

Olfactory nerve

Anosmia. The major causes include high maxillary trauma with cribriform plate or naso-ethmoid fractures, chronic nasal mucosal inflammation and frontal lobe tumours. Hysterical anosmia is described.

Optic nerve

Acuity, visual fields and fundi. In addition to the major opthalmological implications, direct and consensual pupil responses require intact optic nerves for the afferent limb of the reflexes. Orbital trauma, complications of FESS via the middle meatus, demyelination and tumours arising in the pituitary gland and optic cortex result in field defects or blindness. Hysterical blindness is described.

Oculomotor, trochlear and abducens nerves

External ocular movements and pupils. Co-ordinated movement of the globe in all directions requires intact peripheral nerves and a functioning medial longitudinal fasciculus. Diplopia occurs if this mechanism is defective. Congenital squint with amblyopia occurs in children and requires surgical correction in some. Acquired squint with diplopia occurs with orbital fracture and soft tissue tethering ('blow out'), cerebrovascular events and demyelination. The efferent limb of the pupil reflexes requires intact motor pathways.

Trigeminal nerve

Facial sensation, facial pain, taste and secretion. The three major divisions subserve common sensations similar to dermatomal supply in the limbs and trunk. Taste sensation is transmitted in lingual and chorda tympani nerves. Lacrimation and nasal secretion are a function of the parasympathetic systems whose fibres run with branches of the ophthalmic and maxillary divisions. Facial pain syndromes such as trigeminal neuralgia and Tolosa Hunt syndrome usually occur in relation to terminal branches of the trigeminal nerve divisions. Reactionary herpes zoster occurs in a dermatomal pattern and the post-herpetic neuralgia follows suit. Facial anaesthesia or dysaesthesia occurring *de novo* or iatrogenically are well documented. Disorders of taste are uncommon, and many are psychogenic. Post-parotidectomy Frey's syndrome occurs. Disorders of lacrimation are uncommon. Sicca syndrome and drug-induced dry eyes are described. Epiphora and excessive lacrimation are usually post-traumatic or postoperative, where damage to the nasolacrimal duct system has occurred. Nasal secretion, if excessive, occurs in relation to perennial rhinitis or coryza. Post-radiotherapy nasal drying is well documented.

Facial nerve

Facial animation, saliva secretion and taste. The superficial musculature of the face is supplied by the facial nerve. Paralysis results in facial palsy. The common causes include trauma, post-parotidectomy damage, middle ear tumours and cerebellopontine space-occupying lesions such as acoustic schwanoma. Idiopathic Bell's palsy is well described. Upper motor neurone facial weakness occurs after cerebrovascular events and as a complication of cerebral angiography and neck surgery for malignancy involving the internal carotid system in patients whose collateral cerebral circulation is already compromised. The parasympathetic efferent system serving submandibular and sublingual gland salivation and nasal secretion has central connections in inferior salivatory nuclei and lacrimal nuclei respectively. First order efferent fibres travel with the facial nerve until the submandibular and pterygopalatine ganglia respectively.

Vestibulocochlear nerve

Deafness, dizziness and tinnitus. Acoustic neuromas or schwanoma at the cerebellopontine angle produce slowly progressive deafness. Demyelination and inner ear damage may mimic deafness and tinnitus. Menière's disease affects older males typically. Drug-induced damage may affect patients treated with high dose or long-term aminoglycosides such as gentamycin. Eustachian tube dysfunction due to nasopharyngeal lesions occluding the orifice may initially mimic this pattern of symptoms. Rinne and Weber clinical tests will help differentiate the conductive deafness from true vestibulocochlear lesions which cause sensorineural pattern deafness. Post-radiotherapy and maxillectomy symptoms may require grommets. Congenital deafness may occur in Pendred's syndrome in association with thyroid functional disorders. Cleft palate children very commonly have conductive pattern deafness and usually require grommets. Hysterical deafness does occur.

Glossopharyngeal and vagus nerves

Swallowing, speech, pharyngeal sensation and saliva. Co-ordinated activity in the pharyngeal musculature is required during the first and second phase of swallowing. Included in this are the actions of the tongue, floor of the mouth and soft palate muscles. Swallowing disorders due to neuromuscular inco-ordination occur in bulbar and pseudo-bulbar palsies, demyelination and after radiotherapy. Drooling, aspiration and regurgitation may all result. Dysphagia usually results from disease lower in the oesophagus. Speech requires normal motor innervation of the intrinsic muscle of the larynx. The commonest lesion affecting these nerves is iatrogenic recurrent laryngeal nerve damage during thyroid surgery. Pharyngeal sensation is rarely affected alone. The sensation of globus is troubling typically to middle aged women. Pain referral to the ear from lesions in the region of glossopharyngeal sensation is described. Glossopharyngeal neuralgia is disabling but uncommon. First order parasympathetic efferents from the inferior salivatory nucleus travel via glossopharyngeal nerves to the otic ganglion *en route* to the synapse and provision of secretomotor supply to the parotid gland.

Accessory nerve

Shoulder weakness. Sternomastoid and trapezius weakness after neck dissection are well documented. Functional neck dissection preserves this function.

Hypoglossal nerve

Tongue movements. Co-ordinated bilateral action is required for normal control of tongue movement. Space-occupying lesions adjacent to the jugular bulb or iatrogenic damage during submandibular triangle surgery may occur. Demyelination may cause weakness. Lower motor neurone weakness is associated with tongue wasting. Cerebrovascular events affecting the internal capsule may result in upper motor neurone weakness but rarely occurs in isolation.

Upper cervical nerves

Neck sensation, speech, swallowing and breathing. Cutaneous sensation to the supra-clavicular and infra-mandibular regions is subserved by cervical afferents from C2 to C4. Accessory muscles around the hyoid and larynx are important in swallowing and speech, but major symptoms rarely arise from loss of these nerves alone. Accessory respiratory muscles around the neck are innervated, and diaphragmatic motor innervation arises from C2 to C4. Injuries or surgery to upper cervical vertebrae may result in damage. Immediate trauma management must involve use of hard cervical collars to prevent damage to the cervical spinal cord and consequent quadriplegia. Osteoarthritis with osteophyte formation, cervical disc prolapse and cervical vertebral fractures may all result in damage to the cervical cord or peripheral nerves. 'Whiplash' injuries are soft tissue injuries and result in no immediate neurological sequelae. Progression to late osteoarthritis is a matter of dispute. Neurosurgery for cervical disc prolapse may result in iatrogenic damage.

Related topics of interest

Facial nerve (p. 130)
Headache and facial pain (p. 190)

Revision points

Cranial nerve anatomy
Embryology of facial development

OBSTRUCTIVE SLEEP APNOEA

OSA is a poorly named group of conditions in which few demonstrate any true obstructive features. Nevertheless, some respond moderately well to surgery designed to relieve obstruction. The group of conditions includes excessive snoring, Pickwickian syndrome, obesity-related sleep apnoea and true obstructive apnoea. It is possible that the sudden infant death syndrome is a variant of OSA.

The common denominator in all the conditions is that of poor, non-restful sleep due to frequent waking secondary to apnoeic episodes and the sudden restarting of respiratory effort. Some patients report nocturnal paroxysmal cardiac dysrhythmias which contribute to the disturbance in sleep pattern. Day time somnolence, poor concentration and diminished performance in objective cognitive testing are all associated.

Clinical associations

Obesity, narcotic or sedative use, alcohol ingestion, asthma and COAD. The Pickwickian syndrome may be the primary pattern of this disorder. The factors mentioned above being provoking agents for the secondary type. The underlying pathophysiology is postulated to be a relative insensitivity of the chemoreceptors located in the medulla oblongata to arterial pCO_2. This results in a slowly progressive failure of responsiveness to a hypercapnic stimulus so that respiratory effort becomes dependent on the peripheral chemoreceptors, the principal site of sensitivity to pO_2. As fluctuations in pO_2 are of lesser magnitude during normal respiration, they contribute little to the minute to minute respiratory drive. Where pCO_2 sensitivity is reduced, this drive to respiration is ineffective and periods of apnoea result. These are of sufficient duration to allow the patient's pO_2 to fall sufficiently to act as a peripheral stimulus to respiratory effort, so ending the period of apnoea.

The neurological substrate and the propensity for CO_2 retention are adequate to explain the provoking effects of the stimuli mentioned previously, and the periods of hypoxaemia would be sufficient to explain the nocturnal dysrhythmias in sensitive patients.

Investigations

- Baseline screening investigations including ECG.
- Echocardiogram if indicated on clinical grounds
- Upper airways examination and flexible endoscopy, including Müller's manoeuvre.
- Sleep studies including 12-hour recorded pulse oximetry.

- Plethysmography.
- Invasive monitoring of blood gas tensions during sleep–wake cycles is possible.

Treatment options

1. Conservative. Weight loss, reduction in alcohol consumption especially in the evening, nebulized drugs in the evening for asthmatics and domicillary oxygen have all been of suggested benefit. Sleep–wake alarms with a variety of triggered stimuli have been used to provoke respiratory effort in some. These devices have found particular application in the sudden infant death risk babies. Night clothing and sleep positions are thought by some to be important in children but have not been shown to be relevant in adults.

2. Surgery. In snorers, uvulopalatopharyngoplasty (UVPPP) has its advocates and, whilst it reduces the snoring element of the problem to the satisfaction of the patients partner, the very painful nature of the surgery, the risk of velopharyngeal incompetence and the dubious benefit to the apnoeic element make it a questionable option.

3. Other options. The following operations have all been performed with reported benefits in OSA sufferers, but in small numbers in each reported series. It is likely that the functional element is the most prominent in most patients and only in a small percentage is there a clinically definable, surgically correctable oropharyngeal abnormality. In these patients, surgery can be expected to produce a successful outcome. The procedures advocated include tongue reduction, pharyngoplasty, adenotonsillectomy, sagittal split mandibular osteotomy, Le Fort I maxillary osteotomy, nasal surgery including correction of deviated nasal septum and inferior turbinectomy

In all patients, careful psychological screening and counselling of affected relatives and bed partners is important.

Related topic of interest

Osteotomies (p. 297)

Revision points

Respiratory physiology

OCCULT PRIMARY CANCER

Occult primary disease presents as metastatic squamous cancer in cervical lymph nodes but without evidence of a primary lesion. The diagnosis of an occult primary tumour is made only if no primary tumour is detected after careful search, or where evidence of a primary lesion does not appear during therapy. Patients with cervical lymph node metastases histologically related to a previously treated primary tumour as well as patients with lymphomas and adenocarcinoma are usually considered as having a known primary, even where evidence of recurrence is absent.

Three-year survival rates following surgery or radiotherapy for unknown squamous primaries range from 40–50% in N1 patients to 38% and 26% for patients with N2 and N3 disease respectively. In those patients who later develop clinically evident primary lesions, survival rates compared with those patients whose primaries remain occult are approximately half that expected on the basis of their nodal disease alone.

A patient with neck metastases from an undetectable primary should nevertheless be given the benefit of definitive treatment. Despite the poor prognosis of an undiscovered primary, a significant number of patients do achieve cure by both surgical and radiotherapeutic approaches. In some patients, long-term repeat examinations will eventually disclose the primary tumour, and at a treatable stage.

Stage is defined by TNM classification, but there is no tumour classification (T) for occult primary cancer metastatic to neck lymph nodes. The local control and survival rates for squamous cancers of the neck nodes with unknown primary tumour are: N1, 40–50%; N2, 25–30%; N3, 10–15%.

Clinical correlations

The most likely site of the primary lesion is sometimes suggested by the cytological or histological findings from examination of the neck tissue.

(a) *Undifferentiated carcinoma*: the most probable primary site is in Waldeyer's ring, but may be the nasopharynx, base of the tongue or the tonsil.

(b) *Epidermoid carcinomas*: if metastatic to lymph nodes of the upper half of the neck may originate from a head and neck primary site.

(c) *Squamous carcinomas*: if metastatic to the lower neck may represent a primary site in the head and neck, oesophagus, lung or genitourinary tract. Evidence of other obvious metastatic disease, such as lung, liver or bone may be present.

(d) *Cryptogenic nasopharyngeal primary tumours*: these lesions may be secondary to EBV infection, and EBV genomic material may be detectable in cervical nodal tissue after DNA amplification using the polymerase chain reaction.

(e) *Clinical probabilities*: cervical nodal malignancy is the sole presenting symptom with the following primary lesions: nasopharynx (60%), oropharynx (20%), pyriform fossa (10%).

Histopathological correlates

Histological and immunohistochemical techniques, with appropriate, electron microscopy provide guidance for the continuing clinical evaluation. The complexity of the pathological evaluation tends to be inversely related to the degree of differentiation of the nodal disease. Electron microscopy may aid in distinguishing a primary diagnosis not obtained by light microscopy in approximately 10% of cases.

Histological features

1. *Well or moderately differentiated tumours.* The pathological differentiation of an epithelial cancer from lymphoma, sarcoma, melanoma or a germ cell tumour is usually straightforward.

2. *Adenocarcinomas.* Acinar spaces and microacini are seen in many specimens.

3. *Amelanotic melanomas.* Pre-melanosomes may be found.

4. *Neuroectodermal tumours.* Secretory granules are seen commonly.

5. *Gastrointestinal or renal tumours.* Periodic acid–Schiff (PAS) staining may be useful in confirming the diagnosis.

Immunohistochemical features

For poorly differentiated tumours, serum markers and immunohistochemical stains of pathological specimens for β-human chorionic gonadotrophin and α-fetoprotein should be performed. Some of these tumours respond to platinum-based combination chemotherapy in a manner similar to extragonadal germ cell malignancies.

Staining for keratins, leukocyte common antigen and S-100, a neuroectodermal antigen expressed in melanomas, may be performed.

Polymerase chain reaction

DNA amplification of EBV genomes can be used for diagnosis, with tissue provided by fine-needle aspiration biopsy. The presence of EBV in metastases from an occult primary tumour suggests the development of nasopharyngeal carcinoma.

Management

The management has two goals: diagnosis if possible of the site of primary lesion and treatment of the neck. The hunt for the primary site is based on history, clinical examination and baseline investigations.

History and examination

These are not usually revealing unless advanced disease of the infra-clavicular viscera is present. Cough, haemoptysis, weight loss, bleeding per rectum, haematuria or vaginal discharge in a woman may all alert clinical suspicion. Baseline investigations include full blood screen, biochemical function tests of liver and renal indices and serum tumour markers.

Imaging

1. *Plain films of the neck* demonstrate calcification, or obvious soft tissue shadows. Tuberculous nodes, laryngoceles and thyroid shadows may all be seen.

2. *Chest X-rays* are essential.

3. *Sinus X-rays* are commonly indicated.

4. *MRI scanning of the neck* delineates the extent of nodal disease and may demonstrate the primary lesion.

5. *Low level or posterior triangle cervical nodes* may arise from infra-clavicular disease which may be demonstrated by abdominal or pelvic ultrasound, barium contrast studies, IVU or CT scanning. The prognosis for thoracic or abdominal primary lesions with cervical metastases is, however, poor.

Endoscopy

Direct nasopharyngoscopy, laryngoscopy, bronchoscopy and oesophagoscopy should be performed with biopsy of any suspicious area. If no suspicious lesions are found, random biopsies of the nasopharynx, base of the tongue, tonsil and pyriform sinus on the side of the lesion should be performed. If the tonsil is not present, biopsy of the tonsillar fossa should be performed.

The neck mass	An excision biopsy should be carried out to establish a histological diagnosis. Surgical preparation should be for formal radical neck dissection. A frozen section intra-operatively may be used to guide the decision to proceed to neck dissection. Interval neck dissection may be planned.
Histological	*1. If histology reveals squamous carcinoma,* in a single isolated node without extracapsular spread, neck dissection is warranted as the primary lesion is likely to be of head and neck origin.
	2. If multiple nodes or extracapsular disease is present, or if the histology of the lesion is unclear, radiotherapy is preferable. Neck dissection is of less clearly demonstrable benefit.
	3. If adenocarcinoma, anaplastic carcinoma or squamous carcinoma in supraclavicular nodes is present, neck dissection is unlikely to be beneficial. Radiotherapy and attention to infra-clavicular disease is required.

Recurrent metastatic squamous neck cancer with occult primary tumour

The prognosis for any treated cancer patient with progressing, recurring or relapsing disease of the neck is poor, regardless of cell type or stage. Deciding on further treatment depends on many factors, including the specific cancer, prior treatment, site of recurrence as well as individual patient considerations.

Related topics of interest

Endoscopy (p. 127)
Imaging (p. 206)

Revision point

Patterns of lymphatic drainage of head and neck viscera

ODONTOGENIC TUMOURS

There are a wide variety of tumour-like lesions which present in the jaws. They have a spectrum of behaviour from slow growing to aggressive, causing extensive local destruction. Some are cystic, others are myxomatous, but few if any metastasize outside the jaws. There is a widely accepted but frequently modified WHO classification for the odontogenic tumours.

Epithelial

1. Ameloblastoma. These lesions account for almost 1% of jaw tumours. They affect mainly 20–50 year olds, and 80% occur in the mandible adjacent to the angle. They arise from odontogenic epithelial remnants and cause painless expansion of the jaw, tooth drift and exfoliation. They appear radiographically as multi-locular cysts, and should be considered as the main differential diagnosis in primordial or odontogenic keratocyst presentations. There are several histological variants. The commonest, follicular type occasionally produce microcysts. Stromal cysts are also common in the plexiform pattern. Eosinophilic or granular cell variants and squamous metaplasia with keratinization are also described. Malignant variants are described but are extremely rare. Treatment by generous enucleation and follow-up is the preferred method. For large lesions, recurrent lesions and those affecting soft tissue, a wider resection is advised.

2. Adenomatoid odontogenic tumour. Commonest in late teens and 20 year olds, it demonstrates a slight female preponderance. Typically in the maxillary canine region, it may be associated with an ectopic or unerupted tooth. It is clearly encapsulated, may have cystic areas within it but equally common are densely calcified areas. The lesion may arise from a failed enamel organ and the calcified tissue may be more dental in type than osseous. Simple enucleation is usually required.

3. Calcifying epithelial odontogenic tumour. A rare locally invasive lesion arising from odontogenic epithelium. It is commonest after 40 years of age, and the sex incidence is about equal. Seventy five percent affect the mandibular premolar region. An unerupted tooth may be associated. Radiographically it presents as a mixed radiolucent–radio-opaque lesion. Its histology is unusual, with eosinophilic, polyhedral cells in a variable stroma of hyaline material with calcified masses adjacent to the epithelial tissue. Occasional tooth tissue or partially formed dental structures are present. Incomplete excision confers a high risk of local recurrence.

4. Squamous odontogenic tumour. A relatively recently described but uncommon lesion. It is thought to arise from the periodontal cell rests of Malassez. The incidence is about equal between the jaws, and it may be multi-focal. Histology reveals epithelial islands, microcysts and crystalloid material in a chronically inflamed fibrous stroma. If the lesion is extensive, wide local excision is required to prevent recurrence and damage to adjacent structures.

5. Calcifying odontogenic cyst. A painless swelling which can occur in bone or extra-osseous tissues. Always affecting the tooth-bearing tissues, 80% occur in the mandible. These lesions may be cystic or solid, and cells resembling any of those in the enamel organ may be present. Aberrant keratinization may occur. 'Ghost cells' and dystrophic calcification have been described. Inflammation occurs if the keratinous tissues escape into the surrounding tissue. Local curettage is required.

Connective tissue

1. Cementomas. Under the WHO classification there are four types.

(a) *Benign cementoblastoma.* Typically affects young males and is commonest in the mandibular pre-molar region. A dense radio-opacity with a tendency to resorb adjacent teeth due to osteoclast-like giant cells. Simple enucleation is curative.

(b) *Cementifying fibroma.* Typically a solitary lesion in the mandibular molar region of older patients. Often an incidental radiographic finding, this periapical radio-opacity is usually associated with a vital tooth. Enucleation is curative.

(c) *Periapical cemental dysplasia.* Similar in presentation to the cementifying fibroma, this lesion is more usual in the mandibular incisor region and is commoner in women. It may be multi-focal and more sclerotic. Enucleation is curative.

(d) *Gigantiform cementoma.* This is the least common variety. It has a familial predisposition, occurs most often in middle-aged negroid women and affects each jaw equally commonly. It may be multi-focal. Mucosal ulceration and secondary chronic osteomyelitis may be associated. The lesions may become quite large, but enucleation is usually curative.

2. Dentinoma. A rare lesion consisting of mixed odontogenic epithelium and dysplastic dentine. Most lesions are mandibular and affect the unerupted molar of young adults. Local excision is curative.

3. Odontogenic fibroma. A tumour consisting of mature collagenous fibrous tissue, it is thought to originate from odontogenic mesenchyme. An unerupted tooth is usually associated and there have been peripheral gingival lesions described. Complete excision is curative.

4. Myxoma. Originating from odontogenic mesenchyme, this lesion produces a characteristic 'soap bubble' appearance on radiographs. This is due to central bone resorption with sclerotic cortical margins which may be expanded or eroded focally. It is associated with expansion, missing teeth and loosening or displacement of the adjacent teeth. The jaws are affected equally and the tumour is commonest in young patients. Often infiltrative with poorly defined margins, it is a difficult tumour to excise fully. Incomplete removal will usually lead to recurrence.

Mixed origin

1. Odontomes. Hamartomatous rather than neoplastic, these lesions consist of mature dental tissues in a well-organized arrangement (compound odontome or denticle) or in a haphazard array (complex odontome). Mixed patterns are found. An unerupted tooth is associated. Dens invaginatus is a common related developmental abnormality where the enamel organ is persistent as an inclusion in the fully formed tooth. A spectrum of severity from incisor lingual pits to gross deformation of dens in dente or gestalt odontome exists.

2. Ameloblastic fibroma. A true mixed tumour comprising odontogenic epithelium in a mixed connective tissue stroma, it occurs in childhood or teenage years. An array of mixed strands of odontogenic tissues and mixed hyaline and fibrous stroma formation is described. Wide excision is required to prevent recurrence, and very rare reports of sarcomatous change in the stromal elements make this measure essential.

3. Odontoameloblastoma. A very rare lesion similar to ameloblastoma in appearance and behaviour. It occurs in young children more commonly in the maxillary pre-molar region. Wide excision is recommended as recurrence is common.

Other lesions

- Non-odontogenic lesions such as melanotic neuroectodermal tumour of infancy
- Primary bone tumours and tumour-like lesions
- Metastatic deposits from carcinomas of breast or bronchus, kidney, thyroid, prostate and colon
- Tumours of lymphoid origin
- Histiocytoses
- Fibrous and osseous dysplasias
- Jaw cysts.

Related topic of interest

Cysts (p. 123)

Revision point

Embryology of tooth development

ORAL ULCERATION

An ulcer is a crater that extends through the entire thickness of an epithelial surface, involving the underlying connective tissue. The surrounding tissue is infiltrated with inflammatory cells to a varying degree depending on the cause of the ulcer.

Causes of oral ulcers

Traumatic

Ill fitting dentures, poorly finished restorations and rough edges to teeth may all cause oral ulcers. Habits such as tongue thrusting and occupational habits such as pencil or needle sucking can lead to ulcers. Chemicals can lead to burn ulcers; aspirin and eugenol are known to produce ulcers. Thermal burns and cryotherapy have similar effects.

Recurrent oral ulceration (ROU)

Eleven to 20% of the population are affected by ROU. There is a slight female preponderance. Most ROU is of unknown aetiology but in a few people there appears to be a related haematological disorder. This is ill defined, however, and causal relationships are difficult to establish. The conditions sometimes associated with ROU include anaemia, cyclic neutropenia, suggested haematinic deficiencies including iron, zinc, folate and vitamin B12. However, there is a poor relationship between ROU and tissue iron levels in most patients. Other factors important in the assessment of the patient include life style factors and stress, smoking, the relationship with foods if there is a suspicion of allergy and the relationship with the menstrual cycle as ulcers typically occur during the luteal phase of cycle. Evidence of immunodeficiency and granulocytopenia, is important as is family history. There are suggested HLA associations including HLA-A2, Bl 2, Aw-29.

1. Minor ROU. This is the commonest form affecting about 80% of sufferers. The ulcers are shallow, about 2–4 mm in diameter with a yellow necrotic base. They last 7–10 days with up to 6–10 ulcers at any time. The non-keratinized mucosa is commonly affected and ulcers usually heal without scarring. They commonly affect patients in the first three decades of life and tend to recur at 4–12 monthly intervals.

2. Major ROU. These lesions are rarer occurring in crops of 1–6 ulcers. They are typically large ovoid ulcers up to 2 cm in size affecting lips, fauces, tongue and soft palate. They can take up to a month to heal and unlike the minor form may heal with scarring.

3. Herpetiform ROU. These are uncommon and unrelated to herpetic infection. They tend to be small and numerous with up to 100 ulcers present at a time. They may fuse and coalesce to form one large ulcer which may then scar. They are more common in females over 30 years old.

Infective

1. Viral. Herpetic stomatitis, varicella (chickenpox), herpes zoster, hand, foot and mouth disease, herpangina, infectious mononucleosis, and HIV may all be associated with oral ulcers. In ROU, however, there is rarely a proven viral aetiology and aciclovir has no demonstrable benefit in most patients.

2. Bacterial. Acute ulcerative gingivitis, cancrum oris, tuberculosis and syphilis all have typical patterns of associated ulcers. *Streptococcus mitis* is a possible direct pathogen which appears to exhibit cross reactivity with keratinocyte antigenic determinants.

3. Fungal. Candida, histoplasmosis, and blastomycosis have all been implicated in oral ulcers.

Neoplastic

Oral squamous cell carcinoma often presents as an ulcer with a deep indurated crater and sometimes with associated cervical lymphadenopathy. The variant leukaemia, mycosis fungoides infiltrates submucosally and may cause epithelial ulceration.

Dermatological

Erosive lichen planus presents as ulcers superimposed on a reticular or macular pattern of background inflammation. The bullous conditions pemphigus and benign mucous membrane pemphigoid and erythema multiforme have a common end stage lesion in oral ulceration. Dermatitis herpetiformis is associated with inflammatory linear IgA disease and inflammatory bowel disease particularly small bowel Crohn's disease.

Gastrointestinal

Two to 3% of all oral ulceration is estimated to be related to inflammatory bowel disease. Coeliac disease may produce associated ulcers.

Renal disease

Oral ulcers are common especially in patients where anti-basement membrane antibody mediated glomerulonephritis is present. In renal dialysis oral ulcers are a frequent occurrence.

Connective tissue disease

Systemic lupus erythematosus and rheumatoid arthritis may have oral ulcers as part of the symptom complex. Reiter's disease presents with a mixed picture of genital, oral, and ocular lesions with its associated arthritis. It has good prognosis. Evidence of mycoplasmal or sexually transmitted infections should be sought during investigation. Bechet's syndrome has four described clinical subtypes; mucocutaneous, arthritic, neurological and ocular. Oral ulceration is typically part of the mucocutaneous syndrome but may occur in any of the other variants. Bechet's syndrome is rare and affects males more frequently than females in a ratio of about 3:1. The diagnosis requires oral ulceration and at least two other lesions.

Iatrogenic

Lasers, cryotherapy, diathermy, topical agents such as eugenol and drugs such as aspirin may all cause accidental oral mucosal breach, subsequent ulceration and inflammation. Non-steroidal anti inflammatory agents (NSAID) and cytotoxic drug therapy are potentially complicated by oral ulceration. Lichenoid reactions to anti-hypertensives and gold injections are also described. Radiotherapy related mucositis and ulceration is well documented.

Factitious

Occasionally, patients present with ulcers that defy diagnosis and by a process of careful exclusion, self-inflicted ulceration may be diagnosed.

Management

Diagnosis

The clinical presentation is important. A history of a prodromal illness such as URTI or herpes zoster may be elicited. The pattern of onset, whether acute or chronic, and the duration, frequency and pattern of recurrence are all important features.

A history of pain, bleeding or blistering are important. Genital ulcers, ocular symptoms, joint pain or effusions or a rash are features to be noted if present. Associated lymphadenopathy suggests malignancy or local sepsis. Relevant medical history includes detailing allergies and underlying systemic disease. Family and social history including tobacco and alcohol consumption is helpful.

Investigations

1. Baseline haematology and biochemistry including iron studies, haematinics and immunological investigations; ESR, CRP, serum immunoglobulins, C3 and C4, and serum immune complexes are requested. If required on the basis of the history, specific serology is also done. Basement membrane and desmosomal auto-antibodies may be present in bullous disease and in glomerulonephritis associated ulceration. Oral mucosal smear and swabs for microbial culture may be required and VDRL and viral titres may all be done.

2. Imaging. Chest X-ray, abdominal X-ray, contrast studies if dysphagia is associated or ultrasound in renal disease may be required.

3. Biopsy is essential for suspected malignancy or for immunofluorescence in dermatological lesions, connective tissue disease or Crohn's ulceration.

Treatment

1. General measures. Correction of any underlying deficiencies and analgesia is required. Dietary modification is sometimes required typically where a gluten free diet in coeliac patients is needed. Otherwise this step is rarely helpful for most patients.

2. Local measures. Benzydamine oral rinse or spray and chlorhexidine gluconate 0.2% have been tried with success in control of symptoms. The natural history of the ulcers is little altered, however. Carbenoxolone sodium granules 1% are effective in some patients but it is necessary to monitor serum potassium especially in elderly or patients taking digoxin.

3. Topical steroids. Triamcinolone acetonide and hydrocortisone sodium succinate pellets 2.5 mg are widely prescribed. Beclomethasone valerate lozenges or by inhaler (Becotide 100 inhaler) have been used more recently. Prednesol mouthwash (5 mg in 20 ml) is used in more severe cases.

4. Intralesional steroid injections. Triamcinolone with or without lignocaine given in 0.2–0.3 ml per ulcer site and repeated at weekly intervals may prove beneficial.

In patient

Hospital admission may be necessary if pain control and nasogastric tube feeding is required. Occasionally oral ulcers are of such severity to warrant this pattern of treatment. Patients with potentially life threatening bullous disease such as pemphigus may require in patient treatment and high dose parenteral steroids in addition.

ORBITAL SURGERY

Periorbital surgery constitutes part of many maxillofacial operations. The conditions requiring attention during facial surgery include eyelid lacerations, orbital skeleton fractures, and traumatic epiphora. Planned surgery involving the orbit includes orbital decompression, eyelid surgery, facial palsy, temporal artery biopsy and oculoplastic surgery.

Eyelid lacerations

Lid involvement in facial trauma is relatively uncommon but the techniques required for repair are important.

Lid margin   Accurate apposition is essential to prevent ectropion postoperatively.

Tarsal plate   Marginal sutures are placed to allow accurate apposition. The tarsal plate is closed with sutures placed such that the conjunctival surface is not breached.

Lachrimal apparatus   Medial lid injuries place the lachrimal sac at risk. Careful exploration and repair of the canaliculi and sac is required if disabling epiphora is to be prevented. Medial canthal ligament reconstruction in naso-ethmoidal injuries is important in preventing nasolachrimal duct occlusion.

Orbital fractures

Inferior and medial wall fractures are the commonest bony injury affecting the orbit. Blow-out fractures are wall fractures with an intact orbital rim. Previously thought to be caused by an occluding injury with a sudden increase in hydrostatic pressure within the globe, these injuries are now thought to be due to transmitted forces within the bony walls themselves.

Clinical features   Diplopia, enophthalmos, pain and mechanical gaze palsies are fairly constant features. Lateral gaze is restricted with medial wall fractures and upward gaze more so with floor injuries.

X-ray and CT   Evidence of fracture, wall comminution and orbital soft tissue herniation into the sinus system may all be seen. Ethmoid sinuses can be breached in medial wall injuries. Lateral wall and roof injuries are rare and tend to present as part of a more major injury complex.

Principles of management	Conservative treatment in the early phase is advised until the extent of diplopia and globe tethering can be assessed accurately. Initial swelling and periorbital bruising can be allowed to settle.
Surgery	The incision options include skin crease, subciliary or blepharoplasty, subtarsal or fornix pattern. The injured walls are explored in the subperiosteal plane taking care to preserve the lachrymal apparatus medially. Orbital hernias are reduced and the bony defect repaired. The options for repair include alloplastic materials such as Teflon, Silastic sheeting or titanium mesh. Autogenous bone from the frontal outer table, temporal fascia or fascia lata may be harvested for use. Bony rim injuries are repaired with mini plates.

Lachrimal surgery

Indications	Congenital obstruction and stenosis is the preserve of the ophthalmic surgeon. Lachrimal injuries are uncommon in maxillofacial practice and acquired obstructions are due to dacroliths and mass lesions adjacent to the nasolacrimal duct.
Surgery	The operation of dacrocystorhinotomy is often required to overcome these obstructions to prevent persistent epiphora. The operation is done via a high lateral nasal incision over the lachrimal crest. The sac is gently mobilized and retracted laterally and the bony base of the lachrimal groove osteotomized. The posterior wall of the lachrimal sac is incised and the sinus mucosa exposed by osteotomy is prepared similarly.
	Canalicular stents are passed through the upper and lower punctae and passed through the newly fashioned osteum. The anterior wall is then repaired and the skin wound closed in layers.

Eyelid reconstructive surgery

Tarsorraphy	Permanent or temporary, surgical closure of the palpebral fissure may be required during extensive orbital surgery to preserve the corneal epithelium and

reduce drying. In proptosis due to thyroid eye disease it can be useful and should be a considered option in chronic facial palsy, tear film deficiencies and dry eye syndromes. In keratitis or dendritic ulcer healing can be hastened by use in some patients.

Ectropion and enotropion

There are many reconstructive operations described.

Facial palsy

Insertion of lid gold weights and reanimation or sling procedures are all used in some centres to correct the eyelid problems and corneal drying in chronic facial nerve palsies.

Reconstruction

In extensive trauma or after ablative tumour surgery there is occasionally the need for eyelid reconstruction. The important factors are to ensure that the conjunctival surface is repaired without leaving a roughened surface to interfere with the tear film. Attention to the lid margin, tarsal plate and lachrimal apparatus are essential. Direct closure is often possible. Canthotomy or cantholysis is sometimes required in order to achieve this. In other patients, rotational flaps, periosteal advancements and tarsal grafts may be required. Mucosa and skin can be mobilized by rotational flaps or free grafting from the temporal region or from the oral cavity.

Orbital decompression

Trauma and postorbital floor exploration are the situations most likely to lead to retrobulbar haematoma formation. Mass effect from tumours will require decompression. Graves ophthalmopathy can also present as a need for emergency decompression.

In trauma patients the floor must be re-explored and quite extensive inferomedial osteotomy performed in order to preserve optic nerve function. Any alloplastic material should be removed at this point. Lateral orbitotomy may provide better access.

CT scan is usually required and steroids will reduce the oedema and 'buy time' whilst preparations for operation are underway.

OSTEOTOMIES

The use of planned bone cuts and mobilization of different parts of the facial skeleton is common in maxillofacial surgery.

Uses of osteotomies

- Correction of disproportion of the jaws and cosmetic deformities of the face.
- Correction of congenital defects of the head and face, including cleft-associated defects.
- For access during neurosurgery for correction of defects in the upper spinal cord and brain stem.
- To allow access to deeper structures of the neck and skull base.
- To increase access during oncological surgery particularly of the posterior oral floor and pharynx.

The advances in reconstructive techniques designed particularly for use in treatment of complex jaw fractures and improved understanding of the patterns of vascular supply of the jaws has allowed more easy use of elective osteotomies in other branches of head and neck surgery. In planning osteotomy surgery several aspects of the osteotomy need to be considered.

1. The nature of the underlying condition. Preoperative medical status and a history of previous radiotherapy is important.

2. Anaesthetic considerations. Endotracheal tube placement, hypotensive anaesthesia, perioperative analgesia all need preoperative liaison with the anaesthetist.

3. The predicted changes in appearance significantly affect the recovery and psychological well being of the patient. Normal racial characteristics and the effect of surgery on ageing tissues must be considered in planning surgery. Preoperative psychiatric conditions such as disorders of body image and dysmorphophopia need specialist psychiatric assessment.

Preoperative investigation and documentation

- *History* and family history and recording of family characteristics.

- *Soft tissue function.* Particularly of tongue, lips and cheeks should be noted.
- *Speech* disturbances and neurological deficits should be noted.
- *Swallow* diatheses can be recorded. They are uncommon.
- *Dental status.* Particularly intra-oral hygiene, restorative condition and denture wearing or edentulous areas.
- *Intra-oral examination* should record the dental eruptive status and restorative condition. Orthodontic base line data is recorded including centre line discrepancies, crowding, inclination of the buccal and incisor segments and overbite and overjet should be recorded.
- *Upper airways.* In particular nasal breathing and tonsil size is important. Intrusion of the maxilla may adversely affect nasal airway where turbinate hypertrophy is present preoperatively. The competence of the 'sphincters' is important and endoscopy is required where velopharyngeal competence is in doubt .
- *Speech assessment and videofluoroscopy.* These investigations are particularly important in planning osteotomies for cleft patients.
- *Orthopantomograph.* To determine the presence of unerupted and impacted teeth and dentoalveolar pathology.
- *True lateral skull radiographs* allow accurate cephalometric measurements to be taken.
- *Impressions* for study models are essential in the early planning stages for orthognahic and cleft patients. Duplicate models should be made so that model surgery can be performed on articulated casts.
- *Clinical photographs.* As part of serial records during the course of orthodontic and surgical treatment and for medicolegal documentation photographs are increasingly important.
- *Other imaging and records.* 3D reconstructed CT scanning and digital laser imaging of soft tissue form may be used. For straightforward osteotomies however CT scanning is rarely justified or necessary. In complex or high level deformity correction, these

techniques may be useful. MRI scanning will allow more accurate assessment of the soft tissue and may permit prediction of the likely changes to be expected during treatment. This remains an experimental rather than a routine clinical procedure. Cine sequences allow assessment of the role of lip, tongue and swallow actions in the genesis of the facial abnormalities. Again this is rarely performed in routine osteotomy planning.

- *Computerised plotting programmes* using digitized data from lateral cephalometric radiographs are widely used in osteotomy planning and most programmes have a predictive module.
- *For osteotomies designed as access procedures.* Investigations intended to determine the extent of malignancy are important in addition to the preparations for the osteotomy. A chest radiograph and baseline haematology is usually required. CT and MRI or ultrasound scans looking for occult lymph node metastases may be essential and fine needle aspiration cytology and endoscopy aid in determining the extent of the disease.
- *Endoscopy.* Particularly fibre-optic pharyngeal endoscopy is becoming increasingly useful in assessment in cleft cases and before cancer surgery. Where sleep apnoea is to be treated by osteotomy, endoscopic-controlled Müllers manoeuvre is helpful in assessment of the flaccidity of the pharyngeal wall musculature.

Once all these records are available, surgery can be planned either by manual tracing of lateral skull films or by use of digitized tracings and computer-aided analysis and prediction. Use of the photographs as a montage and the articulated plaster models allow planning of surgery and preparation of intra-operative acrylic wafers. All the preoperative investigations and the documentation should be available to a joint planning orthognathic clinic comprising surgeon, orthodontist and if necessary speech therapist and psychologist.

In planning treatment, several phases should be considered. The routine dental care should proceed normally and any underlying medical problems should be treated. Presurgical orthodontics is almost always required. Relief of crowding, correction of tooth alignment, co-ordination of arch dimensions, reduction of the over jet in the class 2 case and decompensation of low incisors are commonly required. Creation of the necessary space is important where segmental osteotomies are planned. Levelling of the occlusal planes is sometimes required. Expansion of the maxilla in late treatment of cleft patients is often required preoperatively.

Investment in equipment is considerable. A department undertaking this sort of surgery usually involves a dedicated computer system attached to a digitiser and plotter as well as investment in the appropriate software. The necessary radiographic equipment should be available if more advanced imaging is considered necessary. In particular the CT 3D reconstruction software represents a major investment. Laser imaging is not widely available but fibre-optic endoscopy facilities should be to hand.

Related topics of interest

PAROTID GLAND TUMOURS

The WHO Classification of parotid neoplasms is the most widely used.

Epithelial tumours
- Pleomorphic adenoma (mixed parotid tumour).
- Monomorphic adenomas.
- Adenolymphoma (Warthin's tumour).
- Oxyphil adenoma.
- Other types.
- Mucoepidermoid tumour.
- Acinic cell tumour.
- *Carcinomas*: adenoid cystic carcinoma; adenocarcinoma; epidermoid carcinoma; undifferentiated carcinoma; carcinoma in pleomorphic adenoma (malignant mixed tumour).

Non-epithelial tumours
- Sarcomas.
- Malignant lymphoma.
- Others.

Unclassified tumour-like lesions
- Benign lymphoepithelial lesion
- Sialosis
- Oncocytosis

Incidence

Salivary gland tumours are relatively uncommon. They have an estimated incidence of between 0.25 and 2.5 cases per 100 000 of the UK population. In European races, salivary gland tumours account for less than 3% of all neoplasms. Over 70% of parotid tumours are pleomorphic adenomas. Adenolymphomas or 'Warthin's tumours' are most often seen in men between the ages of 55 and 65. In about 5% of cases further primary tumours subsequently develop in the same or in the opposite parotid gland.

Benign tumours

Pleomorphic adenoma
Also known as a mixed cell tumour it arises from intercalated duct cells and myoepithelial cells. It is the commonest tumour of major salivary glands and in the parotid gland, it forms 90% of all benign tumours; in the submandibular gland, 50%. The average age at presentation is 40–50 years. It is usually unilateral but a few bilateral tumours have been described. The sex

incidence is roughly equal. About one-quarter of patients with this tumour have vague local discomfort, but it is usually symptomless apart from the lump, and the facial nerve is never paralysed as the tumour is benign. Most of these tumours occur in the tail of the parotid gland. They can also occur in the retromandibular portion of the parotid gland, either as solitary deep-lobe tumours or dumb-bell tumours. They are very rare elsewhere in the parotid gland. On palpation, the tumour is usually smooth, superficial, round and mobile. The capsule is of compressed normal parotid tissue and varies in thickness. Microscopically duct formation, squamous metaplasia, keratin production and fibroblasts, cartilage, bone precursors may all be found. The tumour is highly implantable and the recurrence rate after primary surgery is about 5%. If simple enucleation is performed, the recurrence rate is between 20 and 30%.

Warthin's tumour

This is also known as a papillary cystadenoma lymphomatosum or adenolymphoma. It is considered to be a neoplastic proliferation of epithelial cell rests usually investing perisalivary lymph node tissue. The commonest site is the periparotid nodal system but submandibular gland tumours may also occur. The tumour cells may resemble salivary serous cells and are arranged in basophilic sheets. In parotid lesions, 43% will involve the lateral lobe only and 27% will involve both lobes. Fifteen to 20% exhibit extraglandular extension.

Adenoid cystic carcinoma

This tumour arises in major and minor glands: 25% occur in the parotid gland, 15% in the submandibular gland, 1% in the sublingual gland and the remainder in the minor glands. Seventy per cent of minor gland tumours arise within the mouth. It forms about 40% of malignant tumours at all salivary sites. It accounts for about 2% of all parotid tumours. Adenoid cystic carcinoma is commonly unilobular. It is unencapsulated but appears circumscribed. Microscopically it has a characteristic cribriform pattern. It exhibits a tendency to invade nerves and this accounts for the high frequency of pain. Only 15% will metastasize to lymph nodes. The hallmark is the incidence of distant metastases in the lungs (40%), the brain (20%) and in the bones (20%). Approximately 40% of patients will ultimately manifest distant metastases. The most probable source of the tumour is the intercalated duct cells.

Adenocarcinoma

This tumour forms about 3% of parotid tumours and 10% of submandibular minor salivary gland tumours. The sex incidence is equal and it can occur at any age. It is one of the commoner malignant salivary gland tumours seen in children. It may present as an asymptomatic mass or with typical malignant features. In the parotid, most occur in the deep lobe or extend beyond the gland when first seen. They are highly malignant with a high metastatic rate and the 5 year survival is only about 10%.

Squamous cell carcinoma

This is extremely rare (1%) in the parotid and is only slightly more common (5%) in the submandibular gland. Before the diagnosis of squamous cell carcinoma in a salivary gland raises, the possibility of this being a mucoepidermoid tumour and malignant pleomorphic adenoma must be excluded. Metastases in the parotid lymph nodes from a neighbouring skin tumour or from another head and neck primary site may also present as an apparent parotid neoplasm. Two-thirds of the patients are men and the average age at presentation is in the seventh decade. It is an aggressive tumour and shows no tendency to encapsulation. It grows rapidly, causing pain, facial nerve paralysis, skin fixation and ulceration. About half have metastatic neck nodes when first seen. It has a poor prognosis whatever method of treatment is used.

Sarcomas

These are extremely rare but neurofibrosarcoma, rhabdomyosarcoma, histiocytoma and Kaposi's sarcoma have all been described.

Carcinoma ex pleomorphic adenoma

One per cent of these tumours arises *ab initio*, but most arise from a pre-existing benign pleomorphic adenoma. The benign tumour is likely to have been present for at least 10–15 years before malignant change occurs. About 1–5% of pleomorphic adenomas lasting this length of time are at risk of changing their biological character. When they become malignant they may still be grossly encapsulated; suspicious features are the occurrence of pain, a rapid growth spurt and infiltration at the periphery. Regional lymph node metastases occur in 25% and distant metastases in 30%. The 5 year survival is around 40% and the 15 year survival 19%.

Metastatic tumours

The parotid gland lymph nodes occur within the gland and on its external surface, and can be the site of metastatic tumour deposits. Eighty per cent of these are from skin of the face, temple or scalp, and they are most frequently melanoma or squamous carcinoma.

Recurrent pleomorphic adenoma

There are two problems with treatment of pleomorphic adenomas. The first is recurrence after an inadequate 'lumpectomy' or enucleation for a pleomorphic adenoma. The second is unexpected recurrence after a superficial parotidectomy for pleomorphic adenoma.

The lesion recurs very readily and bursting the capsule during surgery, or opening the tumour to carry out a frozen section increase this risk. These tumours are highly implantable and even after superficial parotidectomy they may implant in the deep or retromandibular portion of the parotid gland and occasionally in the skin. The histology of pleomorphic adenomata exhibits micro 'pseudopodia' which may remain *in situ* after too limited an excision. The operation of choice on first presentation of the tumour should be a superficial parotidectomy. In recurrent disease, relationship to the facial nerve and skin, and the histology to exclude malignant foci within the recurrent tumour are all important factors. Residual parotidectomy or conservative deep lobe excision may be required. If enucleation was performed previously, total conservative parotidectomy may need to be planned.

Related topics of interest

Facial nerve (p. 130)
Salivary gland surgery (p. 340)

Revision point

Anatomy of the parotid gland

PENETRATING TRAUMA OF THE HEAD AND NECK

Modes of injury

Penetrating head and neck trauma is relatively uncommon in the UK. In civilian injuries from USA and South Africa the use of firearms is more frequent and penetrating injuries are therefore more common as a result. In UK civilian trauma this picture is changing with knives, broken beer glasses and bottles increasingly common weapons of interpersonal violence. Military casualties have a proportionally higher rate of penetrating injuries due to projectile impact and shrapnel type wounds.

Anatomical regions of face

- *Zone 1.* From superior orbital rims upwards to include the frontal region and frontal sinuses.
- *Zone 2.* From superior orbital rims to commissure of the lips.
- *Zone 3.* From commissure of the lips to the level of the hyoid bone.

Anatomical regions of neck

- *Zone 1.* From sternal notch to cricoid cartilage.
- *Zone 2.* From cricoid cartilage to lower border of mandible.
- *Zone 3.* From lower border of mandible to skull base.

Management

1. *Resuscitation.* Immediate management of airway, breathing problems and haemorrhage are vital. The precise injury details are of secondary importance to good resuscitation.

2. *Other injuries.* Determining priorities for treatment where multiple system injuries are present is essential.

3. *Zone 1 facial injuries.* Frontal sinus, orbital roof and intracranial injuries may occur. Full neurological assessment with CT scanning is essential. Neurosurgical intervention to remove foreign bodies, repair dural tears, evacuate haematomata and close CSF leaks may be required. Frontal sinus injuries may require exenteration, cavity obliteration and occlusion of the frontonasal duct.

4. *Zone 2 facial injuries.* Structures at risk include facial nerve, parotid duct, orbit, globe, maxillary antrum and buccal tissues. Full neurological and ophthalmological assessments are required. CT or MRI scans of brain, orbits and middle third of the face are essential. Functional assessment of facial nerve function and parotid saliva flow are recorded. Midfacial fractures are treated appropriately and closure of mucosal and skin wounds is performed early. Parotid duct injuries are repaired over an indwelling stent retained *in situ* for 10–14 days. Microneural repair of the facial nerve is performed at an interval of 48–72 hours once the wound is infection free and thoroughly debrided. Cable grafting may be required to make good nerve trunk losses. Sural or greater auricular nerves may be used. Maxillary antral injuries may require fixation of associated midface fractures, exploration of orbitozygomatic injuries and pernasal antrostomy drainage.

5. *Zone 3 facial injuries.* Injuries to the mouth, oropharynx, carotid sheath contents, submandibular salivary gland, facial artery and lower branches of the facial nerve may occur. Full oropharyngeal examination, panendoscopy and if necessary, angiography or duplex Doppler studies for suspected vascular injuries may be required. MRI scanning is a useful investigation in complex injuries to this region. Exploration, repair of aerodigestive viscera and vascular repair may be required. In major vascular injury, emergency shunting is available. Mandibular fractures if associated should be reduced and fixed as appropriate.

6. *Zone 1 neck injuries.* Injuries to the first rib, clavicle, and subclavian vessels may occur. CT scanning and angiography or duplex Doppler scans are required. Major vascular injuries require combined thoracic and cervical surgical approach. Cooling and emergency vascular shunting may be required to permit vascular repair. Injuries to the trachea or oesophagus require endoscopic assessment and surgical repair. The lung apex if injured may result in pneumothorax,

haemopneumothorax or cervical surgical emphysema. Surgical repair is usually necessary.

7. *Zone 2 neck injuries.* Major injuries to the upper aerodigestive tract occur. The larynx, vocal cords, recurrent laryngeal nerve and hyoid bone may be damaged. Vascular injuries may also occur. The decision to explore or manage the injury conservatively is made on the basis of clinical, CT scan and endoscopic findings. Retrieval of bullets, shotgun pellets or missile fragments are frequently required and constitute a strong indication for surgery.

8. *Zone 3 neck injuries.* Assessment and surgery can be demanding. Carotid sheath contents, cranial nerve and mandibular injuries may occur. Expanding para- or retropharyngeal haematomata may present with worsening stridor, drooling and respiratory distress. Wide exposure and mandibulotomy may be required for access. Injuries to the base of skull region may occur in association.

Related topic of interest

Blunt trauma to the head and neck (p. 21)

Revision points

Anatomy of the neck and thorax
Approaches to the different regions of the neck
Principles of neurosurgery
Resuscitation

PRE-PROSTHETIC SURGERY

Pre-prosthetic surgery involves a group of techniques designed to prepare the mouth to receive new dentures or to improve the fit and function of new dentures. There are techniques applicable to full or partial denture construction.

Soft tissue modification

1. Fraenoplasty. Buccal fraenal attachments or lingual fraena can be excised or reduced. Simple incision with closure will elongate the attachment and free an ankyloglossia. Z plasty techniques are equally good at achieving fraenal reduction.

2. Fibrous ridge reduction. Wedge resection and primary closure of leaf fibromas and denture hyperplasia may be required before provision of new dentures.

3. Vestibuloplasty. Insertion of mucosal inlay grafts, split skin grafts or Edlan flaps are effective.

4. Muscle reattachment operations. Repositioning by detachment and reattachment procedures are described.

5. Nerve repositioning. High lying mental nerves may be subject to denture trauma, neuroma formation and may cause the patient considerable pain. The mental foramen can be moved into inferior position away from the alveolar ridge and the nerve trunk sited in the new, lower position.

6. Facial palsy correction. Facial sling operations and a variety of facial reanimation operations including those based on microvascular transfer of neuromuscular grafts are described.

Bony modifications

1. Ridge augmentation. Bone grafts either with rib or vascularized bone is an option. Wisor pattern or sandwich osteotomies may be useful.

2. Ridge reduction. Alveolar bone resorbs once teeth are lost, muscle attachments often become more prominent. The mylohyoid ridge and genial tubercles are examples. Excessive width, sharpness or associated bony undercuts may require reduction. Exostoses may also require reduction.

3. Removal of tori. Midline palatal tori may be of similar thickness and bony dimensions to the remainder of the palatal shelf and may constitute a deformation or abnormality of contour rather than formation of excessive bone. Over-zealous reduction will then result in fistula formation.

4. Osteotomies or orthognathic procedures. Segmental surgery is occasionally performed and sagittal split mandibular osteotomy or Le Fort 1 procedures may be required.

Dentoalveolar procedures
1. Tooth preparations. Undercut reduction, orthodontic tooth alignment or arch alignment and provision of prosthodontic support for planned dentures may be required.

2. Implants. Submucosal frame implants have been described. These designs have all been subject to a high failure rate and are not widely advocated.

3. Osseointegrated implants. The advent of titanium oxide coated alloys has allowed the design of implants which, if placed into alveolar bone, over a period of months integrate with the bone. Placement technique is critical so that overheating is avoided and physiological loading is imposed at the correct time. Loading via a denture superstructure ensures continued alveolar bone integrity once osseointegration has occurred. Complex restorative options have become possible with the advent of this technology and extraoral reconstructon has become possible. Orbital, nasal and auricular reconstruction are now possible once a properly placed osseointegrated stud is placed and allowed to heal.

4. Transmandibular devices. The treatment of the grossly atrophic mandible is always a challenge and there are a variety of options that have been proposed. The transmandibular implant requires a combined extra-oral and intraoral approach with transmandibular abutment insertion secured into a base plate subperiosteally at the lower mandibular border. The superstructure is secured to the transmandibular abutments. Prosthetic reconstruction is supported on transmucosal abutments similar to those used in osseointegrated implant work.

5. *Sinus lifts*. Placement of bone grafts in the antral floor with or without osseointegrated implants in the maxillary alveolus can be performed. This procedure helps the retention and osseointegration of the fixtures by increasing the bone depth available by bone graft placement submucosally in the antral floor. The approach is via a Caldwell–Luc type incision bilaterally.

Other procedures

Lip commissures. Alterations to the width and extent of mouth opening may be required. Scarring, cheilitis and correction of commissural defects after previous lip surgery may be required to permit denture wearing. Excision of oral submucous fibrosis, correction of TMJ ankylosis, coronoidectomy, and revisional lip surgery can all be considered where mouth opening is a significant problem.

Related topics of interest

PRESURGICAL ORTHODONTICS

Most orthognathic surgery requires a period of preoperative orthodontic treatment. This is particularly true were jaw disproportion surgery is performed and in cleft palate cases. Where osteotomies are planned as part of a craniofacial operation or where maxillofacial access is required during neurosurgery there is no need for presurgical orthodontics.

Presurgical orthodontic treatments

The intention is to facilitate orthognathic surgery and produce tooth alignment such that in the immediate postoperative period a stable occlusion can be established.

1. Establish tooth alignment. Correction of incisor imbrication by interdental enamel stripping or of mild malalignments by axial tilts in the incisor region will increase space sufficiently to allow correction and relieve mild crowding.

2. Decompensation. Dento-alveolar compensation for an underlying skeletal base abnormality often occurs. Decompensation by orthodontic proclination or retroclination of the incisor segments is often required prior to osteotomy. This is essential to allow normal occlusion to be established when the skeletal base movements are performed surgically. In the preoperative period these orthodontic tooth movements may accentuate the underlying skeletal base abnormality. In mild class II division I cases the upper incisors are proclined. In more severe class II division I cases upper incisor retroclination may be present in an attempt to compensate for the class II skeletal base relationship. The lower incisors may be proclined in addition. Preoperative decompensation involves correction of the incisor to maxillary or mandibular plane angles to normal. Subsequent surgery usually requires setback and occasionally rotation or impaction of the maxilla in order to reduce the overjet. In class III cases the retroclined lower incisors require axial correction. In addition, upper incisors may be proclined to compensate for the reverse overjet. If long face syndrome is to be corrected at surgery, maxillary intrusion will exacerbate the tendency toward prognathism so over correction in the presurgical orthodontic phase is advised. In class II division II cases, proclination of upper and lower incisor segments is often required. Decompensation corrects the incisor to skeletal base angles in all these patterns of jaw disproportion.

3. Arch coordination. Elimination of localized cross bites is important. Complete arch or hemiarch cross bites can be treated by arch expansion or contraction. The effect of surgery on cross bites should be predicted and any possibility of surgically induced cross bites should be anticipated in the preoperative orthodontics.

4. Elimination of crowding and abnormal spaces. Appropriate dental extractions should be performed early in the preoperative phase. Attention to the third molars is often required.

5. Mandibular anterior segment depression to correct an abnormal occlusal plane and help reduce a deep traumatic overbite is sometimes required.

Cleft orthdontics

1. Post-natal, presurgical orthopaedics. In the early months of life before cleft lip repair, moulding of the alveolus is sometimes required. Feeding appliances are still occasionally made in severe cases.

2. Mixed dentition phase. Guidance for the erupting permanent teeth is often important and secondary alveolar bone grafting are usually required to allow the permanent canine to erupt.

3. Post permanent dentition. Many cleft patients require orthognathic surgery to correct their class III skeletal pattern. The mandibular arch is usually normal and provides a good basis for maxillary arch alignment and for planning any necessary jaw movements and osteotomies.

Orthodontic procedures

1. Appliances. Functional, removable or fixed appliances may be used. In the UK, upper and lower fixed appliances are the preferred method of treatment in presurgical orthodontics.

2. Palatal screw and quadhelix appliances. These are usually required to expand or contract the maxilliary arch prior to orthognathic surgery in cleft patients. Occasional correction of the lower arch lateral dimension is also required.

3. Bite planes. In traumatic deep overbites, flattening of the occlusal plane is often required preoperatively.

Orthodontic surgical aides   *1. Facebow recordings.* In bimaxillary or segmental osteotomies, positioning and orientation of the maxilla based on preoperative predictions can be transferred from articulated study models to the patient using a facebow recording. Acrylic wafers are constructed for use intra-operatively. Their construction requires articulated models which have already undergone the planned surgery and they are essential for transfer of the plotted jaw movements to the patient during the operation itself.

2. Acrylic wafers. Intra- and postoperative wafers are constructed to allow each stage of the operation to conform to the surgical plan. The intra-operative wafer should permit the passage of wire ligatures for firm temporary fixation using the *in situ* orthodontic appliance and the postoperative wafer should have cleats to allow placement of elastics or wires during the early postoperative period if required.

3. Orthodontic – surgical fixation. With rigid fixation using titanium bone plates and screws, fixation for protracted periods in IMF is rarely required. The option should nevertheless be retained in any orthodontic appliance or postoperative wafer designed.

Postoperative orthodontics   On completion of surgery, orthodontic treatment should ensure that the interdigitation is sufficient to ensure stable intra-arch relationships. However final stability is dependent on all the usual orthodontic factors such as soft tissue envelope, jaw movements and swallow pattern. Several specific postoperative problems may require attention.

1. Maxillary intrusion. In class III cases maxillary intrusion allows mandibular autorotation but the possibility of early relapse of the incisor relationship may be a problem.

2. Anterior segment osteotomies. May produce step deformities in the premolar region of the upper occlusal plane.

3. Tilts in the maxillary plane can occur after Le Fort I level osteotomies and may result in anterior open bite with a less stable result than originally intended.

Timing of orthodontics The orthodontic phases of treatment usually require 18–24 months in the initial phase and about 6 months to complete the postoperative phase.

Related topics of interest

RADIOTHERAPY – SOME PRINCIPLES

Exposure of biological tissue to energetic, ionizing radiation results in absorption, molecular excitation, ionisation and serious risk of damage to cellular organelles and biochemical processes.

The initial effects occur in about 10^{-12} sec after exposure. The initial 'ionizing' effects result in formation of very short lived free radicals which in turn cause protein disruption, lipid oxygenation, nucleic acid damage and membrane damage. Secondary formation of other high energy molecular species may amplify this effect. The biological effects of radiation exposure include disruption of cell replication, sublethal genetic damage and mutation, and occasionally interphase death if radiation dose is massive. Exposure to sublethal radiation dose and absorption of associated energy initiates within hours a series of cellular and nuclear repair mechanisms. Success is variable and failure results in late cell necrosis or mutation.

The important factors in determining the response to ionising radiation are tissue type, normal rate of mitosis and cell complexity. Oxygenation and cell maturity are also important factors.

Leucocytes and gametogenic cells are the most radiosensitive of normal tissues. Skin, mucosae and bone marrow cells are similarly radiosensitive. Cartilage, neuronal tissue and fibrous tissue are much less sensitive.

Radiobiological effects

Cellular responses

The direct molecular effects of ionizing radiation and the indirect effects of ionizing radiation due to free radical damage are important. Because mammalian cells are at least 70% water the indirect action of ionizing radiation involves generation of highly reactive free radical-like species derived from water molecules. The macromolecular damage which results includes:

- *Nucleic acids.* Breakage of hydrogen bonds and fragmentation and damage to DNA molecules results in chromosomal protein damage. The teratogenic effects occur as a result.
- *Cell proteins.* Damage to side-chain groups, complex structures such as the secondary and tertiary turns in proteins can be completely disrupted by free radical generation.
- *Lipids.* Formation of lipid peroxides particularly in unsaturated fatty acids is likely to result in cell death.

Intracellular sites that are particularly radiation sensitive include the nucleus, in particular the DNA strands, and the structural proteins.

- *DNA repair processes.* Researched in bacterial strains exposed to germicidal ultraviolet irradiation. Repair mechanisms include excisional repair, S-phase post replication repair and photo reactivation with strand break repair. Damage to the DNA base molecules may occur, base replication will occur after exposure to ionizing radiation and unscheduled DNA synthesis may occur as part of the repair process.

- *The cell cycle.* The effects of ionizing radiation on the progresion of the cell cycle are now well documented. The decline of the number of mitoses indicates interference with the cellular progress between the different stages of the cycle. Cell numbers may be reduced and the mitotic delay is related to falling cell number. A complete but temporary block of progress in the G2 stage is termed G2 block. Cells entering the M or G1 stage after irradiation are less responsive in terms of mitotic delay than those in the G2 phase. The cell cycle after the one in which irradiation occurs is characterised by prolongation of degeneration time, decreased probability of division and frequent appearance of dead and non-dividing cells and those with chromosome abberations.

- *Molecular oxygen.* Required for maximal cell killing. Free radical generation and fixation is proposed as the mechanism. Hypoxia may impede radiosensitivity of tumour cells by a factor of 3. Hyperbaric oxygen therapy demonstrably improves radiosensitivity in some head and neck lesions. Radiosensitizing agents may be of value. Chemical agents effective separately in hypoxic and non-hypoxic conditions are described.

- *Other effects.* Some chemotherapeutic regimens appear radiosensitizing. Alterations in ambient temperature may improve responses to radiotherapy; hyperthermia in particular.

Radiosensitivity

1. Particles and photons. A massive particle travels slower than a lighter one and therefore remains in the vicinity of an ionizable atom for a longer period, the probability of ionization is greater therefore. Heavily charged particles have a relatively short range dependant on their initial kinetic energy and velocity. The change in linear energy transfer of a particle with the distance travelled along its path shows that as a particle slows down it transfers its kinetic energy of motion to the surrounding medium. This release of a large amount of energy in a relatively small volume results in poorer penetrance but greater cell damage.

2. *Linear energy transfer* refers to the energy transferred to the tissue or the absorbing material by the radiation beam by unit length of the beam path. The units are KEVs. Different sorts of ionizing radiation have widely different energy transfer rates. Photons for example can penetrate deeply into tissues but exhibit gradual dissipation of energy. Charged particles have a different charge-to-mass ratio and different velocities such that the energy transfer is different.

3. *As a measure of susceptibilty* of cell populations to injury due to ionizing radiation exposure, a dose required to reduce the replicating cell population to 37% of the initial value is calculated. The decay in cell numbers is exponential and this figure is reflective of this. Cell cycle variations in the degree of radiosensitivity occur. These variations are proportional to type of radiation and their energy transfer rates. Photons provoke cellular responses which are maximal in M and G2 phases. Neutrons, heavy ions and other particles have a high linear energy transfer and the cell cycle variations in response are less marked.

Radioresistance

Reciprocal to radiosensitivity. Dependent on several factors including tumour bulk, degree of central necrosis, rate of clearance of necrotic cells, the rate of cell proliferation, the quantity and biochemical complexity of intercellular matrix and nutritive state of the lesion.

Radiocurability

The importance of the radiosensitivity indices is to permit a clinical estimation of the likely effectiveness of planned radiotherapy. In addition to the tumour biology and the particle physics of the incident radiation there are other patient-related factors which affect clinical outcome and *in vivo* biological behaviour of tumour masses.

Radiosensitive tumours include the lymphoid series of leukaemias and germ cell tumours such as seminoma and most will be controlled with 2000–3000 cGy but neuroblastomas and Wilm's tumours require 3000–4000 cGy. Hodgkin's and basal cell skin carcinoma require upwards of 4000 cGy. Metastatic disease in lymph nodes particularly from squamous cell carcinomas of the head and neck usually requires 5000–6000 cGy.

Therapeutic radiation dose The therapeutic ratio is an estimation of the likelihood of tumour kill over the likelihood of adjacent normal tissues being killed.

The tumour control dose Calculated using the therapeutic ratio and the theraputic response curves of a tumour to different radiation doses.

Clinical uses

Curative Indications for primary radiotherapy include conditions where surgery and radiotherapy are equally effective but function or cosmetics is less damaged by DXT. T1 laryngeal carcinoma or mid-oesophageal carcinoma are examples. Very radiosensitive tumours (Hodgkin's disease) and patient preference to avoid surgery or tumour inoperability are factors.

- *Radical radiotherapy.* DXT as the sole treatment modality applied with intent at achieving cure. In the head and neck, nasopharyngeal carcinomas, craniopharyngioma and some lymphomas are treated in this way.
- *Combination radiotherapy.* Used in conjunction with surgery to achieve cure. DXT may be given pre- or postoperatively. In squamous lesions of the head and neck postoperative radiotherapy is preferred currently.
- *Adjuvant radiotherapy.* DXT in conjunction with chemotherapy or radiosensitisers. Some lymphomas are responsive to this pattern of therapy.

Palliative	Objectives of palliative radiotherapy include pain relief, especially from bony metastases, reduction of neurological sequelae due to intracranial or orbital mass lesions, spinal cord compression, and increased intracranial pressure. Alleviation of obstructive symptoms due to occluding pressure from adjacent tumour masses on structures such as trachea and oesophagus and superior vena caval occlusion due to massive cervical lymphadenopathy is resposive to a short course of DXT.

Treatment planning

- *Planning* requires liaison with other specialist services including surgery, speech therapy and prosthetics. Cancer nursing and psychiatric support services and facial camouflage services are available.
- *Tumour localization;* accuracy is essential. Clinical examination and imaging results are used.
- *Tumour or target volume calculation.* The target volume is determined by clinical and radiographic measurement of macroscopic tumour volume with addition of margins for biological or microscopic tumour clearance and technical plotting of dose errors.
- *Construction of facial mask or shell.*
- *Plotting of isodose curves.*
- *Wedges and compensators.* Multiple external beams intersecting at the point of highest dose are often used. Dose homogeneity across the tumour mass is achieved by wedge placement and use of compensators.

Decisions regarding treatment as inpatient or outpatient will be determined by geography, patients domestic circumstances and family support and general medical condition.

Technicalities

Methods of delivery

1. External beam. Delivered from sources positioned 80–100 cm from the affected site. The HVL value (half value layer; tissue thickness which reduces the applied radiation intensity by 50%) and the linear energy determine the dose. Penetration is proportional to the generating energy.

- *Orthovoltage.* Superficial X-rays (80–140 kV) and orthovoltage X-rays (180–400 kV) may be used to treat skin cancers and superficial lesions. Skin radiation damage and osteoradionecrosis are higher than with other techniques.
- *Megavoltage.* X-rays from ^{60}Co (1.25 MeV) or from linear accelerator (4–30 MeV) may be used to treat intra-cavity and deep seated tumours. Fast neutrons (18–50 MeV) or electrons (5–35 MeV) may be available. High energy photons with good tissue penetration and minimal intra-cavity scatter are available.
- *Different type of radiation* (heavy ions or pi mesons) may be used, most often under experimental conditions. Using the Bragg peak permits delivery of a greater dose within the depths of an internal tumour mass than more superficially. The Bragg peak is a derived quantity detailing the change in linear energy transfer of the particle with the distance travelled along its path. This energy distribution demonstrates that as a particle slows down it transfers its kinetic energy of motion to the surrounding medium. This release of a large amount of energy in a relatively small volume has made various types of particle of considerable interest in radiotherapy.

2. Brachytherapy. Delivered with radiation sources close to the target. Permits high dose delivery to very small tissue volume and minimises unwanted damage to adjacent tissue due to lower scatter and steeper isodose curves. Oral cancers are amenable to this sort of radiotherapy. Interstitial, intra-cavitary or surface placement techniques are described. Intra-oral lesions usually require interstial placement under anaesthesia.

3. Systemic. Parenteral radiotherapy may be given with injectable isotopes. Radio iodine (^{125}I) may be used in treatment of thyroid carcinoma.

Modern techniques

1. Accelerated DXT. Multiple daily treatments with dose regimens identical to conventional fractionation. Theoretic reduction in tumour cell escape by increasing the intensity of the course and consequent reduction in recurrence rates is achieved.

2. Hyperfractionation. Multiple smaller doses per day with the same total dose given in major fractions over the same time as for conventional DXT. Adjacent tissue damage is reportedly reduced.

3. CHART (continuous hyperfractionated accelerated radiotherapy). Reportedly combines the benefits of acceration and hyperfractionation.

Complications and side-effects

Damage to normal tissues is inflicted with DXT. Clinical effects are determined by the cell turnover time, the dose and stem cell damage and the number of normal surviving clonogenic cells.

Stem cells   Cell recovery and repair mechanisms are decreased particularly where fractionational split dose techniques are used and genetic effects of irradiation are expressed at subsequent mitoses. Marrow and skin stem cells are very sensitive.

Mucosal damage   Oropharyngeal mucositis, loss of intestinal villi, and cilia in respiratory epitheum are marked.

Parenchymal cells   Damage to hepatocytes, thyroid parenchma and renal tubular cells may result in delayed organ failure manifest over weeks or months depending on cell turnover times.

Vascular damage   Vascular occlusion, endarteritis with stromal inflammation events is common.

Glandular damage   Xerostomia after salivary gland damage is almost universal in head and neck irradiation. Pilocarpine and synthetic saliva preparations may help.

Specific organ damage   Visceral damage to GI tract and bladder occurs with ulceration, haemorrhage and stricturing are well documented. Adhesions may occur. CNS cellular depletion due to endovascular occlusion and demyelination occurs.

Radiation carcinogenesis

Development of metachronous primaries and leukaemias is well described. Solid tumours induced by radiation exposure include breast, thyroid, lung and digestive tissues. The age at exposure and latent period, the interaction betwen host and environmental factors such as hormonal influences and exposure to other carcinogens such as cigarette smoke may play a significant role in second tumour induction.

Radiation teratology

The developing fetus is highly susceptible to radiation. The most radiation sensitive age for the human fetus is between 6 and 12 weeks post-conception.

Revision point

Radiation physics

RECONSTRUCTION – SOME PRINCIPLES

The ability to reconstruct a major surgical defect is important and the use of complex reconstructive techniques is increasingly required in the fields of cancer surgery, in burns patients, and for those suffering major trauma.

The principles of reconstruction in maxillofacial surgery include recontouring both hard and soft tissues to restore function and aesthetics. The options include primary closure, skin, fascia or bone grafting, flap transfer and free tissue transfer with microvascular anastomosis. Rehabilitation requires comprehensive access to maxillofacial specialist technical support as well as to speech and physiotherapy.

Primary closure

1. Careful placement of excision margins can greatly aid sound wound closure at the end of the operation. The position of incisions must be consistent with sound oncological surgery, however. Straight incisions and incisions crossing natural lines of cleavage or wrinkles should be avoided and primary closure which results in over tight tissue around the operative site should also be avoided.

2. Judicious undermining of oral mucosa will often allow a very large area to be closed primarily. The resultant problems with tethering and disturbance of function particularly in lips and tongue may be considerable and should be considered especially if any large trans–mid line defect has been created. Clearance of the tumour should not be compromised in the desire to obtain primary closure, however.

3. Mucosal advancement after lip shave or excision of the vermilion border of the lip for carcinoma *in situ* or for a T1 lesion of the lower lip is a technique which is well described with good cosmetic results post-operatively.

4. Scar modifying skin closure techniques. 'Z' plasty lengthens the scar and interrupts the relatively poor cosmetic effect of a linear scar. Multiple 'Z' plasties may be performed to revise an unsightly established scar. 'W' plasty is a good method for breaking up the linearity of a scar. 'VY' closure lengthens and 'YV' shortens a scar.

Tissue expansion

Insertion of soft silicone tissue expanders into a subcutaneous tunnel in the weeks prior to a planned reconstructive procedure permits the elevation of much more extensive soft tissue flaps than would otherwise have been possible. Insertion of expanders in the scalp and in the post-auricular area is well described and pinna reconstruction is more readily completed with the latter technique than with non-expanded skin. Haemorrhage, sepsis and extrusion are complications.

Skin grafts

Removal of skin from one anatomical site and grafting it onto another is a fundamental part of reconstructive surgery. Skin grafts are bereft of their blood supply and their 'take' requires a healthy, non-infected granulating recipient bed and that skin alone without subcutaneous fat is transferred to minimize the barrier to vascularization from the recipient site. Accurate apposition and gentle pressure for 10–14 postoperative days increase the uptake of the graft to the recipient bed.

1. Split thickness skin grafts. Harvested from the lower limb or buttocks, large areas of skin can be provided to cover an orofacial defect. The pliability of such grafts is usually good but the poor colour match and presence of skin adnexae such as hair are disadvantages. Split skin grafts can contain variable thickness of dermal tissue and wound contracture is reduced by use of a thicker graft. Donor sites heal from their margins and from retained skin adnexae in the donor wound base. This pattern of graft is harvested using a hand held dermatome or 'Humby' knife or by use of a power driven blade or drum dermatome.

2. Full thickness skin grafts. Full thickness skin grafts may be used to replace small areas of tissue after tumour excision such as at the nasal tip and pinna of the ear. Treatment of ectropion may require use of a Wolfe graft. It requires freshly cut tissue and a well vascularized recipient bed and placement of such grafts on granulating surfaces is not likely to lead to success. The donor site must be closed primarily as there are no residual skin primordia from which regeneration can take place. This limits graft size. The advantages of full thickness grafts are the better colour match and inhibition of wound contracture at the recipient site.

3. Pinch and mesh grafts. Although widely used in orthopaedic and general surgery these techniques have not found particularly wide applications in head and neck surgery.

4. Dermal grafts. The deep subcutaneous tissues can be used to protect vascular pedicles and neurovascular anastomoses. Their use in head and neck surgery is not common as muscle transposition is more widely used for such purposes if required. Dermal fat grafts can be used to provide padding or subcutaneous contouring where facial hollowing or flattening is present.

5. Deep fascial or myofascial grafts. Temporalis fascia is widely used in ENT surgery. A number of tissues can be fashioned from it including tympanic membrane and fascial strips are used in the treatment of the cosmetic defects resulting from facial nerve palsy. It has been described in use for closure of large oro-antral and oro-nasal fistulae.

6. Graft failure. Causes include haematoma, seroma, poor immobilization, poor quality recipient bed and infection. Meticulous haemostasis, pressure dressing and tie overs, avoidance of grafting directly onto cartilage, cortical bone or exposed tendon are important practical steps. Beta haemolytic streptococci will cause graft necrosis.

Flaps

1. Local flaps. This pattern of flap depends on musculocutaneous perforator vessels for its blood supply. Its length is therefore limited and the ratio of base to length is important in flap design. They are random in pattern. The geometry of these flaps is very variable and can be quite complex. Advancement, rotational and transposition designs are all described.

2. Regional flaps. Although random flap designs are described, larger regional flaps are usually pedicled on a large arterial vessel and elevated in the line of this vessel. They are therefore axial and they are capable of being of much greater length than a random flap.

3. Myocutaneous or composite flaps. Using a muscle segmental artery, a flap comprising muscle and its overlying skin may be raised. The skin depends on the perforator vessels penetrating the transposed muscle for its supply.

4. Myofascial flaps. It is possible to redesign well described axial flaps to be raised excluding the skin component. For example a pectoralis major flap may be raised using the same pedicle vessel but transferring only the pectoralis muscle and not the overlying skin which may then be closed primarily. This reduces the donor site morbidity and for intra-oral reconstruction, the graft is rapidly covered in oral mucosal epithelium.

Free tissue transfer

Free flaps are designed as axial pattern flaps and transferred to the recipient bed after complete separation from the donor blood vessels. Immediate re-anastomosis to prepared vessels in the recipient bed ensure immediate re-vascularization of the flap.

Bone grafts

Bone grafts are widely used in head and neck surgery. Grafted bone can be non-vital or vascularized. Non-vital grafts can be in the form of cortical chips, cancellous harvest or as anatomically intact bone. Common sources include iliac crest, rib, fibula and hard palate. Microvascular techniques allow vascularized bone transfer from the hip where the deep circumflex iliac vessels serve as the pedicle. The upper limb girdle may serve as a donor site where the circumflex scapular vessels allow transfer of scapular bone with its vascular supply. Free composite grafts comprising bone and associated soft tissue may be raised from the hip, scapula, fibula and radial regions. The bone is of varying quality depending on the donor site. Radial bone is of poorer quality for intraoral reconstruction than fibula or iliac crest bone. Uses of bone grafts include closure of defects after trauma, secondary clefts of the alveolus, and in cancer surgery.

Other tissues	Cartilage, dura mater and subcutaneous fat all have their uses in restoration of contour and closure of defects. Cartilage can be used to close orbital floor dehiscences after fracture. Autogenous tissue can be harvested or bovine materials can be used. Fat can be used to restore facial contours in a variety of congenital abnormalities and in the postoperative correction of flattening after other reconstructive techniques. Muscle can be harvested for use in closure of chronic CSF leakage and to close the wound after transsphenoidal hypophysectomy.
Alloplastic implants	In the immediate perioperative period reconstruction plates and trays may be used to restore mandibular continuity and to allow cortical bone chip grafting. In the longer term, the use of osseointegrated implants allows restoration of the dentition, construction of high quality orbital prostheses after enucleation of the eye and reconstruction of the external ear after excision for cancer.

Related topics of interest

Bone grafts (p. 25)
Free flaps (p. 156)
Microvascular surgery (p. 256)

Revision points

Healing of bone, fractures and soft tissues
Principles of plastic surgery

RHINOPLASTY

Surgical correction of functional or cosmetic defects in the shape or structure of the nose is an increasingly common procedure. Patient selection should be performed with particular care as this is one cosmetic operation which is a potential source of disagreements and litigation. Preoperative psychological status of the patient should be assessed carefully to screen out those for whom surgical correction of their nose is unlikely to answer their expressed unhappiness with face or bodily form. Frank dysmorphophobia is a contraindication to surgery.

Indications for rhinoplasty

Post-traumatic
After nasal or midface fracture the form of the nose is often unsatisfactory. Early correction of obvious deformities at the time of trauma obviates the need for later revision.

Orthognathic
During maxillary orthognathic surgery changes in nasal shape occur. During the planning phase of midface surgery, the likely effect of surgery on the nasal form should be considered and appropriate steps to correct any predicted iatrogenic problems should be incorporated in the planned procedure.

Cleft palate associated
Palatal clefts are almost always associated with major functional and cosmetic defects of Eustachian tube function and and nose shape. During the adolescent years the need for orthognathic surgery in cleft palate patients is common. Rhinoplasty may be performed in conjunction with orthognathic correction or later as a separate procedure.

Pure cosmetics
The nose is often the focus of a patient's unhappiness with their body image and as such the subject of requests for surgical alteration. There is a significant risk of the surgeon becoming the focus of the patient's unhappiness in place of their dissatisfaction with the preoperative appearance of their nose.

Preoperative assessment and surgical planning

Precision in diagnosis will improve subsequent surgical planning and outcome. Age and race are important factors and racial norms should be respected in treatment planning but severe age related changes in the nose are rare. Only limited reversal of age related changes in facial appearance should be attempted in a single operation. Records are essential and full documentation of all planning and treatment stages is mandatory. A complete collection comprises comprehensive notes, X-rays, clinical photographs and plaster casts.

Facial analysis

1. Frontal. Clinical and radiographic assessment of intercanthal distance (normal 35 ± 2 mm) for telecanthus and the presence of uncorrected dysmorphic syndromes is essential.

2. Midline relationships. The relationship to other facial structures such as chin and vertex should be assessed and the degree of septal deviation recorded. The coincidence of the centrelines of nose, philtrum, dental arches and chin allows determination of the degree of nasal skeletal and cartilaginous nasal tip deviation.

3. Facial 'thirds'. The height of the nose in relation to upper lip and forehead is important and lower facial height assessment will allow variation from the 45%:55% ratio of the classical facial norm to be determined.

4. Profile planning and lateral relations. The nasofrontal angle ($N = 30 \pm 5°$) and the nasolabial labial angle ($N = 90 \pm 3°$ in men and $105 \pm 3°$ in women) are important. If the nasofrontal angle is $> 105°$ a previous nasoethmoid fracture should be suspected and if the nasolabial angle is $< 90°$ a history of prevous septal surgery should be sought. If the nasal defects are part of a larger midface disproportion, full profile planning is required.

5. Cleft related nasal problems require particular attention to both profile and the frontal appearance. Maxillary retrusion, nasal 'beaking' and shortening of the columella and lip to nasal sill distance may all require correction.

6. Sub nasal or basal X-ray views. Clinical and photographic views allow alar anatomy and septal deviation to be documented.

7. Skin and subcutaneous tissues. A realistic assessment of the likely outcome of skeletal surgery on the overlying soft tissues must be made. Preoperative tissue expanders may be of use in some patients.

Upper airway function and pathology

1. Assessment of the upper anyway function by examination and fibre-optic nasendoscopy to determine nasal deviation, rhinorrhoea, and sinus related symptoms is required.

2. Pre-rhinoplasty correction of the nasal airway may be required if there is a risk that the rhinoplasty may compromise the volume, and pattern of airflow across the nose. Where compensatory turbinate hypertrophy has occurred, turbinectomy may be required. Polypectomy and control of allergic symptoms is undertaken where required before nasal cosmetic surgery.

3. Lesions such as sarcoidosis, Wegener's granulomatosis and syphillis are sometimes associated with nasal deformity.

Psychiatric assessment

Dysmorphophobic patients assessment, clinical neurosis, family pressures and frank psychosis all require appropriate psychiatric referral before the surgery at least in the first instance. Such patients can present very severe problems postoperatively.

Surgery

There are several classical operations described with many modifications and eponymous variations. However, there are a number of distinct surgical elements to each of these operations.

Surgical elements

1. Incisions. The commonest approaches in rhinoplasty use one of intercartilaginous, transcartilaginous, rim, hemi and full transfixion incisions. Septal incisions, either of Killian or Freer patterns are well described and an alar rim approach is favoured by some surgeons. External or open rhinoplasty involves an incision in the columellar skin in addition to the mucosal incisions and permits wider soft tissue degloving.

2. Nasal tip surgery. Tip lowering is achieved by separation of medial and lateral crura from septum and upper lateral cartilages respectively. Nasal ridge augmentation will simulate a tip reduction operation. Medial scoring of the dome cartilage may be a useful adjunctive technique.

Elevation of the tip is often best simulated by reduction of a dorsal hump. An interpositional cartilage button graft to provide a columellar strut may aid in tip elevation.

Shortening of the nasal tip is achieved by cephaladad rotation after separating upper and lower lateral cartilages and excising a margin at the contacting edges.

Lengthening a nasal tip which has been shortened by previous surgery or by naso-ethmoid fracture is simulated by dorsal grafting and broadening a narrowed tip using a cartilage graft may overcome notching and alar contraction.

3. Septal surgery. If cartilaginous deviation is present, septoplasty via a hemi transfixion incision is the operation of choice. Where cartilage ridges or spurs are present they are almost always the result of previous nasal fracture. Therefore severe nasal fracture should be considered for septal surgery in the acute stage. Several patterns of post-fracture related septal pathology are described.

4. Dorsal ridge surgery. Reduction or augmentation is commonly required. Simple reduction using scalpel or scissors or rasp is effective. Where augmentation is necessary, there are many options for implantable materials. Tragal cartilage, bone or alloplastic materials such as Silastic and hydroxyapatite have all been used with varying success.

5. Nasal osteotomy. Immediate reduction of nasal fractures is important. Late residual deviations require osteotomy performed narrowing or broadening can be achieved with the correction of any bony displacements from earlier trauma.

6. *Alarplasty.* Wedge excision of alar cartilage will narrow the ala margin but Z plasty allows greater reduction if required. Ala widening can be simulated by tip lowering procedures and Le Fort I maxillary advancement.

7. *Nasal angles.* These angles can be altered significantly by augmentation bone grafting and maxillary or premaxillary osteotomies.

8. *Associated skeletal surgery.* Genioplasty may improve apparent nasal prominence in microgenia. Orthognathic correction of jaw disproportion or asymmetry usually has consequences for nasal form and these changes are predictable. Orthognathic surgical planning should account for the need for rhinoplasty either at the time of the facial operation or at a later stage. Cleft palate patients have functional and cosmetic problems in proportion to the severity of their original cleft and the method of its closure. Rhinoplasty is often required as part of the late corrective surgery in these, usually teenage patients.

9. *Soft tissue surgery.* Blepharoplasty, procerus muscle repositioning to alter the nasofrontal angle, upper lip augmentation, implant placement to correct nasolabial angles and dermabrasion of facial skin may all have their place in the correction of poor facial aesthetics in association with rhinoplasty.

Complications

Approximately 10% of all patients undergoing rhinoplasty present with complications. These include acute septal haematoma, tip irregularities and persistent deformities in the later postoperative period.

SAGITTAL SPLIT MANDIBULAR RAMUS OSTEOTOMY

One of the most versatile mandibular ramus operations, the sagittal split mandibular ramus osteotomy allows both forward and backward movement of the mandibular dentition and a measure of rotation with respect to the maxillary teeth. It is not a good operation for treatment of anterior open bite unless a simultaneous maxillary osteotomy is planned in conjunction. It is very easy to introduce unplanned rotations in the occlusal plane and the inferior alveolar neurovascular bundle is at risk of damage.

Historical review

Trauner and Obwegeser (1957)
- The horizontal cut is made just above mandibular foramen on medial side of ramus.
- The vertical cut is taken down anterior border of ramus.
- Avascular necrosis of the mandibular angle due to extensive stripping of the pterygomasseteric sling is described.

Dalpont (1961)
Modified the sagittal split operation by advancing the oblique cut towards the molar region and the vertical cut through the lateral cortex.

Hunsuck (1968)
Shortened the cut through the medial cortex of the ramus by taking it only as far as the bone immediately posterior and superior to the mandibular foramen. The medial cut runs forwards toward the mylohyoid line.

Bell and Schendel (1977)
The anterior vertical cut of the lower border is sectioned through and the split is kept more lateral by directing fine osteotomes down the inner surface of the lateral cortex to produce easier splitting and greater protection for the inferior dental nerve.

The vascularity of the the ramus is preserved as elimination of need to strip the pterygomasseteric sling.

Epker (1978)
The lower mandibular border is preserved unsplit and the inferior part of the split runs above the level of the lower border.

Technique
1. The incision, is taken from high on the external oblique line in the cheek and runs medially and

inferiorly towards the posterior end of the last standing molar tooth. A buccal triangular based flap is therefore raised and a generous skirt of mucoperiosteum is left to facilitate suturing at the end of the operation.

2. The exposure. Allows access to the buccal plate as far forward as the first molar tooth and upwards onto the ramus to the posterior margin buccally and lingually. The soft tissues are reflected anteriorly up the coronoid process. Lingual retraction above the level of the lingula is required and buccal channel retractors are placed in the vestibular part of the flap. Light source channel retractors are available to aid with this part of the dissection. Identification of the neurovascular bundle above the lingula as it enters the mandibular canal is essential to prevent injury at this point.

3. The horizontal osteotomy is made on the lingual aspect of the mandibular cortex which must be cleanly sectioned with a fine drill or oscillating saw under adequate cooling. Ramus anatomy is such that outward flaring of the lingual plate occurs which makes the most posterior aspect of the horizontal cut difficult. The modified techniques make this stage of the operation a little more straightforward. In the Dalpont and Hunsuck techniques the vertical part of the split is placed more anteriorly on the medial cortex of the ramus than the original Obwegeser operation.

4. The vertical osteotomy. A buccal channel retractor is placed vertically adjacent either to the second or first molar depending whether a forward slide or posterior movement is planned. Complete section of the cortex is required and it is essential to ensure that the cut goes cleanly through the lower border of the mandible. Inadequate section through the lower border may result in fragmentation when the osteotomy is completed. The Epker modification preserves the lower border.

5. The sagittal osteotomy. The horizontal and vertical limbs are joined by an osteotomy parallel with the internal oblique line. Each of the osteotomy limbs is then connected in such a way to ensure that all cortical bone is sectioned cleanly. The split is then performed using half inch osteotomes and with a gentle twisting action. It is essential to ensure that the inferior dental bundle is not damaged during this procedure and that on completion of the split the neurovascular tissues remain on the lingual aspect of the section. The operation is easier and the results more stable when the mucoperiosteal envelope is completely stripped through the completed osteotomy. The muscle attachments are usually preserved, however.

6. *A mirror image osteotomy*, is performed on the opposite side. On completion the tooth bearing fragment of the mandible should be completely free.

7. *Fixation.* Rigid fixation using plates and screws or lag cortical screws is preferred although semi-rigid wiring is still favoured by some. On some occasions inter-maxillary (IMF) fixation may be required.

8. *Postoperative care.* Monitoring the airway is essential during the immediate postoperative hours. Analgesia demands are not usually excessive and antibiotics are advised. Some surgeons advocate steroids in the early postoperative period.

Related topics of interest

Le Fort I osteotomy (p. 218)
Mandibular surgery (p. 238)
Osteotomies (p. 297)
Segmental osteotomies (p. 346)

SALIVARY GLAND DISEASE

Developmental

1. Aplasia or agenesis. Very rare, usually affects the parotid glands but can affect all major salivary glands.

2. Atresia of ducts.

3. Hypoplasia. Occurs as part of Melkerson–Rosenthal syndrome. This may occur secondary to atrophy of parasympathetic nervous system.

4. Aberrance. Very common. May occur in the neck, middle ear, mastoid bone or as a Stafne's bone cavity in the lingual cortex of the mandible.

5. Accessory ducts and lobes. Very common. Occurs in about 50% of parotid glands and most are asymptomatic.

Inflammatory

1. Bacterial. Acute suppurative sialadenitis arises due to ascending infection following major surgery, dehydration, cachexia or duct obstruction.

2. Signs characteristically include an enlarged gland, periductal inflammation with pus exudate and constitutional symptoms. Causative organisms include *Streptococcus viridans*, *Streptococcus pyogenes*, *Staphylococcus aureus*.

3. Investigations. Full blood count, plain radiography, pus samples for microbial culture and antibiotic sensitivity are useful and blood cultures if the patient is toxaemic. Sialography is not performed in the acute stage as infection may be spread up the duct system but ultrasound scanning may be helpful. The treatment is high-dose antibiotics and intravenous rehydration.

4. Viral infection. Mumps is the commonest cause of viral parotitis and is the most frequent cause of acute swelling of salivary glands in children. Adult mumps may be complicated by pancreatitis, orchitis, oophoritis or meningoencephalitis.

5. Recurrent parotitis of childhood. Typically affecting pre-adolescents between the ages of 5 and 9 years with a male to female incidence of about 2:1. It is commonly a recurrent condition and resolves at puberty. Sialography shows a characteristic punctate sialectasis ('snow storm' appearance). Epstein–Barr virus has been implicated. Structural damage to gland acini occurs and they are then susceptible to ascending infection. Episodes are characteristically unilateral and last about 10–14 days. The clinical picture is one of general malaise with a swollen, tender parotid gland. Antibiotics may reduce the length and severity of acute episodes.

6. Post-irradiation parotitis. Acute onset of parotid swelling occurs within hours of starting radiotherapy and then subsides within a few days. The duct cells are more resistant to ionizing radiation than surrounding gland parenchyma and normally survive and proliferate. Xerostomia is almost universally present and is a long-term problem in irradiated patients.

7. Sialadenitis of minor salivary glands. Sarcoidosis, Sjögren's syndrome and stomatitis nicotina may all exhibit minor gland sialadenitis.

8. Acute necrotizing sialometaplasia affecting the hard palate in tobacco smokers resembles squamous cell carcinoma.

Obstruction and trauma

1. Papillary obstruction. Rough edged teeth or restorations, denture flanges, and parafunctional habits may all cause ulceration around the papilla.
Chronic trauma is a cause of stricture and stenosis. The treatment is papillotomy.

2. Sialolithiasis. The commonest cause of recurrent, painful gland swelling at meal times. Recurrent episodes of acute suppurative sialadenitis are frequently associated. Submandibular glands are more commonly affected than parotid glands. Parotid stones may occur as staghorn calculi and are usually radiolucent.

3. *Obstruction in and around the duct wall.* Stricture formation is often secondary to chronic calculus formation. Submandibular calculi, if chronic usually require excision of the gland. Direct trauma to the duct, masseteric hypertrophy involving the parotid duct at the anterior border of the muscle and tumours may all present with salivary gland obstruction.

4. *Mucocoele.* Mucous extravasation cysts arise due to mechanical damage to the duct or to a minor gland with salivary leakage. Mucous retention cysts are due to obstruction to saliva outflow producing a balloon like dilatation of the obstructed gland. Ranulae are sublingual gland mucous retention cysts and maybe superficial, deep or plunging.

5. *Salivary duct fistula.* The causes include gunshot wounds, animal bites, and post-surgical following parotidectomy and rhytidectomy.

6. *Frey's syndrome.* The incidence is reported to be 2–6% after parotidectomy due to aberrant reinnervation of sweat glands by postganglionic parasympathetic fibres normally supplying the parotid gland. It may also follow the pre-auricular approach in temporomandibular joint surgery, or subcondylar fracture or drainage of a parotid abscess.

Bilateral gustatory sweating may be a sign of diabetic autonomic neuropathy. Treatment with antihidrotic gel or spray may be helpful Re-exploration and introduction of a fat or fascial membrane may be beneficial in a few patients.

Degenerative

1. *Sjögren's syndrome.* Classically a triad of xerostomia, keratoconjunctivitis sicca and rheumatoid arthritis (66% of patients). Salivary or lacrimal gland enlargement may be a feature. Aggressive Sjögren's syndrome may be associated with a benign lymphoproliferative lesion. The incidence of Sjögren's syndrome is reported as affecting 15% of patients with rheumatoid arthritis, 30% with SLE and almost 100% with primary biliary cirrhosis. Lymphomatous change affects approximately 5% of patients with Sjögren's syndrome.

Metabolic

2. *Investigations.* Raised plasma viscosity, elevated circulating autoantibodies and raised serum IgG are typical findings. Rose Bengal staining, salivary scintigraphy and labial biopsy have all been used to establish the diagnosis. Immunological screening may demonstrate anti-ro or anti-la, autoantibody status. Schirmer's test may be positive in keratoconjunctivitis and sialography may demonstrate chronic salivary gland disease.

Sialosis. A non-neoplastic and non-inflammatory enlargement of salivary glands. The causes include dietary fadism and anorexia nervosa and chronic alcoholics have a higher incidence than expected. Hormonal aetiology is suggested in diabetics and post-oophorectomy. In some patients there is a drug-induced salivary lesion. Cystic fibrosis or mucoviscidosis is associated with thickened mucus and retention of inspissated saliva which in turn causes a chronic sialosis.

Related topics of interest

Parotid gland tumours (p. 301)
Xerostomia (p. 431)

Revision point

Physiology of saliva production

SALIVARY GLAND SURGERY

Superficial parotidectomy

The operation is performed for benign tumours or end stage inflammatory disease of the superficial part of the gland. Several incisions are described. The commonest in the UK is the pre-auricular approach with reversed 'C' relieving limb inferiorly. The skin flap is developed anteriorly in the subcutaneous plane.

1. Preservation of the facial nerve is mandatory. Posterior dissection is commenced anterior to the perichondrium of the cartilaginous external auditory meatus. The landmarks of the facial nerve's main trunk are several.

(a) *tragal pointer*: the main trunk is 1 cm deep, medial and inferior to the tragal apex;

(b) *McEwan's triangle*: the main trunk bisects the triangle formed by the posterior belly of the digastric, the posterior border of the mandible and the tympanic plate;

(c) *buccal branch dissection*: in glands previously operated on, or after radiotherapy, the anterior gland margin is dissected and the buccal branch traced posteriorly until it joins the main trunk.

2. Mobilization. The posterior margin of the gland is freed from the auditory meatus and the inferior aspect from the sternomastoid. Careful forward dissection proceeds to dissect the parotid tissue of all the branches of the facial nerve.

3. Preservation. The structures encountered during the dissection are the auriculotemporal nerve, which should be divided close to the gland and the terminal branches identified should subsequent cable grafting to facial nerve be required.

4. The parotid duct. The duct is identified anteriorly and ligated before the gland is delivered.

Complications

1. Nerve injury or transection. Treatment is by immediated microneural anastomosis or nerve grafting. About 6–12 months is required for full functional recovery.

2. *Frey's syndrome.* Occurs in about 2% of cases and is due to secretomotor parasympathetic fibre regeneration and regrowth into auriculotemporal sheaths.

3. *Ear numbness.* This arises due to greater auriculotemporal nerve section. Slow recovery usually occurs.

4. *Salivary fistula.* In non-irradiated tissues, spontaneous resolution can be expected.

Deep lobe parotidectomy

This is done for deep tumours or deep lobe recurrence after previous surgery. Superficial parotidectomy is performed first. A decision regarding the preservation or sacrifice of the facial nerve must be made. If compromise of the oncological operation will not result, the nerve may be retracted out of the operative field and preserved.

Extended total parotidectomy

Where nodal metastases are demonstrated secondary to a malignant parotid tumour, neck dissection may be required as well as gland excision.

Reconstructive techniques

Primary neural or microneural anastomosis and nerve repair are performed as required. Auriculotemporal or sural nerves may be used. Muscle fibre grafts using either fresh autologous tissue or freeze-dried homografts may be used. Sternomastoid rotation will obliterate the hollow which almost always follows parotidectomy.

Rehabilitation techniques

After facial nerve section, several techniques for rehabilitation are available. They include tarsorrhaphy, lid margin implants and weights, fascial sling procedures, muscle implants and temporalis flaps.

Submandibular gland removal

Indications for removal
- Recurrent infection
- recurrent stone disease
- as part of neck dissection
- as part of Wilkies' operation for persistent drooling
- for tumour (uncommon)

Investigations
- Ultrasound scan

	• sialography if gland not acutely infected
	• orthopantomograph (OPG)
Operation	A *skin crease incision* preserving marginal mandibular branch of facial nerve is used and deepened through platysma and deep fascia.

Dissection proceeds to free the gland from the facial vessels, the posterior belly of digastric, the deep venous plexus around hypoglossal nerve and lingual nerve.

The posterior belly of mylohyoid is retracted and the deep lobe of the gland is drawn into the wound. The duct is dissected free and lingual nerve then retracts in to the floor of the mouth.

Sublingual gland removal

Indications	• Ranula
	• chronic infection
	• tumour (rare)
Operation	*Incision* via a floor of mouth approach.

Important structures protection of the lingual nerve and submandibular duct medially is required.

For plunging ranula a submental approach is described. This is only rarely necessary as only rarely does abnormal tissue penetrate mylohyoid and even if this does occur it is suggested the removal of the gland via an intra-oral incision will permit involution of any tissue deep to mylohoid.

Related topics of interest

Neck dissection (p. 267)
Parotid gland tumours (p. 301)
Salivary gland disease (p. 336)

Revision points

Anatomy of the facial nerve
Anatomy of the floor of the mouth

SECONDARY CLEFT DEFORMITIES

The evaluation of secondary or residual cleft deformities is the assessment of the aftermath of surgery performed during the early years of the patient's life. It is a potentially good audit tool and requires ongoing follow up of an individual patient into early adulthood before the full effects of childhood operations can be accurately and fully appreciated.

Clinical assessment

Alveolus

- Quality of bone grafted alveolar cleft.
- Maxillary growth.
- Profile and severity of maxillary hypoplasia.
- Dental status and position of missing or unerupted teeth.

Lip

- Total quantity of lip tissue.
- Vermilion visibility.
- Vestibular depth and freedom of lip from alveolus.
- Bulk and muscular function and alignment.
- Cupid's bow development.
- Notching and quality of primary repair.

Nose

1. Anteriorly. Alar bases, upper lateral and lower lateral cartilages, width and depth of bony pyramid.

2. Profiles. Nasolabial angles, condition of septum, length and visibility of columella, and the relative position of the nasal tip.

3. Inferior. Nares form, septal deviations, vestibular form and anatomy of alae.

4. Superior. Straightness and centrality of nasal midline, position of cartilages and alae.

Lip

Residual scars. Surgery in young people often results in florid scarring. Correction is commonly required. 'W' or 'Z' plasties or use of buried, de-epithelialized margins to increase depth and improve form of lip landmarks is required. Scar revision corrects skin defects but correction of associated muscle and mucosal deformities should proceed simultaneously.

Vertical lip excess. Uncommon other than with Le Mesurier primary repairs. Requires horizontal excision either at horizontal limb of primary scar or at level of alar base. Excessive rotation during a Millard lip repair leaves a long lateral segment which requires excision of a sub alar 'C' flap.

Vertical lip deficiency. The vertical limb of the primary scar contracts and each element, skin muscle and mucosa all exhibit shortening. Most techniques of primary repair produce a degree of shortening. 'Z' plasty, transpositional flap techniques and conversion to a functional type of lip repair will each improve the lip depending upon severity of the shortening.

Horizontal tight lip deficiency. In non-cleft patients the upper lip is capable of protrusion in front of the lower lip and of pouting. Shortened lips are drawn taut over the maxillary teeth. Correction requires cross lip Abbe flap insertion. If the donor position of the lower lip is the central portion, a simulation of the normal Cupid's bow may be achieved in the lengthened upper lip.

Orbicularis oris abnormalities. Inadequate muscle reconstruction results in poor speech, facial expression, whistling and chewing. The early signs in inadequacy of muscle repair include scar widening, and increasing disparity in lip fullness between upper and lower lips. Dissection of orbicularis oris and paranasal muscles permits 'functional' pattern reconstruction. If failure of previous muscle repairs has occurred, 'Z' plasty may be required. Percutaneous, mucosal and transvermilion approaches have all been described.

Philtrum. Cupid's bow, vermilion deformity and vestibular deformities may all require correction.

Lip–nose	*Columella.* The columella height is often deficient and correction in conjunction with septal surgery or tip rhinoplasty is often required. Whether one pattern of lip repair produces greater columella shortening than another remains a subject of much debate.
	Alae. Flattening and asymmetry of the upper lateral cartilages is common and tip rhinoplasty often via and external approach may be required.
	Nasal sills and base. Broadening is a more common defect than sill narrowing in cleft patients. Alar separation at the level of the nasolabial groove permits revision of the alar base width.
	Septum. Deviation and dislocation is common and septorhinoplasty is then necessary for correction.
Fistulae	*Oro-nasal fistulae* may occur at the level of the hard palate, anteriorly at alveolus or posteriorly affecting the soft palate. The site of previous palate closure is a common site. Post-fistula repair, breakdown is common and repeat surgery offers diminishing benefits.
Maxilla	*1. Residual alveolar clefts.* Repeat bone grating may be required. This may be performed in conjunction with maxillary osteotomy if required.
	2. Maxillary retrusion. The options for surgical treatment include: onlay bone grafts; osteotomies (Le Fort I, Le Fort II, segmental maxillary osteotomy).
Jaw disproportion	Common in cleft patients who may in addition have defects in mandibular development. The options include mandibular osteotomies, genioplasty or bimaxillary osteotomy.

SEGMENTAL OSTEOTOMIES

The segmental operations are performed at the subapical level and may used to move the dentoalveolar tissues in any direction which is permitted by the available angulation of the opposing teeth and the soft tissue envelope. Anterior, posterior and total dentoalveolar mobilization is possible.

Mandibular segmental osteotomies

The lower labial segmental osteotomy (Köle subapical osteotomy)

Indications

- For levelling an abnormal curve of Spee.
- For correction of isolated dentoalveolar segment causing occlusal dysharmony.
- When orthodontic treatment is inappropriate or not acceptable to the patient.
- To produce a change in the angulation or proclination of the anterior mandibular teeth.
- To correct a deep overbite and increased overjet in class II division l cases.
- Some anterior open bites may be corrected by a segmental operation.

Technique
Pre-molar extractions are usually necessary to create space for planned segmental movement. A labiobuccal degloving incision is made and dissection proceeds in the subperiosteal plane. To the lower border anteriorly but to the gingival margin only at extraction sites. This permits space for vertical osteotomies. Vertical osteotomies are made in region of pre-molar extractions. Horizontal subapical cuts unite the vertical osteotomies. The osteotomized segment is pedicled on the lingual mucoperiosteum. Bone grafting is occasionally required and may increase stability. Fixation with an interpositional wafer and IMF or full coverage acrylic splint is required. Orthodontic fixation is satisfactory. Miniplate fixation may be used.

Modifications. The Sowray–Haskell modification incorporates a symphysis splitting osteotomy which allows narrowing or in occasional cases broadening of the transverse distance across the lower dental arch.

Anterior mandibulotomy

In patients with short lower face heights, the clinical need for segmental mandibular surgery may be present but a subapical approach may not be possible due to the inadequate amount of bone between the apices of the anterior teeth and the lower mandibular border. The approach requires the vertical osteotomies to be continued from alveolus down to the lower mandibular border bilaterally. The segment mobilized therefore includes the chin and anterior basal bone in addition to the dentoalveolar segment. The effect on the chin button must be planned in addition to the change in the occlusion.

Anterior mandibuloplasty

A combined segmental dentoalveolar osteotomy with genioplasty can be performed. This may produce a greater change in the profile and a greater improvement in the final facial appearance.

Posterior subapical mandibular surgery

1. Indications
- For correction of cross bites.
- For correction of an abnormal curve of Monson.
- To correct severe linguoversion or buccoversion.
- For closure of cheek teeth spaces.
- For levelling of over erupted posterior teeth.

2. Techniques

- A horizontal vestibular incision developing a mucoperiosteal flap. The mental nerve is located and protected.
- Dental extractions are performed as required.
- Vertical osteotomy cuts are made from buccal to lingual direction protecting the lingual soft tissues. The subapical cortical bone on the buccal side is divided and the osteotomy is completed. The osteotomy fragment is pedicled on the well vascularized lingual tissues.
- The planned movements are performed and the final position determined by using an inter-positional acrylic wafer.
- Fixation with rigid plating and where required, bone grafting may be used.

Total subapical mandibular surgery

1. Indications

- To increase mandibular height or dental vertical dimension.
- To level the occlusal plane.
- For simultaneous advancement of mandibular dentoalveolar tissues with surgical levelling of curve of Spee.
- For simultaneous advancement with lengthening of the lower third of the face.

2. Techniques

- A buccal vestibular degloving incision is made from third molar to third molar region. Degloving down to the lower mandibular border is required and protection of both mental nerves is essential.
- The anterior border of the ascending ramus up to the coronoid process should be exposed. The lingula should be visualized on both sides.
- The horizontal osteotomies are placed subapically protecting the inferior dental bundle. Extension of these cuts at the anterior portion of the ramus of the mandible and through the lingual cortex similar to that for sagittal split osteotomy.
- The entire mandibular dentoalveolar segment is mobilized and placed into the planned position. Inter-positional acrylic wafers are required. Simultaneous inter-positional bone grafting or genioplasty may be performed.
- Rigid miniplating is usually required. IMF may also be required.

Segmental maxillary surgery

Principles

The maintenance of as much palatal or labial mucoperiosteum as possible is required to ensure the vitality of the osteotomized segment.

Osteotomies are designed to produce as large a fragment as possible as bone–bone contact and stability is easier to establish than with a small fragment.

Inadvertent apicectomy results in progressive pulpal fibrosis and degenerative change.

1. Single tooth osteotomy. Vestibular or vertical incisions are used and subapical osteotomy is performed in addition to the interdental bone cuts. The mobilized single dental unit is repositioned and maintained by splint or fixed orthodontic appliance.

2. Corticotomy. To correct isolated premaxillary protrusion resulting in a class II division 1 malocclusion. Vestibular incisions are used and interdental osteotomy is performed between each of the maxillary anterior teeth. Heavy orthodontic traction provides the force to reposition the teeth and a means of fixation.

3. Anterior segmental osteotomies. Wassmund (1935) described a procedure to mobilize the maxillary anterior segment and the six anterior teeth. Through vestibular and sagittal palatal incisions he performed tunnelling osteotomies both buccally and transversely across the palate having extracted the first maxillary pre-molars. The nasal septum and lateral nasal walls are then mobilized via a sub-labial incision.

Wunderer (1963) described a modification in which the palatal mucosa is incised transversely rather than sagittally in the midline. Epker and Wolford (1980) performed a similar osteotomy from a short buccal vestibular incision similar to that used in Le Fort I osteotomy. All osteotomies are performed via this incision including the nasal and palatal bone cuts. The palatal mucosa must remain intact.

4. Posterior segmental osteotomies

- For correction of lateral open bites and buccal cross bites.
- Closure of space in the dental arch.
- To correct molar over eruption.

5. Techniques: Schuchardt (1959) and its Kufner modification (1968). These procedures are performed through a horizontal vestibular incision. Osteotomies are made in vertical and subapical bone buccally. Palatal osteotomy via the buccal incision is performed ensuring palatal mucosa remains intact. Fixation using orthodontic appliance or full coverage splint is required. Rigid miniplate fixation is an option.

6. Horseshoe osteotomy: Wolford and Epker (1975). This procedure is performed through a Le Fort 1 pattern buccal vestibular incision. The dentoalveolar segment of the maxilla is mobilized as a 'horseshoe'. The palate remains *in situ* in an attempt to preserve the volume and form of the nasal airway. The horseshoe segment may be intruded and fixed with miniplates or IMF and splints. There are few if any advantages over the Le Fort 1 osteotomy.

Related topics of interest

Le Fort I osteotomy (p. 218)
Mandibular surgery (p. 238)

Revision points

Muscle attachments to mandible
Nasal anatomy
Sinus anatomy

SPEECH AND SPEECH DISORDERS

Normal speech requires intact oral, velar, pharyngeal and laryngeal anatomy. In addition, hearing, neurological pathways and social interaction are required for completion of development of adult speech patterns. Experience with cleft palate children illustrates the need for normal oropharyngeal anatomy at an early age for development of unimpaired speech patterns. The native language spoken appears to be unimportant; people of all nationalities will have impaired speech if cleft palate repair is performed late.

Developmental milestones and language acquisition

If speech development appears delayed, the child should be assessed for causes of deafness, the commonest cause of childhood speech delay. Major neurological or psychiatric illness may be present.

- 9–15 months   First words spoken
- 18 months   20 word vocabulary
- 24 months   Word combinations used
- 36 months   Sentences used

Aetiology (all age groups)

- Cleft syndrome related speech problems.
- Tongue lesions.
- Denture problems.
- Larynx problems (nodules, tumours).
- Neurology (bulbar and pseudobulbar palsies, peripheral nerve lesions).
- Psychiatric conditions.

Elements of speech

- Nasals (n, m).
- Labials (l).
- Fricatives (f, th).
- Plosives (p, b).
- Sibilants (s, ts, z).
- Dentals (t, d).
- Non-nasal vowels (a, o, u).

Speech pathology

1. Dysphasia. Difficulty in the understanding, assimilation or production of language. This condition is the result of damage to the dominant cerebral hemisphere. The common causes include cerebrovascular disease or tumour.

- Receptive (sensory) dysphasia. Difficulty in comprehension of language.

- Expressive (motor) dysphasia. Speech comprehension is normal, but central induction and production of language is impaired.
- Mixed pattern dysphasia. Mixed receptive and expressive dysphasia frequently occur together; in such cases, one type usually predominates. Cerebrovascular disease typically causes this pattern of dysphasia.

2. Dysarthria. Difficulty in articulating and enunciating words correctly. Dysarthria is commonly due to disorders of the neuromuscular control of articulation. Dysarthria may be sub-classified in several ways.

- Spastic dysarthria. Upper motor neurone damage (pseudobulbar palsy). Lesions must be bilateral before there is significant dysarthria. Causes include motor neurone disease, multiple sclerosis, amytrophic lateral sclerosis, and brainstem tumours. Slurred and indistinct speech usually results from these lesions.
- Extrapyramidal dysarthria. Rigid and stiff muscles are the clinical result of extrapyramidal disease. Such lesions are typical of Parkinsonism. Speech is typically monotonous, words merge and tonality, inflection and accent are all absent.
- Ataxic dysarthria. Cerebellar lesions result in muscular incoordination due to a defect in proprioceptor input processing. Speech is typically irregular and slurred. Jerky variation of timing and volume also result.
- Bulbar dysarthria. Lower motor neurone damage may result in flaccid dysarthria. It then causes problems with individual words and sounds. Tongue paralysis affects a large number of sounds and causes the most profound speech disturbance. Palatal paralysis produces nasal speech.
- Peripheral dysarthria. Abnormal articulation due to abnormalities of the tongue, lips, teeth or palate or due to difficulties with dental prostheses cause a very varied pattern of abnormal speech patterns.

3. Dysmetria. This type of disorder reflects an abnormality in the normal rhythmic generation of controlled pulses of airflow across the larynx. It is, however, a central disorder rather than peripheral. It is typified by the condition of stammering. Disturbance of the normal rhythm of speech occurs with sudden interruption of flow and repetition of sounds. There is rarely any other neurological abnormality detectable, but occasionally it is a manifestation of a mild dysphasia. Cerebellar lesions may also affect respiratory muscles as well as articulatory musculature and so disrupt normal speech rhythm.

4. Dysphonia. Impairment of pitch, quality or loudness of voice is usually due to an abnormality within the larynx, or its innervation. Psychogenic disorders may mimic true dysphonias and hysterical dysphonia is described. Hysterical hoarseness may also occur. Brain stem lesions may cause spastic dysphonia giving the unmistakable pattern of 'Donald Duck' speech. True bulbar palsy may result in a coarse dysphonia. Complete absence of phonation is termed aphonia. In those aphonic patients who can cough normally, a psychogenic or hysterical origin should be suspected.

Revision points

Physiology of proprioception
Physiology of speech
Vascular supply to the brainstem and higher centres

SURGICAL ENDODONTICS

Surgical approaches to the dental root surface or periapical region can be used to overcome difficulties or therapeutic failures with orthograde root filling techniques.

Apicectomy and retrograde root filling

Indications for surgery

1. Failed conventional endodontics. Underfilled or overfilled root canal, root perforation laterally or apically, and undiagnosed or unfilled canals all constitute indications for surgery. Endodontic instrument fracture in the root canal may require apicectomy.

2. Impossible conventional endodontics. Sharp root curvatures and multiple roots with poor coronal root canal access.

3. Dental indications. Current or planned use of tooth as an abutment for restorative dentistry.

4. Apical indications. Extensive periapical or periradicular pathology, need for biopsy and tissue diagnosis and recurrent apical lesions all demand surgical exploration.

Contraindications

1. Pre-radiotherapy. The risk of subsequent osteoradionecrosis is considerable if dental extraction is required after radiotherapy.

2. Pathological. Where a suspicious apical lesion or extensive sepsis is present tooth extraction is often preferable.

3. Impossible repair. Lateral perforations where palatal access would be required for satisfactory repair.

4. Whole mouth considerations. Extensive tooth loss elsewhere in dental arch; whether actual or planned, single unit preservation may not be wise or justified. Retention of a dental useless unit where no intra-arch contact or functional occlusion will be achieved by retention.

Techniques

1. Incision. Gingival envelope or semilunar patterns.

2. Bone removal. By conventional water cooled round bur. Care with adjacent roots and intimate structures such as antral lining.

3. Curettage. Apical granulation tissue removed in entirety. Suspicious tissue or cystic lesions are submitted for histological examination.

4. Apical section. Oblique with bevelled root face towards operator.

5. Toilet and cavity protection. Thorough saline irrigation and bone coverage with ribbon gauze or bone wax to prevent subsequent amalgam tattooing.

6. Filling material. Retrograde root fillings are still prepared using dental amalgam.

7. Review policy. One week and 12 weeks for repeat intraoral films.

Hemisection and root resection

Root resection

Extensive mucoperiosteal flap elevation and bone removal is required. Subcoronal root section is performed and the affected root extracted with as little trauma to the remaining dental tissue as possible. Sound root fillings are required in the remaining canals and the periodontal support must be adequate to bear the increase in occlusal loading that will result from loss of a root. Complex restorative therapy is inevitably required and must be planned in conjunction with the surgery. The dental unit should be suitable for use as a bridge abutment or for placement of a full crown after healing of the surgical wound is complete.

Molar hemisection

If crown destruction due to caries is extensive and associated with pulpal death it is occasionally possible to consider complete dental hemisection. Mucoperiosteal flaps and bone removal must be adequate for root amputation and excision. Stability must be considered during treatment planning and subsequent use of the tooth to support a crown or as an abutment for advance restorations should be possible.

Tooth transplantation

If destruction of a posterior tooth is sufficiently advanced to make restoration even with the aid of surgery impossible, extraction may be planned in conjunction with removal and reimplantation of a healthy, viable tooth. Third molars are good options for replacement of more anteriorly positioned molar teeth. A cast acrylic splint or preformed arch bar is prepared and the two teeth removed. No socket preparation is performed as drilling the bone of the recipient socket is likely to result in osteocyte death and subsequent failure of the transplant. Insertion, fixation for 6 weeks and occlusal relief are usually required. Long term success frequently requires root canal therapy in the transplanted tooth and this is sometimes performed extraorally before reimplantation. Long term retention of transplanted teeth is between 40 and 60% at 1 year.

Tooth extraction

Honest appraisal is required. If the prognosis is so poor that surgery offers little improvement it is often better to offer extraction and short term denture replacement. In other patients, osseointegrated implant placement may be required after suitable period for socket healing and alveolar remodelling to occur.

Root fractures

Root fractures may be transverse, vertical, oblique or spiral in pattern. Horizontal or transverse fractures are treated depending upon the quantity of coronal root remaining above the fracture.

1. *Apical third fractures.* Apicectomy and retrograde root filling placement is required. Restoration by conventional means is possible with a good prognosis.

2. *Middle third root fractures.* May be root filled across the fracture site and subsequently stabilized by

placement of a conventional post crown. The apical portion of the root fragment is removed surgically. Mobility and periodontal conditions dictate whether retention of the coronal part of the tooth is possible without further intervention or whether a diodontic implant is required. This pattern of treatment carried a poor prognosis but this improved significantly with the advent of titanium based alloys which permit osseointegration.

3. Coronal third root fractures often entail loss of the tooth or retention of the larger apical segment with complex restorative procedures required to fit a functional crown. Loss of the whole tooth may require space maintenance and implant planning.

4. Vertical, oblique and spiral root fractures. Although attempts may be made to conserve such teeth the prognosis is very poor and early loss with space maintenance is advantageous in many cases.

Tooth avulsion

Reimplantation is possible if the tooth is undamaged, non-carious and previously vital or successfully root filled. Transport in isotonic saline or milk is advised and immediate reimplantation and splintage are necessary. Inevitably devitalized, these teeth commonly require endodontic therapy and restoration to overcome the progressive discolouration which occurs.

SURGICAL INSTRUMENTS

Diathermy

Principles

Diathermy is a technique in which high frequency AC electric current is passed through tissue. Use of mains frequency AC (50 Hz) would result in neuromuscular stimulus and electrocution at high current. Increasing the frequency permits increased current strength (mA) to be used. Heat generation results from energy passage through the tissues and the temperature at the instrument tip may exceed 1000°C. Surgical diathermy commonly uses AC frequencies in the range 400 kHz–10 MHz.

Monopolar diathermy

The current generated is passed via the instrument tip and takes a short route through the patient and is earthed via the adhesive common electrode plate. Metal parts of the operating table must not be in contact with the patient's skin as preferential earthing may occur and a localized burn will then result.

Bipolar diathermy

The diathermy current passes from one instrument tip to the other via a very small volume of tissue. No earth plate is required. No cutting of tissue is possible. Use of bipolar diathermy adjacent to nerve trunks is possible as minimal 'scatter' occurs.

Cutting diathermy

This technique uses monopolar diathermy with high voltage and continuous current output. An arcing effect between the electrode tip and the adjacent tissue results in tissues being cut by localized destruction.

Coagulation diathermy

The use of monopolar diathermy set to generate a pulsed current reduces tissue disruption and cutting effect. Tissue desiccation and vessel sealing is greater than with continuous current output.

Blend diathermy

Modern diathermy generators permit a variable blend of pulsed and continuous current output. This device setting permits tissue cutting with a greater degree of haemostasis. It is very useful in head and neck surgery.

Problems

1. Burns. Burns occur only with poorly earthed monopolar diathermy. Precautions required include use of an adhesive common electrode plate, careful positioning of the patient on the operating table to prevent metal to skin contact. Regular diathermy generator maintenance is essential.

2. Pacemakers. Monopolar diathermy should be avoided if possible but bipolar diathermy is usually relatively free of problems.

3. Caution in appendages. Fingers and genitalia are at risk with excessive diathermy use as vascular occlusion can occur.

4. Intracavity use. Gas accumulation in the peritoneal cavity may be inflammable.

5. Skin preparation. Spirit based agents may prove inflammable.

Laser

Acronym: Light Amplification by Stimulated Emission of Radiation. A laser device produces a highly collimated, coherent, monochromatic and 'in phase' beam of electromagnetic radiation.

Principles

1. Requirements include a lasing medium, a source of electromagnetic energy and system of optical amplification and delivery system.

2. Lasing media. Crystalline, liquid or gaseous. The medium determines the wavelength emitted and therefore the colour or visibility.

Lasing media

1. HeNe (helium neon). A laser producing low power (milliwatts) red light (630 nm) used as a guide light for infrared lasers, or experimentally for biostimulation.

2. CO_2. CO_2 lasers emit invisible infra-red radiation (10600 nm). Rapidly absorbed by water the laser exhibits little tissue penetration. Useful for superficial surgery. The colour permits extensive superficial stripping as well as cutting to be performed. Charring occurs and lasing through charred tissue increases the local burn effect of the laser. The wavelength makes the CO_2 laser particularly suitable for microscopic, 'no touch' and endoscopic procedures such as microlaryngoscopic surgery.

3. Nd:YAG (neodymium: yttrium–aluminium–garnet). Devices use a crystal which emits light at the near infra-red range of the spectrum (1060 nm). The laser emission therefore has a wavelength one tenth that of CO_2 lasers. The light emitted is transmitted well through fluid filled media such as the ocular humours and the colour determines that good light absorption occurs with dark tissues. This laser therefore coagulates well. It causes more extensive tissue damage than CO_2 lasers. When used in tissue contact via a sapphire probe it finds a wide range of medical uses.

4. KTP (Potassium titanyl phosphate). KTP is a crystal used to change the wavelength of a Nd:YAG laser from 1060 nm (near infra-red) to 532 nm (green). The green colour exhibits a useful specificity for haemoglobin and melanin. Coagulation and destruction of coloured skin lesions are effectively performed.

5. Tunable dye lasers. The lasing medium is one of a range of organic media which confer the colour of the emitted beam. Elements permitting wavelength tuning are incorporated in the medium. The light source used is usually an argon laser. Pulsed dye lasers with different wavelengths are used in photocoagulation of vascular skin lesions and to fragment kidney stones.

6. Excimer lasers. Excited dimeric lasers are a class of device which use a dimeric molecule which is stable in its excited state but which dissociates with the loss of a photon to achieve its resting state. The light is near ultraviolet in wavelength. Argon fluoride, krypton fluoride and xenon fluoride are the commonest media in medical use. The laser devices are naturally pulsed, precise in their cutting action and used in ocular surgery. Their potential in intraoral surgery is considerable.

7. Semiconductor diode lasers. LED like in action these devices emit a continuous light. Photocoagulation is their principal medical use.

Tissue effects of lasers

The effects of incident light on biological tissue is determined by the amount that is reflected, scattered, transmitted or absorbed. The absorption of laser light results in a heating effect. Local heat generation results in warming, followed by coagulation, protein denaturation, desiccation, vaporization and carbonization.

1. Cutting. Results from tissue vaporization due to heating the cells to boiling point at the point of maximum laser absorption.

2. Coagulation. Protein denaturation results in cell death and haemostasis. The destruction of tumours is theoretically possible by this means and laser coagulation is similar to that achieved by diathermy.

3. Hard tissue surgery. Super pulsing will permit a non-thermal cutting effect and research suggests that bone cutting may be possible with new generation excimer lasers. Cutting by vaporization is less effective in bone than in soft tissue owing to the much lower water content in calcified tissue.

Advantages of lasers

- Dry surgical field.
- Reduction of blood loss.
- Reduction of postoperative oedema.
- Reduction in fibrosis and postoperative pain.
- Possible reduction in intra-operative seeding of metastases.
- Option of fibre-optic delivery to operative site.
- Minimal interference with anaesthetic monitoring equipment.
- Induced sterility of the operative site.

Disadvantages of lasers

- Cost.
- Complexity of equipment.

- Health and safety issues in use, maintenance and staff training.
- Costly maintenance.

Cryotherapy

Cryotherapy is a technique in which tissue denaturation using application of cold medium is employed. Liquid nitrogen by direct application or cryoprobes are used. The cryoprobe operates by temperature reduction due to the cryomedium passing across an internal venturi system and as a result, progressively reducing the temperature at the probe tip.

The technique is particularly effective in treating fluid-filled lesions. Application of the probe in a sequence of freeze–thaw cycles results in formation of an 'ice ball'. Intracellular ice formation results in expansions of the cell volume and disruption occurs on thawing. Repeated cycles result in reduction of lesion cell mass.

Optical and imaging enhancements

In maxillofacial surgery there are several useful techniques for optical enhancement. Magnifying loupes and operating microscopes are widely used in microvascular surgery. Fibre-optic technology is used as a diagnostic tool in endoscopy and as a delivery tool in laser surgery. Rigid endoscopes and 'Storz' rods find wide application in FESS and pharyngolaryngoscopy and permit biopsy and microscopic surgery to be performed.

Intra-operative video and X-ray image intensification are not as widely used but there are potential applications in head and neck surgery.

SURGICAL NUTRITION

Patients in hospital have a high risk of nutritional disorders. Disease related and iatrogenic malnutrition or nutritional complications of surgery exhibit a risk that increases with increasing length of hospital stay. Although minor degrees of protein calorie malnutrition do not appear to affect the outcome of surgical operations, major nutritional disorders undoubtedly jeopardise recovery.

Patients at particular risk include surgical patients with septic complications, medical patients with chronic illness or who require prolonged inpatient care, patients with malignant disease, malabsorption syndromes and a history of previous gastrointestinal surgery. A kwashiorkor-like malnutrition characterized by a low serum albumin concentration, muscle wasting, and water retention is the typical picture in septic patients but postoperative starvation presents as a more mixed picture resulting from starvation, increased catabolism, and reduced anabolism. Malnutrition in surgical patients is accompanied by an increased risk of postoperative complications.

Diagnostic criteria of malnutrition in inpatients include

- Recent unintentional weight loss weight < 80% of ideal for height.
- Albumin less than 30 g/l.
- Lymphocyte count of less than $1-2 \times 10^6$/l.

Diagnostic information includes measurements of body weight, arm muscle circumference, skin fold thickness and serum albumin concentration. Nutritional treatment is important in the preoperative phase for patients due for resection of head and neck malignancy if they are malnourished. Many exhibit concomitant malnutrition as their lifestyle (ethanol abuse in particular) often predisposes them to anorexia and malnutrition. Nutritional therapy will not be effective in the presence of active sepsis.

Surgical patients can be fed by enteral or parenteral means. Their oral disease may prevent oral feeding or dysphagia may make oral supplements inappropriate.

Enteral nutrition

Supplemental feeding is needed for many patients with malignant disease to combat the cachexia which is associated with the condition. An easily taken nutrient preparation to supplement intake of normal food is required. Total enteral nutrition is primarily indicated for patients who cannot eat or drink.

Indications for total enteral nutrition

- Prolonged unconsciousness
- Neurological dysphagia
- Oesophageal obstruction
- Inflammatory bowel disease
- Short bowel syndrome
- Post-traumatic weakness
- Postoperative weakness
- Post irradiation weakness
- Head and neck surgery
- Chemotherapy
- Burns
- Old age

Enteral nutrients and supplements

There is a wide range of enteral preparations, the principal differences between them being the way the proteins and calories are presented. Liquid whole protein regimens are cheaper and more palatable than those based on oligopeptides and amino acids. The oligopeptide and amino acid preparations appear to be better absorbed, especially in patients with shortened or diseased bowel. The energy content of the diet is offered as glucose, oligosaccharides, maltodextrin, corn syrup, medium chain triglycerides and sunflower oil. Other essential nutrients, such as electrolytes, minerals, trace elements, and vitamins, are added in varying quantities depending on the preparation. Five hundred millilitres of a typical enteral regimen provides 20 g of protein (3–15 g of nitrogen), and 500 kcal in 2–3 l of fluid. The proportion of energy provided by fat should be about 30–40%. The mixture should contain minerals, trace elements and vitamins. Voluntary oral nutrition supplementation may prove ineffective and intervention may be required.

Administration of total enteral nutrition

- Nasogastric tube (NG) feeding.
- Pharyngostomy.
- Percutaneous endoscopic gastrostomy (PEG).
- Open gastrostomy.
- Feeding jejunostomy via minilaparotmy or laparoscopic jejunostomy.

In some patients who cannot eat because of dysphagia the normal diet may be liquidised and swallowed in the usual way. Alternatively a commercially prepared liquid food may be used. Patients who cannot swallow or those with continually high losses from stomas or fistulas will need tube feeding.

Modern feeding tubes are fine bore and made from polyurethane or silastic. They can remain in position for long periods without damaging the oesophagus. Fine bore tubes preclude their use for the administration of liquidised food. In patients with total oesophageal obstruction or upper intestinal fistulas the diet can be infused directly into the jejunum through a gastrostomy or jejunostomy.

Complications of total enteral nutrition

- Gastric retention
- Hyperosmolar coma
- Electrolyte disturbances
- Aspiration
- Hyperglycaemia
- Nausea and vomiting
- Tube misplacement
- Diarrhoea
- Oesophagcal erosions
- Dehydration
- Infection
- Nasal septal erosions with NG tubes

Parenteral nutrition

Intravenous administration of nutrients is indicated when patients cannot be fed by mouth, by nasogastric intubation, or by gastrostomy or jejunostomy. The principle indication for parenteral nutrition is intestinal failure. In head and neck surgery the indications are relatively few. Patients with low hypopharyngeal cancer who are planned for a pharyngo oesophagectomy and gastric pull up procedure are not candidates for PEG and although a jejunostomy may be inserted at operation, preoperative intensive nutritional support may require parenteral techniques. Burns, and head injured patients may benefit.

Intestinal failure may be acute and reversible, for example, until a enterocutaneous fistula closes or a segment of short bowel adapts. Alternatively it may be chronic, as in cases of short bowel syndrome, where virtually all ileum and jejunum have been removed.

Principal causes of intestinal failure

- Reduction in absorbtive surface of small bowel – short bowel syndrome.
- Premature loss of enteric content – intestinal fistula.
- Disorder of peristalsis – chronic idiopathic intestinal pseudo-obstruction.
- Parenchymal disease of small bowel – Crohn's disease or radiation enteritis.

Technique of parenteral nutrition

Access

- Peripheral venous feeding; isotonic solutions; tend to thromboses veins readily; appropriate only for short-term use.
- Central venous feeding; medium term intravenous feeding; subclavian commonest route; less rigourous demand for isotonicity in feeding solutions.
- Tunnelled central venous catheter; in subcutaneous tissues of the anterior chest wall; long-term or permanent parenteral feeding.

Strict asepsis is essential.

Central venous catheters are advanced into the superior vena cava.

Feeding lines are not used for purposes other than administering TPN.

Initially a constant infusion is given.

Once stabilised, nocturnal feeding only is possible.

Catheter care is important; flushing and filling with heparin saline when not in use permits patient mobility.

Nutrients are administered from a 3 l bag, prepared in the pharmacy under sterile conditions.

Regular rate of infusion is ensured by using a constant volume infusion pump with alarms to warn of air in the infusion system and changes in the flow rate.

Some complications of total parenteral nutrition (TPN)

- Catheter infection, fracture, tip malposition in pleura or subclavian artery.
- Catheter-induced venous thrombosis.
- Air embolism.
- Fluid overload.
- Metabolic derangement, for example hyperglycaemia.
- Trace element deficiency.

Nutrients used in parenteral feeding

The regimen used is tailored to the individual's requirements. A stable patient requires about 2500 kcal (5–10 Mj) of energy and 12 g of nitrogen as crystalline amino acids in 2500 ml of fluid. Energy is provided using glucose and lipid emulsion. In the United Kingdom lipids are supplied by soya bean oil emulsion as it exhibits similar biochemical properties to chylomicrons. Amino acid provision includes all the essential amino acids, and a wide range of non-essential ones. Egg albumin provides an appropriate ratio of amino acids. The normal daily requirement of electrolytes, trace elements, and vitamins is added to the daily bag. Treatment with parenteral nutrition continues until the underlying condition has resolved and enteral nutrition can be reintroduced.

Ambulatory home enteral and parenteral nutrition Where restoration of enteral nutrition is likely to be delayed or in those committed to lifelong support by parenteral feeding the advantages of home parenteral nutrition should be considered. Patients can be taught the techniques of catheter care and intravenous infusion. This enables them to leave hospital and return to the community. Most of these patients, by feeding themselves overnight, can live an active social life and return to work.

SURGICALLY INDUCED OSTEOGENESIS

Distraction osteogenesis

1. The concept. Lengthening long bones by post-osteotomy distraction is not a new idea. For close to a century, many surgical disciplines have attempted applications of the concept. In orthopaedics, long bone lengthening was first achieved by carrying out an oblique osteotomy and then applying acute and intense distraction to steel rods driven into the proximal and distal portions of the osteotomized limb. Once lengthening had taken place the limb was stabilized with a plaster cast. A modification of this approach was suggested by Ilizarov. Gradual traction applied to an induced callus produced similar lengthening in a less traumatic fashion. Interestingly, Ilizarov's intention was to use external compression to bone ends in order to treat cases of fracture non-union. A patient who had failed to grasp the instructions given, turned the screw of the compression appliance the wrong way and ended up distracting rather than compressing their bone ends. Ilizarov noticed new bone being formed. Based on this observation he was subsequently able to treat several cases of osteomyelitis without the use of antibiotics.

2. Surgical technique. Post-fracture or post-osteotomy callus formation is a well recognised phase in bony healing in a healthy skeleton. Distraction forces applied to the proximal and distal bone ends during this phase is known as distraction osteogenesis. It relies on prolonged, progressive and gradual distraction which does not disrupt the local bone vascular supply. The osteotomy is usually carried out in the subperiosteal plane and a latent period of about 5 days is allowed before beginning distraction. Application of a distraction force requires modified external fixators. At the end of the distraction period the bone is allowed to consolidate under function into cortical and medullary phases.

3. This technique can induce callus formation and bone depsition such that growth is induced in multiple directions. It can also be used at an early age. This is significant since previously the options were to operate early and risk scarring or wait until growth had ceased in late adolescence. The advantage of producing a normal mandible and facial appearance at an early age is obvious. In unilateral craniofacial microsomia it is important to correct the mandible in both vertical and anteroposterior directions. If this is not achieved then the maxilla fails to develop and a maxillary osteotomy may be needed in adult life to correct the resulting occlusal cant.

4. Internal distraction devices to distract the maxilla and lengthen the mandible have been described. With intra-oral space limitations, they are difficult to activate. Osseointegrated implants have been used as abutments and then a connector used to distract the mandible. Subperiosteal onlay may also be used.

5. Force application. The daily rate of distraction is dependent on patient compliance. Rates below 0.5 mm each day may lead to premature osteotomy union and distraction of above 1.5 mm each day to formation of fibrous union or occasionally to non-union. Motorized devices can be used to provide a gradual distraction. The alternative is that the patient is instructed to adjust the appliance to give separate lengthenings of 0.25 mm each at different times during the day up to a total of 1 mm of opening each day. This slow distraction is relatively painless and in some cases bones have been lengthened by up to 100% of the original length. Succesful induction of as much as 18 cm of new bone has reportedly been produced in limb long bones. Simultaneous correction of shortening at several sites in the same limb is described.

6. Soft tissues. The effects of bone distraction on the soft tissue envelope is poorly understood. Where lengthening is less than 10% of the initial bone length, soft tissues can adapt. Resting neuromuscular tone is important in shaping bone architecture. Whether the use of soft tissue expansion prior to osteogenic distraction would prove practicable and beneficial remains to be demonstrated. This technique is usually used for production of excess skin prior to elevation of local flaps during reconstructive soft tissue surgery. Whether insertion of tissue expanders beneath the periosteal envelope would encourage or induce the necessary soft tissue adaptation is not yet clear.

7. Complications. Pin track infection, premature consolidation, neuropraxia or scarring are all described. Distraction pain is experienced by some patients and a recent series suggested that 20% had major complications such as deformity of the new bone requiring a repeated traction episode or even subsequent grafting.

Application of distraction osteogenesis to craniofacial problems

Orthodontists are experienced in the use of mechanical forces in the dento–alveolar complex to induce new bone in sites of tension. This has been extended to the palatal suture and new bone formation after rapid maxillary expansion is well documented. As an extension of this experience, distraction osteogenesis has been used to lengthen the mandible, advance the midface and augment the mandibular–alveolar ridge; this latter approach provides a welcome development in the treatment of postextraction alveolar bone atrophy. Cleft lip and palate patients with midface retrusion due to the anomaly itself or following childhood cleft surgery. Correction of this midface retrusion has often required orthognathic surgery but the possibility of using distraction osteogenesis is an attractive option.

Some indications for distraction osteogenesis

- Mandibular hypoplasia related to early tempromandibular joint ankylosis or juvenile chronic rheumatoid arthritis.
- Pathological bone loss or osteopaenia.
- Unilateral and bilateral craniofacial microsomia.
- Micrognathia.
- Treacher–Collins syndrome.
- Calvarial expansion in craniosynostosis.
- Dwarfism or skeletal dysplasia where there is a congenital limb length discrepancy.
- Lengthening of the phalanges, metacarpals, tarsals and metatarsals is also possible.

Costochondral grafting

In young patients whose mandibles are still growing actively, damage to the condylar growth centres due to trauma, fracture, sepsis or juvenile chronic arthritis can result in very marked unilateral condylar and hence hemimandibular hypoplasia. In some children this condition may be bilateral. Severe micrognathia can result and during the adolescent growth phase, the failure in mandibular growth becomes more noticable against the relatively normal maxillary maturation.

The option to harvest a rib with its costochondral cartilage and implant it after excision of the damaged condylar head provides a replacement for the growth potential otherwise lost to the mandible. This procedure can be performed bilaterally if necessary. The results are acceptable growth in 60–70%. In about 20% growth still fails to keep up with the maturation of the maxilla and the rest of the face. In about 10–15% excess growth of the grafted hemimandible occurs.

The problems include, haematoma, sepsis and facial nerve palsy as a result of the condylar procedure and pneumothorax due the rib harvest, particularly in young children.

Osseointegration and bone grafting

Placement of titanium oxide intra-bony fixtures not only stimulates osseointegration but in some patients florid callus formation adjacent to the insertion site. This observation has raised the suggestion that use of implants with or without bone grafting may provide an option in augmentation of atrophic mandibles or maxillary alveoli.

Other measures

The role of bone morphogenetic protein and subperiosteal soft tissue expanders has yet to be proven.

Revision points

Bone growth
Fracture healing

SYMMETRICAL FACIAL DISPROPORTION

In this group of disorders, the appearance from the frontal or anterior aspect of the patient's face may reveal no asymmetry and may be acceptable. These patients nevertheless have antero–posterior discrepancies of facial dimension most apparent on examination of the profile. In discrepancies of the vertical dimension the frontal facial appearance provides the most useful diagnostic view.

Mandibular conditions

1. Sagittal (AP) mandibular excess (mandibular prognathism). Mild cases exhibit edge to edge incisor relationships or mild reverse overjet with compensatory proclination of maxillary incisors and retroclination of mandibular incisors. The sagittal length of the mandible may be the principal abnormality and may be corrected by posterior movement using sagittal split ramus osteotomies. Commonly the disproportion exhibits a degree of maxillary hypoplasia in association. A bimaxillary operation is then more appropriate. Attention to the chin prominence may also be required.

2. Sagittal (AP) mandibular deficiency (retrognathism). There is a wide range of clinical presentations. The causes include congenitally short mandibles, bilateral childhood mandibular trauma and severe juvenile chronic arthritis or Still's disease.

Mild degrees are represented by upper incisor proclination, increased labiomental groove due to the lower lip being caught beneath the upper anterior teeth. There is an incisor class II division 1 relation. The ANB difference documents the degree of skeletal base discrepancy. The more severe degree of this pattern is the bird face deformity usually resulting from childhood condylar trauma or agenesis. Treatment involves incisor decompensation followed by ramus osteotomy to perform mandibular set forward. Segmental mandibular osteotomies may be a suitable alternative. Bird face deformities may require ramus lengthening by distraction osteogenesis or by inverted L osteotomy and bone grafting. Advancement, genioplasty and rhinoplasty are commonly required in the most severe cases.

3. Low angle mandibular deficiency. Reduced lower face height due to anterior direction to mandibular growth. The gonial and SN–MP angles are both reduced. These patients require advancement and increase in subapical bone height.

4. High angle mandibular deficiency. Mandibular growth occurs principally in the vertical and posterior directions. Bimaxillary surgery with genioplasty is normally required.

5. Vertical mandibular excess (long face). Rare as an isolated clinical problem. Usually associated with mandibular asymmetry. The component parts of the affected mandible are the ramus and the anterior segment. Increase in anterior face height is a common finding with an increase in subapical bone. The contribution to the long face syndrome is significant in these patients. It may be associated with anterior open bite and maxillary deformities are usually associated.

6. Bilateral masseteric hypertrophy. Muscle enlargement results in secondary skeletal changes. Transverse mandibular dimensions are increased. Pain, impaired function and trismus may result. Cosmetic improvement may be achieved by muscle reduction.

Maxillary conditions

1. Sagittal maxillary excess. Incisor proclination must be distinguished from dentoalveolar protrusion. Class II division 1 incisor relationships result. Orthodontic or segmental osteotomy will correct isolated anterior deformity. If posterior vertical maxillary dimensions are increased or a high angle or anterior open bite is present, a bimaxillary operation may be required.

2. Panmaxillary hyperplasia. All dimensions are increased and panfacial surgery may be required for correction.

3. *Vertical maxillary excess.* Alveolar growth is excessive in downward direction. Tooth and upper gingivae are visible and the upper lip may be short. Le Fort I impaction osteotomy may be required for correction.

4. *Vertical maxillary deficiency.* Uncommon in non-cleft cases. A long upper lip and prominent chin prominence with little dental or gingival visibility are typical features. Nasal deformities may co-exist. Correction requires Le Fort I advancement often with rhinoplasty. Short face syndrome occurs and the clinical features include a short square face, prominent nasolabial folds and a broad alar base. Reduced anterior face height and deep reverse overbite are associated. Bimaxillary surgery may be required.

5. *Nasomaxillary hypoplasia.* Nasal foreshortening and adjacent maxillary hypoplasia are the hallmarks. There are four patterns described. Dentoalveolar, Binders syndrome, cleft related and panfacial hypoplasia.
    High level maxillary advance or Le Fort II osteotomy is often required.

6. *Other groups of mid face disproportion.*

- Lateral maxillary deficiency.
- Malar deficiency.
- Total mid facial hypoplasia.
- Syndromic associations; Crouzon's, Apert's and the Pierre–Robin sequence are examples.

Bimaxillary conditions

Deep overbite

1. *Class II division l.* Depending on the quality of the profile, a segmental mandibular setdown (Köle osteotomy) may be the only procedure required to establish sound occlusion. In poor profiles, mandibular advance with or without maxillary impaction in addition to Köle osteotomy may be required.

2. *Class II division 2.* Incisor decompensation followed by segmental mandibular osteotomy is corrective if the profile is otherwise good. In poor profiles, orthodontic decompensation converts the problem to a Class II division 1 relationship. Treatment is as described above.

Bimaxillary protrusion

Orthodontic correction is acceptable if dentoalveolar skeletal base relations are satisfactory. Bimaxillary anterior segmental osteotomies are otherwise corrective. Anterior open bite may be associated.

Long face syndrome

Vertical excess in both the maxilla and chin may coexist. The vertical position of the maxilla may be caudal, the angulation of the maxillary occlusal plane may be tilted down posteriorly and the upper lip length may be short. Le Fort I osteotomy permits impaction, tilt correction and vertical repositioning of the maxilla. If present, the mandibular element of the disorder may be corrected by ramus osteotomy. The chin point may be corrected by autorotation or reduction genioplasty.

Short face syndrome

These patients are usually treated cleft patients. The condition may be predominantly midface or predominantly lower face or a combination of both.

1. Lower facial deficiency is treated by anterior mandibular segmental setdown or by orthodontic occlusal plane correction in association with mandibular advancement. Augmentation or sandwich genioplasty may also be required.

2. Midfacial disproportion is treated by Le Fort I osteotomy with interpositional bone grafting. Other cleft related problems may require attention.

Anterior open bite

Dentoalveolar open bite may be corrected by orthodontics or bimaxillary anterior segmental osteotomy. Skeletal base open bite requires Le Fort I osteotomy with posterior impaction and mandibular autorotation. Relapse rates are high if treatment by ramus mandibular osteotomy alone is used as soft tissues of the pterygomassetric sling place severe limits on the change in form which may be imposed on the skeletal tissues.

Soft tissue problems   Tongue enlargement may be associated and surgical reduction has been proposed. This is not commonly performed during orthognathic surgery.

The chin

Progenia   Isolated prominence of the chin point without occlusal or other patterns of facial dysharmony is readily corrected by reduction genioplasty.

Retrogenia   Lack of forward projection of the chin may be associated with other features of facial syndromes or may occur as an isolated feature. The first pattern requires correction as part of a comprehensive orthognathic treatment plan. In many such patients an augmentation or advancement genioplasty will be incorporated into the surgical planning. In isolated retrogenia, advancement or augmentation genioplasty alone achieves good cosmetic results in most patients.

SYNDROMES OF THE HEAD AND NECK

Apert's syndrome

An uncommon craniosynostosis. Typified by oxycephaly and syndactyly affecting hands and feet. There is variable impairment of IQ, palatal clefts and macroglossia.

Takayasu's syndrome

There are two patterns. The first type characteristically affects young women. Inflammatory non-specific arteritis, mild toxaemia at outset and pulseless upper extremities including head and neck are typical clinical features. Chronic cases exhibit orthostatic syncope, epilepsy, facial atrophy, diffuse facial pain, and visual disturbance.

The second pattern affects elderly patients of both sexes and presents as non-inflammatory vascular occlusion. It is typically an atheromatous or rarely syphilitic vasculitis. It is similar in clinical presentation to the younger type.

Chediak–Higashi

Oropharyngeal ulceration associated with tendency toward recurrent mucocutaneous pyogenic infections. Hepatosplenomegaly and lymphadenopathy are associated. Neutrophil functional disorders with failure of intracelluar bacterial lysis and formation of intreacelluar lysomal inclusions occur.

Ellis van Creveld

Ectodermal dysplasia, affecting cutaneous adnexa. Hyperhidrotic dysplasia affecting nails, teeth, and hair. Associated with limb abnormalities including long bone malformations and polydactyly. Occasionally associated with congenital cardiac abnormalities. Autosomal recessive inheritance.

Facial clefts

Oblique facial clefts have been recently classified in detail by Tessier. Some are associated with other congenital abnormalities. Cleft mandibles do occur but are rare. Transverse facial clefts with or without macroglossia are described.

Chromosomal syndromes

1. Autosomal syndromes. Down's (trisomy 21), Cri du Chat (trisomy 18) and Patau's (trisomy 13–15) are well documented. Down's occurs due to several different genetic abnormalities. Chromosome translocations and deletions are documented. The trisomy pattern is associated with mental retardation, short stature, short neck, abnormal ear pinnae, nasal malformations including flattening of the bridge and alar base widening. Ocular abnormalities include telecanthus, stabismus, nystagmus and cataract formation. The skull is typically brachycephalic, with flattened occiput. Obligate mouth-breathing and macroglossia are well described. Palates may be attenuated, high arched and associated with bifid uvulae. A range of dental abnormalities is noted.

2. *Sex chromosomes*. Turner's syndrome (XO). The genital abnormalities and body habitus pattern of this condition are well documented. The oro-facial manifestations include palatal high vaults and occasional clefts, hypoplastic mandibles, cervical webs, microsomia and skull asymmetries.

3. *Klinefelter's syndrome (XXY)*. There are rarely any head and neck stigmata of this condition although the rare variants XXXY and XXXXY are increasingly associated with mandibular prognathism.

Cleidocranial dysostosis

Clavicular agenesis and delayed or complete failure of dental eruption. Hypodontia may be associated.

Waardenburg's syndrome

Congenital sensorineural deafness, laterally displaced medial canthi, broad nasal bases, white forelock, heterchromatic irides and hyperpasia of the medial portion of the eyebrows. Vitiligo in Negroid races is described in addition. Autosomal dominant.

Ehlers–Danlos syndrome

Typified by cutaneous fragility, hyperelasticity, articular and ligamentous hyperelasticity, and formation of skin pseudo tumours. Capillary wall fragility and postoperative haemorrhage are associated,

Epidermolysis bullosa

There are simple and dystrophic forms. Both types exhibit vesicular eruptions and bulla formation. The simple pattern is non-scarring and essentially non-destructive. Dystrophic forms are destructive and scar inducing. They are associated with growth impairment and mental retardation. The recessive pattern is more marked in the severity of developmental impairment and may be rapidly lethal.

Felty's syndrome

A triad of hypersplenism, rheumatoid arthritis and neutropenia. Painful aphthous pattern oral ulceration is common. Refractory hypochromic anaemia is also common.

Gorlin–Goltz syndrome

Classically expressed as multiple basal cell naevi, odontogenic keratocysts, and rib and vertebral abnormalities.

Osler–Weber–Rendu syndrome

Hereditary haemorrhagic telangectasia. Widespread capillary and venous dilated malformations affecting skin and mucous membranes. Spontanous haemorrhage is typical. Oral, gingival and nasal mucosa are affected.

Hunter's and Hurler's syndromes

Mucopolysaccharidoses. There are several related enzyme defects. All exhibit variable degrees of skeletal and facial malformation, mental retardation, hepatosplenomegaly, corneal opacification, sensorineural deafness, and congenital cardiac abnormalities. Oro-facial manifestations include thickened lips and gingival tissues, macroglossia and reduced TMJ mobility. Two genetic patterns; autosomal recessive and X-linked recessive.

Hypertelorism

Rare with an incidence of 1:100 000 live births. There may be associated midline abnormalities including clefts of lip and palate. The skull form is otherwise acceptably normal. However, prominent frontal and bitemporal eminences are described. Craniosynostoses often exhibit a degree of hypertelorism. The severity may be accurately documented using canthal index (medial canthal distance/lateral canthal distance × 100).

Hypohidrotic syndromes

Classically these conditions present as hypohidrosis, hypotrichosis, hypodontia. Most exhibit X-linked recessive inheritance. Rare autosomal patterns exist. Facies exhibit frontal bossing, depressed nasal bridge, protuberant lips, prominent pinnae and thinning hair. Heat intolerance due to poor sweating is described but is usually incomplete. Dental abnormalities include hypodontia and conical teeth.

Caffey's syndrome	Previously considered to be congenital hyperostosis affecting long bones and mandible. In recent times the association at least in some cases with non-accidental injury has been documented.
Marcus–Gunn syndrome	Unilateral ptosis with elevation of affected lid on voluntary jaw movement toward the affected side. Reverse Marcus–Gun syndrome is also described.
Klipper–Feil syndrome	Fusion of variable numbers of cervical vertebrae associated with painless limitation of neck movement. A low posterior hairline is also associated. Occasionally thoracic vertebrae may be involved as may spina bifida, cervical ribs and a wide range of neurological abnormalities. There are no constant oral findings although palatal abnormalities are described.
Treacher–Collins syndrome	Mandibulofacial dysostosis. This syndrome is considered to be an abnormality of first branchial arch derived tissues. Typical facies include antimongoloid slant of palpebral fissure, malformed pinnae, mandibular hypoplasia, hypoplastic malar prominences and occasional arch non-fusion. The mastoids are poorly pneumatized, paranasal sinuses rudimentary, and occipital protruberance is marked. A variety of other skeletal abnormalities is occasionally associated. Unilateral or bilateral macrostomia and severe malocclusion is common. It is probably inherited as autosomal dominant.
Marfan's syndrome	Arachnodactyly, excessive and disproportionate skeletal growth, ectopia lentis and aortic aneurysm formation are characteristic. Other cardiac problems are reported. Most commonly aortic valve regurgitation. High arched palates are typical.
Melkersson–Rosenthal	Unilateral facial palsy, transient facial oedema, tongue fissuring and plication and swelling. In addition granulomatous chelitis is associated in some patients.
Moebius' syndrome	Congenital and usually bilateral facial paralysis. Paresis of the lower cranial nerves is associated and trunk and limb paralyses are also described.
Peutz–Jeghers syndrome	Mucocutaneous melanosis, intestinal polyp formation and occasional intussusception. Autosomal dominant

inheritance. This condition must be distinguished from Addisonian pigmentation.

Von Recklinghausen's syndrome

Multiple neurofibromatosis. Many neurofibromata and *café au lait* lesions are typical. Lipomata and subperiosteal cysts are also associated. Oral tissues may be involved but uncommonly. Rare sarcomatous change is described.

Gardener's syndrome

Multiple osteomas, epidermal inclusion cysts, cutaneous and mesenteric fibrous tumours and intestinal polyposis. Autosomal dominant inheritance.

Goldenhar's syndrome

Epibulbar dermoids, auricular malformations and vertebroskeletal abnormalities are characteristic. Skull asymmetry with a degree of frontal bossing and nares atresia is described. Mental and malar hypoplasia, microtia and fistula formation are features. Micrognathia, macrostomia, and bifid uvulae are occasionally associated.

Papillon–Lefevre syndrome

Palmoplantar hyperkeratosis, is associated with aggressive destruction of supporting tissues of primary and adult dentitions. Possible autosomal recessive.

Fragilitas ossium syndrome

Osteogenesis imperfecta, dentinogenesis imperfecta, blue sclera, otosclerosis and ligamentous laxity.

Albright's syndrome

Polyostotic fibrous dysplasia, cutaneous and mucosal pigmentation, endocrine dysfunction and sexual precocity. Early menarche in female is the most striking of the endocrine dysfunctional findings. Enlargement, expansion and destruction of the maxilla is the commonest of the jaw findings.

Romberg's syndrome

Progressive hemifacial atrophy. Often accompanied by trigeminal neuralgia and contralateral temporal lobe epilepsy. Tongue hemiatrophy may occur.

Pseudoxanthoma elasticum

Cutaneous thickening and formation of xanthomata, recurrent gastointestinal haemorrhages, failing peripheral pulses, and retinal angioid streaks with failing vision are typical features. Paget's disease also produces retinal angioid streaks.

Kartagener's syndrome

Cilial motility disorder. This condition results in recurrent pan-sinusitis, bronchiectasis and is associated with situs invertus. The maxillary antrum is typically involved. Hypoplasia or agenesis of the frontal sinus is described. Nasal polyps are frequent and atopy is common.

Sturge–Weber syndrome
A venous capilliary haemangioma formation affecting the leptomeninges associated with ipsilateral haemangioma of the facial skin. Intracerebral calcification associated with epilepsy, contralateral hemiplegia and mental retardation are described. Buccal mucosae and lips may exhibit vascular hyperplasia and intraoral naevus formation. Gingivae may be similarly affected. Tongue hemihypertrophy is described.

Williams syndrome
The triad of elfin facies, supravalvular aortic stenosis and idiopathic hypercalcaemia. The facial features include ocular hypertelorism, wide mouth, protruberant lips, pointed chin and a variable pattern of malocclusion.

Tuberous sclerosis
One of the neurocutaneous syndromes. Epilepsy, mental retardation and adenoma sebaceum formation are characteristic. Fifty percent demonstrate autosomal dominant inheritance.

Heerfordt's syndrome
Uveoparotid fever. Fever, parotid enlargement, facial paralysis and uveitis are associated. Granulomatous lymphadenitis is associated with the condition. Underlying sarcoidosis is the usual cause.

THIRD MOLARS

Removal of third molar teeth is one of the five commonest surgical procedures performed under NHS inpatient services. It is easy for surgeons to under estimate the morbidity of such surgery and there has recently been much debate about indications for removal of third molars. In the USA the widely quoted NIH Consensus has formed the framework for most research into appropriate use of this opertaion and indications for it.

Indications for removal

1. Recurrent pericoronitis. Definitions and disagreements about clinical course hamper discussions about this condition. Nevertheless it is common. Where true pericoronitis has occurred particularly around a lower tooth, the risk of recurrence is demonstrably enhanced and the presence of a partially erupted contralateral lower third molar is associated with an increased risk to this tooth also.

2. Advanced periodontitis. As with any tooth whose periodontal support is destroyed, removal of the tooth is a viable treatment option.

3. Caries in second or third molar. Restorability is often an issue associated with abnormal interdental contacts due to impaction and partial eruption of the third molar.

4. Pericoronal pathology. Apart from chronic or recurrent infection and operculum ulceration, failure of complete eruption is associated with an increased risk of pathological change in the retained follicular tissue. Follicular cysts and occasionally soft tissue neoplasms are all described. There is a suggested clinical association with the tonsillitis of infectious mononucleosis although both pericoronitis and IM are independently common occurrences in the most at risk age group.

5. Apical pathology. The mandibular angle is the site of predilection of many odontogenic tumour like lesions and the basal bone may be affected by primary bone pathology. Sequelae of dental pulp necrosis may also present associated with partially erupted third molars.

6. *Alveolar bone lesions.* Inflammatory, cystic and neoplastic lesions are all described and third molar removal constitutes a part of the management of these lesions.

7. *Fracture related.* The presence of unerupted third molars may, arguably constitute a site of weakness and increased risk of fracture at the mandibular angle. This site is one of the commonest sites of fracture whether there is a third molar present or not. Nevertheless the retention of a third molar adjacent to or in the region of a fracture carries an increased risk of infection and non-union so removal is usually advised during open reduction and fixation of such injuries.

8. *Orthodontics or orthognathic surgery.* Where complex tooth movements and osteotomy are being planned, early removal of third molars is advised to allow good bony infilling of the sockets prior to the definitive surgery.

9. *Prosthodontic treatment.* Partially erupted teeth, including third molars can impede the production of well-fitting dentures and complicate the construction of more complex restorations.

10. *Dental transplant donor.* Where advanced carious destruction of an isolated tooth elsewhere in the arch has occurred, a sound but impacted third molar may be harvested and splinted into the socket created by removal of the carious unit. This treatment is less commonly performed with the advent of osseointegrated implant technology.

11. *TMJ related.* In the presence of partially erupted third molars it is all but impossible to determine the precise cause of symptoms arising in the region of the TMJ. Therefore, under such circumstances it is common clinical practice to remove such teeth as part of a

treatment plan designed to alleviate TMJ related symptoms or at least contribute to the diagnosis of such problems.

12. Medical indications. The requirement for removal of teeth in patients undergoing cardiac surgery is largely historical althogh careful review by the dentist prior to such surgery is advisable. Before DXT of adjacent orofacial or neck tissues any suspect teeth should be removed as subsequent extraction carries a very high risk of osteoradionecrosis.

13. Occupational. It may be argued that a more radical policy of removal of third molars should be employed in certain occupational groups. Servicemen and missionaries are examples where prolonged deployment in remote parts of the world make the problems of subsequent symptoms and of finding adequate treatment sufficient to justify removal of relatively symptom-free teeth.

14. Prophylactic. True prophylactic removal of four completely asymptomatic third molars is rare. Neverthless, recurrent pericoronitis becomes recurrent more frequently than it resolves and the risk to contralateral teeth is significant after one or more such episodes. The risks of multiple GA must be considered in patients undergoing removal of fewer than their full complement of third molars.

15. Recognized complications. Dry socket or localized osteitis is associated as with dental extractions elsewhere in the arch, with tissue trauma, operator inexperience, prolonged surgery, excessive or non-cooled bone removal and diabetes mellitus. Smoking puts a patient at a much greater risk of developing this complication.

16. Neuropraxias. Inferior alveolar, lingual and occasional mylohyoid nerve damage has been reported. The lingual nerve damage rate is consistently reported as between 0.5 and 1.0%. Lingual retraction is associated with a higher incidence of this problem.

17. Fracture. Well described as a complication with angle fractures of the mandible and tuberosity fractures in the maxilla being noted. Recognition and immediate treatment are required.

18. Uncomplicated surgery. By far the commonest clinical outcome. After the immediate postoperative pain and swelling has subsided few patients report long-term problems.

Further reading

The debate about indications for third molar removal in particular of those considered as prophylactic operations.
Definitions of pericoronitis.
Aspects of operative technique.
Cost–benefit ratio.
Use of intra-operative local anaesthesia, steroids and peri-operative antibiotics.

THYROID AND PARATHYROID GLAND SURGERY

The indications for thyroidectomy are tumour, failed medical therapy for benign goitre and for cosmetics in patients concerned about an enlarged but non-functional thyroid gland. Complete thyroidectomy is rarely required and commits the patient to lifelong oral thyroxine replacement therapy.

Partial or subtotal thyroidectomy

Preoperative preparations   Cervical and chest X-rays to show any calcification or tracheal deviation and indirect laryngoscopy to detect any recurrent laryngeal nerve paralysis are important measures. If required, medical treatment for thyrotoxicosis until the resting pulse rate is below 100 per min is essential before administering general anaesthetic. Untreated thyrotoxicosis is a contraindication to surgery until fully controlled.

Anaesthesia and positioning   General anaesthesia with neck hyper-extension is required. A sandbag between the shoulders and horseshoe ring below the head is normal.

Procedure   *1.   A collar incision* in a skin crease is first marked and then incised midway between the suprasternal notch and the upper border of the thyroid cartilage. The incision is deepened through the platysma on both sides to the anterior sternomastoid borders.

2.   Flaps are developed by sharp dissection to raise the upper flap until the thyroid notch is reached and the lower flap down to the suprasternal notch. Joll's self-retaining retractor is inserted.

3.   The deep fascia is incised and the strap muscles are parted until the thyroid isthmus is exposed. The strap muscles on the opposite side are also raised if a bilateral operation is being performed.

4.   Isolation of the recurrent laryngeal nerve commencing low in the neck is the essential next step. It lies in the tracheo-oesophageal groove. Once isolated the gland dissection can proceed from below upwards ensuring that the nerve is preserved at each stage.

5. *Gland mobilization* by sharp dissection will deliver the lateral lobe into the wound. If necessary, to improve exposure, the strap muscles may be divided between forceps at the level of the cricoid cartilage. This should preserve their nerve supply from ansa cervicalis below. Dissection laterally and posteriorly to the lobe of the thyroid will identify the inferior thyroid artery and recurrent laryngeal nerve if not already located. The nerve is very close to the terminal branches of the inferior thyroid artery which is ligated well away from the gland to avoid recurrent laryngeal nerve injury.

Mobilization of the upper pole and ligation of the superior thyroid vessels is important as this vessel is the major pedicle. It is divided close to the gland to avoid injuring the external branch of the superior laryngeal nerve. This nerve supplies cricothyroid muscle and damage causes hoarseness of the voice.

6. *Dissection deep to the gland* separates it from the trachea and division of the inferior thyroid plexus of veins freeing the pyramidal lobe, if present, further mobilizes the lobe. If total or subtotal thyroidectomy is to be performed, the contralateral lobe is dissected similarly. If partial lobectomy is performed division of the gland substance is performed by applying forceps across the gland parenchyma and cutting the dissected portion free. The clamped margin is oversewn to secure haemostasis.

7. *Although most of the lateral lobes,* the whole of the isthmus and pyramidal lobe may be removed it is preferable to leave some functioning thyroid tissue even in patients with malignancy. As a minimum, two small posterior portions of the gland should be left on either side of the trachea. Preservation of the parathyroids is essential. If total thyroidectomy is deemed necessary, at least one parathyroid gland should be identified, dissected clear of the operative specimen and re-implanted in a subcutaneous site, usually in the forearm.

8. *Closure.* All cut edges of gland parenchyma or isthmus are oversewn. The deep fascia is closed, the platysma is approximated and the skin sutured or stapled. Vacuum drainage is necessary.

Postoperative complications   *1.   Early*

- *Haematoma.* Needs immediate evacuation or aspiration.
- *Respiratory obstruction* may be due to tense haematoma, laryngeal spasm, unilateral or bilateral recurrent nerve paralysis, or rarely to collapse or kinking of the trachea. Respiratory distress may need endotracheal intubation, or occasionally tracheostomy. Ventilation is rarely necessary.
- *Recurrent laryngeal nerve paralysis.* May be unilateral or bilateral, complete or partial, transient or permanent. Superior laryngeal nerve paralysis leads to hoarseness of voice only.
- *Thyrotoxic crisis* occurs occasionally in poorly prepared previously thyrotoxic patients. It is treated by rehydration, antipyretics, steroids and propranolol 20 mg 6 hourly.

2.   Intermediate. Parathyroid insufficiency after 2–5 days. This may occasionally be delayed for 3 weeks. It is treated by calcium therapy.

3.   Late. Wound infection, keloid scar formation and thyroid insufficiency may occur. Thyroid replacement may be required and late onset postoperative myxoedema may be delayed in onset for up to 2 years. Recurrent thyrotoxicosis may occur. Recurrent tumour is a problem with papillary and follicular carcinomas.

Parathyroidectomy

Surgical technique   *1.   Exposure* is made through a collar incision similar to that employed for thyroid operation. The middle thyroid vein is ligated and divided and the space between the carotid sheath, thyroid gland and trachea is opened. It is essential to identify the recurrent laryngeal nerve.

2. *Although preoperative localization* is increasingly accurate, all parathyroid glands should be sought in a systematic manner. Exploration of each side of the neck in turn and identification of all four glands should be carried out before biopsy or resection of any.

3. *The superior parathyroid gland* is more constantly located where the recurrent laryngeal nerve passes to the larynx and the inferior thyroid artery enters the parenchyma of the thyroid glands.

4. *The interior parathyroid gland* is usually found adjacent to the lower pole of the thyroid, lying in the thyroid capsule or embedded within the thymic fat.

5. *Although parathyroids are often closely applied to the capsule of the thyroid gland,* true 'intra-thyroid' parathyroid glands are found in approximately 0.5–3.0% of cases. Although rare, the intra-thyroid hyper-functioning parathyroid tissue is a potential cause for failure of parathyroid surgery.

6. *Intra-operative frozen sections* may aid determination of the presence of parathyroid tissue in resected tissue. The glandular substance is often encapsulated in fatty tissue and enucleation may not be obviously complete. The interpretation of frozen sections may be difficult. Although the microscopic appearance of parathyroid tissue is characteristic, it is often impossible to reliably distinguish between adenomatous and hyperplastic tissue.

Indications for parathyroidectomy

An obviously enlarged parathyroid gland should be resected and the remaining three glands identified. The sites of the remaining glands should be recorded, and preferably marked with a non-absorbable suture or metal clip. If two or three glands are enlarged these are excised, and the remaining glands marked. A less radical approach involves identification of the enlarged gland and if one gland is obviously enlarged and the ipsilateral gland is normal, the abnormal gland may be resected, biopsies of the ipsilateral gland taken and the remaining two glands allowed to remain unidentified.

In approximately l0% of cases all four glands are enlarged due to clear cell or chief cell hyperplasia. This group of patients is at particular risk of persistent or recurrent hypercalcaemia and operative management remains controversial. Resection of three and a half glands (subtotal parathyroidectomy) gives unpredictable results. Reports suggest that at 1 year after operation, 11% of patients have residual hyperparathyroidism and 15% have permanent hyperparathyroidism. One surgical alternative is to resect all four glands and implant a graft of one gland into easily accessible muscle; usually deltoid or brachioradialis. If disordered calcium metabolism recurs, further surgery can be performed easily without the morbidity of re-exploration of the neck.

Identification of all four glands may be difficult if one is located in an ectopic or unusual position. An apparently 'missing' upper parathyroid may be found deep to the posterior surface of the thyroid gland, in the tracheo-oesophageal groove, or even in the posterior mediastinum. Occult lower glands may be encountered on the anterolateral surface of the thyroid lobe, or encased within the thymus. Occasionally glands have been reported in the pharyngeal muscles, carotid sheath or pericardium.

Postoperative care

The plasma calcium is the most accurate marker of successful surgery. Serial assays are required. The serum alkaline phosphatase may rise and indicates healing in patients with known bone disease. Many patients develop mild symptomatic hypocalcaemia on the second and third postoperative days. This does not usually require treatment. In some patients with profound hypocalcaemia it may be necessary to infuse calcium gluconate intravenously and start oral calcium supplements and calciferol or 1 α-hydroxy-cholecalciferol. Permanent hypocalcaemia is rare, occurring in less than 5% of cases.

Persistent and recurrent hypercalcaemia

Following cervical exploration for presumed primary hyperparathyroidism, 90% of patients will be cured and return of plasma calcium levels to normal occurs. Persistent elevation of plasma calcium may be due to inappropriate operation for non-parathyroid disease, the presence of supernumerary glands, or failure to identify an abnormal gland in an ectopic site. This problem rarely arises when the hypercalcaemia is associated with a solitary adenoma, but is more frequently seen in the presence of multiple adenomas or hyperplasia of all four glands or where resection has been inadequate. This problem has been noted in up to 15–18% of patients operated upon for hyperplasia and may occur as late as 20 years after the original operation.

Re-operation

The indications for operation in patients with persistent or recurrent hypercalcaemia are similar to those for primary disease. In asymptomatic patients an expectant policy is wise. Re-operations are technically more difficult, less likely to cure hypercalcaemia, and have significantly greater morbidity than primary explorations. These are particularly difficult cases to manage and CT arteriography and selective venous sampling for parathormone levels is necessary. CT scanning may occasionally pick up an unsuspected mediastinal adenoma, but is usually unhelpful in identifying small cervical glands. Selective arteriography may identify up to 70% of abnormal parathyroid glands and has the advantage that it may be possible to embolize ectopic adenomas and avoid further operation. Selective venous sampling can usually lateralize a tumour, but can only accurately localize it in about 50% of cases. If preoperative localization studies fail to identify a mediastinal gland, it is likely that the abnormal gland had been overlooked at the time of primary operation and lies within the neck. A second neck dissection is often difficult due to obliteration of tissue planes. In cases where a fourth parathyroid gland is still not found after a thorough search, ipsilateral thyroid lobectomy may be required.

Following re-operation approximately 20% of patients remain hypercalcaemic and up to 30% may be rendered permanently hypocalcaemic.

THYROID GLAND

Thyroid gland disease is common. Hypothyroidism is diagnosed in about 4% of females in UK and for malignancy, there are about 400 deaths per annum from thyroid tumours of all types. The metabolic rate of many tissues is controlled by the thyroid hormones and over activity and under activity of the gland are common clinical problems. The thyroid gland consists of two lateral lobes connected by an isthmus. It is attached to the thyroid cartilages and to the upper end of the trachea, and thus moves on swallowing. Embryologically it originates from the base of tongue and descends in the neck to its adult pre-tracheal position.

Biochemistry

Thyroxine (T4) and triiodothyronine are both produced by successive iodination of a tyrosine rich protein precursor in the follicular tissue. Most gland production is T4 but peripheral conversion to T3 is the main means of action at the tissues. Deactivation by conversion to reverse T3 (rT3) occurs. Thyroid hormone is 99% protein bound in plasma. Control of thyroid secretion is mediated via the hypothalamic pituitary thyroid axis. Hypothalamic TRH secretion stimulates anterior pituitary production and release of TSH. Peripheral blood TSH levels are inversely related to the levels of thyroid hormones released and this forms the basis of many thyroid function tests.

Thyroid function tests

Thyroid hormone uptake tests, TSH measurement and TRH test are the main aspects of functional testing in thyroid investigation. Immune screening for lytic or stimulating antibodies is also important. Interpretation of these tests can be complicated by chronic, intercurrent disease, pregnancy and the oral contraceptive pill, and certain drugs. These effects are due to changes in protein affinity and hormone binding as well as interference in production and secretion of the hormones. Examples of factors increasing TBG levels include pregnancy, phenothiazine and acute hepatitis. Factors resulting in depletion of TBG levels include androgens, corticosteroids, nephrotic syndrome and chronic liver disease. Altered protein affinity is associated with phenytoin and NSAID use.

Clinical management problems

Congenital abnormalities   *Dyshormonogenesis.* This may occur due to an inherited defect in production of one of the enzymes required in the pathway of hormone synthesis. Syndromic associations include Pendred's syndrome where congenital sensorineural deafness is associated with dyshormonogenesis. Treatment by hormone replacement is required.

Ectopia. Failures in migration of the thyroid primordia give rise to several anatomical abnormalities. Lingual thyroids, thyroglossal cysts and mediastinal goitres are all described.

Lateral aberrant thyroid. No longer considered to be a discrete entity, this condition is probably due to lymph node metastases from a well differentiated papillary thyroid carcinoma.

The solitary thyroid nodule

The management of the solitary nodule is aimed at exclusion of thyroid malignancy. Indirect or fibre-optic laryngoscopy to determine the condition of the vocal cords and hence of recurrent laryngeal nerve function is essential preoperatively. Investigation should include functional testing of the gland, ultrasound scanning, radionuclide scanning to ascertain the functional status of the nodule and FNA for cytology.

Functional solitary nodule If the patient is euthyroid with a functioning nodule on Te scanning the lesion can be kept under observation. Where the patient is thyrotoxic with a hot nodule the likely diagnosis is a toxic benign adenoma. Where the patient is clinically euthyroid with a warm nodule a policy of observation can be made. Where the nodule is non-functional the suspicion of malignancy is raised and further investigation is necessary.

Cold solitary nodule In addition to the above investigations a cold nodule should be subjected to ultrasound scanning and FNA cytology. If ultrasound scanning demonstrates the lesion to be cystic and FNA allows it to be emptied such that it becomes impalpable, a policy of observation and review can be adopted. If a cystic lesion cannot be emptied during FNA or if it recurs after 4–6 weeks resection should be planned. Thyroid lobectomy or hemithyroidectomy is the operation of choice.

If the lesion is non-cystic the differential diagnosis is benign follicular adenoma or carcinoma.

Intra-operative confirmation of diagnosis and the use of frozen section can help with refinement in surgical planning. If a solitary nodule is discovered to be multiple or multinodular at surgery, most surgeons would proceed with subtotal lobectomy. Frozen section of a confirmed solitary nodule can reveal a variety of non-malignant pathology. Benign adenomata of several cellular types can occur. Papillary, follicular, Hurthle cell and fetal patterns are all described. Local areas of focal cystic degeneraton (false adenomata) can also occur. Autoimmune thyroiditis and secondary malignancy can also present in this way.

Thyroid carcinoma

Several histological types of thyroid carcinoma are described.

Papillary carcinoma
Accounts for 70% of all thyroid tumours and occurs in young patients, usually within the first 30 years of life. Relatively slow growing it has a predilection for local and adjacent node metastasis. Lung and bone are also sites of predilection. It has a good prognosis after resection with a 5 year survival of 90% and little reduction of this figure at 10 years. Thyroid hormone replacement is important postoperatively to suppress residual tumour growth. It is debatable how radical the excision should be. The options are subtotal thyroidectomy with re-implantation of parathyroid or less radical lobectomy and partial lobectomy on the contralateral side.

Follicular carcinoma
About 20% of thyroid tumours are of this type. Its commonest age of presentation is 30–50 years and it is more frequent in females. It carries a 5 year survival of about 60% and a 10 year figure of about 50%. Earlier venous spread than with papillary carcinoma is the case with these lesions and lung metastases are commoner. A more radical approach is justified due to the rather poorer prognosis with total thyroidectomy and neck dissection if there is lymph node metastasis clinically or on CT scanning. Parathyroid re-implantation and postoperative radioiodine to suppress residual thyroid tumour tissue is normal.

Anaplastic carcinoma	Accounting for less than 5% of tumours this lesion carries a very poor prognosis and palliative surgery to prevent respiratory obstruction may be required. External beam DXT is the usual treatment but the prognosis is little altered. This is a tumour of older patients.
Medullary carcinoma	A tumour arising in the parafollicular, calcitonin secreting C cells this lesion accounts for about 5% of thyroid tumours. These lesions usually secrete and high serum calcitonin can be used in diagnosis and postoperative follow up. It can occur sporadically as an isolated lesion or as part of the multiple endocrine neoplasia syndrome (MEN II or Sipple syndrome). The risk of associated phaeochromocytoma and neurofibromata affecting skin, tongue and GI tract tissues constitutes this syndrome and the dangers of phaeochromocytoma should be considered in surgical treatment planning.
	The thyroid lesion, whether isolated or Sipple syndrome related is an aggressive tumour and subtotal thyroidectomy with parathyroid preservation and neck dissection is advocated for both sorts although the sporadic sort is considered the more aggressive pattern. Five year survival is less than 50%.
Lymphoma	Although commoner in older patients, primary lymphoid malignancy can affect any age group. It is usually seen in association with longstanding autoimmune, Hashimoto's thyroiditis. It responds well to radiotherapy with adjuvant chemotherapy. Its prognosis is dependent on its histological subtype and the clinical stage at presentation. Surgery should be reserved for relief of respiratory compression or obstruction.

Multinodular goitre

Differentiation of the various patterns of goitre is necessary. Physiological goitre refers to the benign reversible thyroid enlargement associated with adolescence particularly in females and in pregnancy. Endemic goitre in geographic regions of low iodine levels in the public water supply do occur and too rapid replacement of dietary iodine supplement may provoke thyrotoxicosis. Sporadic goitre may occur in non-goitrous regions and is unrelated to iodine deficiency. Dietary substances decreasing the bioavailability of iodine have been identified but in most patients the cause of their goitre is unknown. There is a slightly increased risk of carcinoma in these patients. Drugs such as sulphonylureas can induce goitre formation and acute thyroiditis, autoimmune thyroid disease, as well as simple colloid cysts can all induce gland enlargement. Rarities such as tuberculosis and sarcoidosis can present in this fashion.

The commonest thyroid enlargement is the multinodular or non-toxic nodular goitre. It is commoner in older women and requires investigation if thyroid function is abnormal or respiratory tract compression occurs. Poor aesthetics may prompt referral for treatment. Investigation therefore involves radiography for tracheal compression and mediastinal extension, biochemical and immunology screening and radionuclide functional testing to isolate cold areas which arouse suspicion of malignancy. Ultrasound and FNA cytology of such areas is warranted and surgery may be required if suspicious cytology is found or if tracheal compression requires it.

Disorders of thyroid function

Hypothyroidism

Hypothyroidism can be primary or secondary. The causes of primary hypothyroidism include congenital gland agenesis or presence of ectopic thyroid remnants, defective hormone synthesis due to drugs, iodine deficiency or dyshormonogenesis, autoimmune disease such as graves or Hashimoto's diseases, infection, surgery and neck irradiation, and tumour infiltration. Secondary hypothyroidism can arise due to hypopituitarism or TSH deficiency.

Symptoms of primary hypothyroidism include tiredness, malaise, weight gain, anorexia, cold intolerance, poor memory and cognitive defects, depression, psychosis (myxoedema madness), coma, deafness, poor libido, dry hair and coarse skin, arthralgia, myalgia, constipation, menorrhagia or oligomenorrhoea. Symptoms of other autoimmune diseases may be present.

In addition, other abnormalities may be present and include organ specific antibodies to other tissues, a resistant normocytic, normochromic anaemia, although the anaemia may be macrocytic if pernicious anaemia is present in association or iron deficiency pattern in women with menorrhagia. Increased ADH secretion and hyponatraemia may be present and liver enzymes particularly AST may be elevated.

Treatment with replacement hormone therapy is required in most patients The adequacy of this therapy is assessed by clinical examination and T3, T4 and TSH estimations. Slow initiation of replacement is required in patients with ischaemic heart disease.

Screening for infantile hypothyroidism is routine in UK using the Guthrie test. The incidence is about 1:3500 live births and undiagnosed can lead to severe neurological and growth impairment.

Hyperthyroidism

Two to 5% of females are affected but occurrence in males is rare. Most cases arise due to primary thyroid disease and secondary lesions due to pituitary causes are very rare. The causes include Graves autoimmune thyroid disease, toxic nodular adenoma, multinodular goitre, acute thyroiditis, and factitious hormone excess, HCG secreting tumours or ovarian teratomas.

Symptoms include weight loss, increased appetite, anorexia in some, irritability, restlessness, malaise, muscle weakness, tremor, choreoathetosis, breathlessness, palpitations, heat intolerance, vomiting, diarrhoea, goitre, oligomenorrhoea, loss of libido, gynaecomastia, onycholysis, tall stature (in children). The ophthalmopathy of hyperthyroidism occurs only with Graves disease.

Thyroid crisis is a rare condition of rapid worsening of the hyperthyroid state with hyperpyrexia, tachycardia and severe restlessness. It carries a mortality of 10% and can occur postoperatively. Immediate administration of propranolol, potassium iodide and steroids is life saving.

Treatment includes antithyroid drugs, such as carbimazole and use of β blockade for symptomatic relief of cardiovascular problems (except in asthmatics). Agranulocytosis in some can complicate the use of carbimazole. In patients where a large goitre is present, or who suffer toxic effects of antithyroid medication or in whom recurrent symptoms occur in spite of maximal medical therapy, subtotal thyroidectomy can be considered. The patient must be euthyroid immediately preoperatively. Radioiodine retains a place in the management of hyperthyroidism. Graves ophthalmopathy may require surgery. Tarsorraphy, or orbital decompression may be required.

Autoimmunne thyroid disease

1. Autoimmune thyroiditis results in lymphoid infiltration of the gland and follicular architecture destruction with a variable degree of fibrotic scarring. A spectrum of severity is recognized. Hashimoto's thyroiditis can result in severe damage to the gland parenchyma but with a very variable pattern of functional disturbance. Most frequently a mild hypothyroid state exists. Graves disease is related to thyroid stimulating humoral factors presumed to be antibodies. A direct causal role of the autoantibodies in gland destruction is unlikely but their occurrence is an epiphenomenon. The stimulating effects of the humoral antibodies in Graves disease is well established.

2. Riedel's thyroiditis. A very rare presentation of dense thyroid fibrosis, it is reported to present with compressive symptoms. Although associated with sclerosing cholangitis a definite autoimmune basis is disputed.

3. Subacute (DeQuervain's) thyroiditis. Preempted by an acute flu like illness with neck and ear pain and a thyroid gland that is tender to palpation this disease is usually self limiting. Presumed to be of viral origin, a transient hypothyroid state is sometimes associated with it. Occasionally it runs a recurrent course and steroids are reported to reduce the severity and frequency of recurrence.

TISSUE SAMPLING TECHNIQUES

Microscopic examination of isolated cells or excised tissue samples is central to the diagnosis of many surgical conditions. Exclusion of malignancy is the principle reason for most such investigations. Microbial identification and determination of drug sensitivity is also important.

Cytology

1. Fine needle aspiration cytology (FNAC). Blind or guided by ultrasound, CT or MRI imaging techniques. Readily performed under LA. Soft tissue masses, salivary gland lesions, suspected lymph node metastatic disease and tumour recurrences may all be diagnosed by this means. The fear of seeding malignant cells into the needle track is much less than with core needle biopsies. The technique is therefore widely applicable to head and neck lesions.

2. Brushings and scrapings from superficial mucosal lesions may yield useful diagnostic data.

3. Aspiration of tissue fluids, pus or fluid collections can be submitted to cytological examination. After neck surgery particularly in malignant disease, postoperative fluid filled collections can be tapped and the presence of malignant cells identified.

4. Endoscopic aspiration or surface brushings or washings are used extensively in respiratory and upper gastrointestinal disease but less commonly as yet in oropharyngeal lesions.

5. Salivary washings and imprint cytology are readily applied to head and neck lesions.

Biopsy

1. Comparison with FNAC. Biopsy techniques provide cells with retention of normal tissue architecture. Abnormal cellular form and mitoses may be identified as with FNAC but so may invasion and breach of normal tissue planes and barriers such as basement membranes. Permeation of lymphatics, perineural spread and venous invasion may all be diagnosed by biopsy rather than using FNAC. Biopsy is a more invasive technique and may require open operation if salivary or lymphoid tissue is required. Anatomical planes may be breached and tumour spread may result if biopsy is performed far in advance of the opportunity for definitive treatment of malignant disease. Histological and cytological examination require different skills in pathological staff. Frozen section techniques are available to permit intra-operative determination of disease extent and marginal clearance of tumour.

2. Biopsy techniques. Punch, drill and core needle techniques ('TruCut') are all described.

When using core techniques, track markers may be placed although FNAC techniques are preferred in head and neck surgery. Guidance for sampling deep tissues such as lymph nodes may require screening X-rays, ultrasound or CT scanning.

Microscopy

1. Microbiology. Visual identification of micro-organisms, supravital staining of fresh slides, identification of pus cells and mononuclear lymphocytes are all possible and useful in diagnosis of infective disease from samples of body fluids, fluid collections and pus. Evidence for infections caused by bacteria, fungi, protozoa and tuberculosis may be available from microscopic examination of cultures or cultured micro-organisms. Gram staining is capable of rapid exclusion of life-threatening organisms such as *Neisseria meningitidis*. Thick and thin films are required for identification of malarial organisms. Live protozoal infestations may be diagnosed from microscopic examination of facial skin scrapings. Phase contrast or dark ground microscopy permit visualization and identification of spirochaetal organisms in syphillis.

Microbial storage, transport and culture media require specific attention if evidence of specific organisms is not to be destroyed. Staining and demonstration of sensitivities to antibiotics are important.

2. Immunopathology. Immunocytochemical staining of mucosal samples in patients with inflammatory lesions may demonstrate autoimmune damage. Benign mucous membrane pemphigoid, pemphigus vulgaris, erythema multiforme may all exhibit adsorption of antisera to autoantibodies. Anti-basement membrane, anti-desmosomal and anti-nucleolar antibodies are often sought. A more complete profile of autoimmune disease is possible and serum assays should be performed concomittantly. Demonstration of cell-surface antigenic determinants and the use of RIA and ELISA techniques is of relevance in patients with hypersensitivity or atopy. Monoclonal antibodies in diagnostic work are increasingly important.

Lymphoma subclasses are determined by use of immunocytochemical staining.

Electron microscopy

Visualizing viral particles requires high-resolution microscopy and high magnification. Preparation of tissue for electron microscopy requires microtomed sections and coating with metallic film. Transmission or scanning techniques are available.

Subcellular organelles may be visualised and autoradiography is used for research purposes.

Flow cytometry

Analytical techniques for determination of DNA content and maturity of malignant cells include flow cytometry and gel elctrophoresis. Polar blotting assays and use of restriction fragment length polymorphisms permits DNA 'fingerprinting'. Increasing use of new molecular genetic techniques is becoming relevant to head and neck surgery and management of patients with head and neck malignant disease.

Clinical genetics

Karyotyping is relevant from buccal mucosal scrapings or from peripheral blood lymphocytes in diagnosis of chromosomal abnormalities. Genetic counselling is only accurate with the availability of this sort of data.

TMJ DYSFUNCTIONAL DISORDERS

This group of TMJ disorders are those without demonstrable joint pathology but marked symptoms. They comprise masticatory muscle dysfunction and disc interference disorders.

There have been many descriptions, classifications and theories about functional masticatory disorders. The determinants of normal occlusion, resting muscle fibre length, mandibular rest position and pattern of masticatory movements have all been extensively investigated. Activity of the masticatory system can be functional, adaptive or parafunctional.

Normal functional activity May be summarized as mandibular closure occurring with the condyles starting in the most infero–anterior position with the discs properly interposed generating even and simultaneous dental occlusal contacts without interference. Rest position involves positioning the condyle in its most superior position, with freeway space between dental occlusal surfaces and with masticatory muscle fibres at the optimum fibre length. Muscle spindle activity will then be minimal.

Adaptive function Occurs when the 'perfection' of the normally functioning system is perturbed but the patient remains symptom free and function continues without deterioration in the masticatory tissues. Whether adaptation carries a significant risk of long term damage and arthritic consequences is not clear.

Parafunctional disorders Occur where oral habits or grinding occur and abnormal movements are performed frequently and repeatedly. Nocturnal bruxism is a good example. Increased force in occlusal contact, eccentric mandibular closing and non-physiological isometric muscle contraction characterize parafunctional activity.

The muscle disorders

Reflex muscle splinting *Protective trismus.* A clear antecedent history is usually present. History is acute, short in duration and muscle tenderness to palpation is obvious. Muscle fibre hyperactivity and muscle stiffness with secondary occlusal abnormalities may be apparent. No mechanical

	obstruction to mandibular movement is demonstrable. Analgesia and reassurance is often all that is required.
Trismus or myospasm	Trauma, local sepsis and chronic pain all contribute to the genesis of trismus. Where local conditions inducing pain responses are occurring, for instance dental pain or pulpitis, treatment of these factors will usually resolve the masticatory muscle disorder.
Myofascial pain or trigger point syndrome	Regional muscular ache with hypersensitive areas or trigger points. Continuous dull pain is typical. Localized tenderness in specific muscle groups and trigger zones may be demonstrable. Association with parafunctional habits or recent trauma may be present. The association with URTI or nutritional deficits is less clearly defined. Treatment of trigger zones with coolant sprays, TENS or injected local anaesthesia and sometimes physiotherapy are all of documented benefit in some patients.
Myositis	Inflammation of muscle is uncommon. It may be associated with neck space or fascial plane infection or localized dentoalveolar sepsis. Connective tissue disease may have an element of chronic myositis associated with it. Treatment of sepsis by antibiotics or surgical drainage is usually curative in patients with neck or facial abscesses. Supportive therapy with anti-inflammatory drugs and occlusal disengagement may help in the initial phase. Steroids and anti-rheumatic agents may be required in connective tissue pattern myositis.
Contracture	Painless limitation of mandibular excursion. Fibrosis and scarring occurs. Chronic spasm, sepsis, radiotherapy, ischaemia and surgery may all be associated.
Hypertrophy	Painless generalized enlargement of muscle fibres. Minimal interference or limitation of mandibular movement only. Cosmetic request for treatment may be reason for the patient's presentation. Surgical reduction is possible.
Neoplasms	Uncommon. Myxoma, rhabdomyoma, rhabdomyo-sarcoma may all occur. Muscle malignancy carries very poor prognosis.

Disc interference disorders

Functional derangement of the condyle–disc complex occurs because the supporting ligaments are stretched, ineffective. The disc itself may be atrophic. The commonest cause is trauma; either associated with facial injury or with chronic occlusal dysharmony. Class II malocclusions are more often associated than other patterns.

There are three basic patterns of disc interference disorder described. Disc displacements, disc dislocation with spontaneous reduction and disc dislocation without reduction. Some include the derangement in meniscal behaviour due to adhesions in this group of TMJ disorders.

Clinical findings

The chief clinical stigmata are loud joint noises sometimes associated with restricted movements or 'locking'. There are numerous descriptions of the detailed patterns of joint sounds heard during mandibular movement in patients with different patterns of disc interference disorders. The reliability of very detailed diagnosis based on joint auscultation as the principal tool is likely to be suspect. MRI imaging has not proved to be as accurate an investigational tool as was first thought likely.

Treatment

There are many described treatments, each of which has its advocates, its evangelists and its detractors. The mainstay of any therapy is drug treatment to aid resolution of the acute phase and simple appliance therapy to overcome the malpositioning of the condyle–disc complex in relation to the glenoid fossa. The details of the particular appliance used are dependent entirely on the surgeon's preference. Surgery is only rarely required in this group of patients and it cannot be guaranteed to produce full symptomatic relief in all those offered an operation. Some may be worse postoperatively.

TMJ – INTERNAL JOINT DERANGEMENT

Organic disease of the TMJ may arise from the effects of trauma, inflammatory lesions and structural joint abnormalities. There is considerable overlap with the disc interference pattern disorders and an element of dysfunctional pattern symptomatology may be associated with these conditions.

Causes

Effusions and haemarthroses *1. Traumatic effusions* may occur in relation to mandibular trauma. Associated condylar neck fractures should be excluded. Occasionally if tense and marked limitation of mandibular opening is present, an aseptic aspiration of the effusion will produce pain relief and quickly restore a degree of function.

2. Haemarthroses. Either traumatic in origin or related to a clotting diathesis.

Structural abnormalities of the articular surfaces The TMJ has a superior and inferior joint compartment. Congenital abnormalities of condylar head anatomy are described but are rare. Bifid condyles are described for example. Meniscal abnormalities occur and the most common is a traumatic perforation. Glenoid fossa abnormalities may present as recurrent dislocation or an arthropathy if the articular eminence form is excessively flat or if osteophyte formation occurs. In children impairment of mandibular growth may occur. In adults dysfunctional symptoms are commonly associated. The definitive treatment is usually surgical. A variety of different patterns of arthroplasty are described and meniscal disease may be treated by repair or excision. Meniscectomy is a radical option and reconstruction using a temporalis muscle flap or alloplastic implant may be considered.

Intracapsular adhesions Adhesions may occur after haemarthrosis, after joint surgery or as a result of another structural derangement such as a meniscal perforation. Disc–condyle adhesions and posterior disc to glenoid adhesions are described. The diagnosis is suggested by a history of abnormal pattern of mandibular movements. Physiotherapy may help and a variety of appliances are described in an attempt to restore a normal path of mandibular excursion. Occasionally surgery for adhesiolysis may be required.

Arthropathies

1.   Inflammatory joint disease may present in the TMJ. Rheumatoid disease affects the TMJ in about 15% af patients but rarely affects the joint in isolation. Juvenile chronic rheumatoid arthritis (Still's disease) may produce severe arthritis and mandibular growth retardation. Secondary arthritis may occur in relation to inflammatory bowel disease, dermatological disease such as psoriasis, other connective tissue disorders and occasionally with sexually acquired infections. Syndromes such as Beçhet's are associated with a 'flitting' arthropathy and acute arthritis may occur in association with rheumatic fever or endocarditis.

2.   Osteo-arthritis may affect the TMJ particularly as an end stage condition as a result of trauma, chronic dysfunctional or parafunctional damage or inflammatory disease.

3.   Osteochondritis. Occasionally the TMJ may be affected by osteochondritis dessicans. This condition typically affects younger people and causes joint discomfort and limitation of movement. Occasional effusions occur in association. The presentation of loose bodies within the joint may suggest that a 'burnt out' osteochondritic process.

4.   Crystal deposition arthropathy. This group of conditions includes monosodium urate deposition (gout), calcium pyrophosphate and hydroxyapatite deposition diseases. Acute gout may be precipitated by surgery in hyperuricaemic patients, by chemotherapy in malignant disease, by starvation or dietary excess, or dehydration and some drugs such as thiazide diuretics. Although classically it affects the joints of the extremities, gout of the TMJ is described. Allopurinol given under cover of a NSAID such as indomethacin is the drug treatment of choice. Weight loss, dietary modification, withdrawal of thiazides and salicylates are required in conjunction.

Differential diagnosis

Preauricular pain presumed to arise from TMJ disease must be diagnosed only after exclusion of other pathology.

- *Odontogenic.* Dental alveolar pain may mimic TMJ pain. OPG aids exclusion of lesions of the mouth or jaws and their treatment is required as part of the management of the presenting condition.
- *Otological.* Although the concept of Costen's syndrome (ear pain and dizziness related to TMJ dysfunction) is not universally accepted, if ear disease is present, particularly chronic inflammatory otological disease, pre-auricuar pain almost indistinguishable from TMJ related pain may be present.
- *Salivary glands.* Parotid tumours particularly adenoid cystic carcinoma must be excluded before making the diagnosis of TMJ disease. Inflammatory parotid lesions may cause similar pain to TMJ dysfunction.
- *Vascular.* Migrainous pain may occur in the midface. Although classically periodic migrainous neuralgia affects the periorbital region, it may also present with episodic pre-auricular pain. Giant cell arteritis may cause masticatory claudication and should be excluded by arterial biopsy if suspected.
- *Neurogenic.* Trigeminal neuralgia of the maxillary division of the trigeminal nerve may occur and although different in character from dysfunctional TMJ pain may be less easy to distinguish from a severe arthritic episode.
- *Referred pain.* Pain referral to the ear and pre-auriucular region may occur from infiltrating malignancies of the oral floor, tongue base, tonsillar fossa and supraglottic larynx. Arthritic changes in the joints of the cervical spine may cause a mid or lower facial pain sometimes confused with TMJ like pain.

Diagnosis

In addition to clinical examination of the head and neck specific diagnostic investigations may be required.

Serology   Laboratory investigation of the inflammatory and crystal deposition arthropathies requires appropriate biochemical and immunological investigations.

Imaging   *1.   Plain TMJ films.* Several views are available. Transpharyngeals in both open and closed views, transorbitals and reverse Townes views may reveal gross bony pathology around the joint but are relatively crude diagnostic instruments.

2. MRI scanning. Although good soft tissue images may be obtained, the concern is repeatedly expressed about the apparent poor correlation of MRI appearances with symptoms or operative findings. It is uncertain how useful this investigative tool will turn out to be once sufficient experience with its use for TMJ investigation has been gained.

Arthrography   Less widely performed than MRI scanning. The images obtained by sterile introduction of a radio-opaque dye into the joint spaces are nevertheless good diagnostic information.

Arthroscopy   TMJ arthroscopy requires dedicated rigid endoscopes and a significant investment in equipment, training and commitment to development of this sort of service. Diagnostic and interventional arthroscopy is possible and access to both joint spaces is described. Whether the very high incidence amongst patients with TMJ pain of dysfunctional rather than frankly organic disease should suggest that frequent use of arthroscopy is wise or not remains an open debate.

Treatment

Conservative   *1.   Medical.* Analgesia, muscle relaxant therapy and NSAIDs all find uses.

2. Appliances. Many designs are described. They are less useful in this group of patients than in those with dysfunctional symptoms.

3. Physiotherapy. Short wave diathermy, local heat and exercise regimens may all be of benefit.

Surgery

1. Arthrocentesis. Joint lavage with sterile saline may have the effect of reducing the intrasynovial concentration of inflammatory mediators and so reduce symptoms. It may be more effective in this group of patients than in others. Infiltration of the joint with a mixture of corticosteroids and local anaesthesia after lavage produces long term benefit in some patients.

2. Meniscal surgery. Repair of perforations, plication or excision may be performed depending on the precise diagnosis. Open or arthroscopic approaches are described.

3. Condyle surgery. Removal of tissue from the condylar head, whether a limited articular reduction, condylotomy or condylectomy, is arguably more justified in patients with demonstrable internal joint derangements than in those with pure dysfunctional symptoms. It is the use of surgery to the condyle in this latter group of patients which has led to TMJ surgery acquiring the stigma of an inappropriate therapeutic approach.

4. Joint replacement. Much less commonly performed in the UK than in the USA, this technique has associated with it some very widely publicized problems; most notably the catastrophic failures and demands by many patients for removal of their prostheses in the USA.

Related topics of interest

TMJ dysfunctional disorders (p. 403)
TMJ mobility disorders (p. 411)

Revision point

Anatomy and embryology of the TMJ

TMJ MOBILITY DISORDERS

This group of disorders includes those which limit mouth opening and those which result in excess mandibular excursion. Haematoma, local sepsis and mandibular trauma all limit the range and extent of mouth opening that is possible. Trismus is reflex muscle spasm and usually occurs as a response to local injury or infection. Periarticular disease with sepsis, haematoma formation, mandibular neck fracture or injection of local anaesthetic solution into muscle may all provoke and trismus.

Ankylosis

True joint pathology with fibrous or bony union of the condyle to the glenoid denotes ankylosis.

Definitions

1. Ankylosis. Fusion of the bone joint and articular surfaces occurs. Severe limitation of mouth opening results.

2. Pseudoankylosis. More commonly due to extra-articular lesions. Fibrous capsulitis, depressed zygomatic arch fractures and myositis ossificans may cause this pattern of ankylosis.

3. Trismus. Reflex muscle spasm due to trauma, sepsis, intramuscular haematoma or adjacent fracture.

Aetiology

1. Childhood trauma. The well-recognized sequence of blunt trauma to the chin followed by intracapsular 'burst' pattern fracture and long term growth impedance may be associated with TMJ ankylosis. Condylar neck fracture if treated by immobilization carries an increased risk of ankylosis.

2. Still's disease (juvenile chronic arthritis) and rheumatoid arthritis. Juvenile oligarticular rheumatoid disease results in chronic joint damage and deformity and consequent limitation of mandibular growth. Adult rheumatoid arthritis affects the TMJ in about 50% of patients.

3. Joint infection. Septic arthritis and tuberculous arthritis in the tropics are important causes of ankylosis.

4. TMJ tumours. Villonodular synovitis is only rarely associated with joint hypomobility. Malignancy may provoke trismus and occasionally radiotherapy may be a cause of ankylosis.

5. Mastoid disease. Although of historical interest only, mastoiditis is associated with severe trismus.

Classification
- Type I – flattened condylar head and limited joint space.
- Type II – bony fusion at outer articular margins.
- Type III – bone fusion between mandibular ramus and zygomatic arch.
- Type IV – entire joint replacement by bone tissue.

Treatment

Surgery is the mainstay of treatment.

Incisions
A pre-auricular approach is generally preferred. Post-auricular or endaural approaches are described but are less frequently used.

Gap arthroplasty
Either a condylar neck osteotomy or high condylar osteotomy increases the vertical dimension of the joint space and creates a new 'joint cavity'.

Excision arthroplasty
Block excision of a bony ankylosis effectively destroys the articulation but permits movement. Extensive bone resection may be required and the risks to the adjacent carotid vessels may be significant. Correction of bony ankylosis may expose the middle cranial fossa as the glenoid requires re-fashioning.

Interpositional grafts
Where meniscal damage has occurred or resection has been necessary, interpositional grafts are a well described means of preventing re-ankylosis. Silastic, pinna cartilage, temporalis muscle and fascia lata have all been used.

Prosthetic joint replacement Several proprietary prosthetic TMJ systems are available.

Costochondral grafts
In childhood ankylosis with evidence of progressive growth impedance, a functional, growth permitting replacement for the mandibular condyle can be

fashioned from a costochondral graft. Bilateral costochondral grafts may be required in juvenile chronic arthritis to ensure symmetrical mandibular growth. Once *in situ*, normal mandibular growth can be expected in about 50–60% of cases. A few patients exhibit excess mandibular growth and in about 25% the mandible fails to grow at all.

Coronoidectomy

Excision of the coronoid process may be required during surgery for TMJ ankylosis. Usually performed via an intraoral route, improvement in net mandibular movement can be gained in excess of that derived from the primary joint operation.

Adjuncts

Physiotherapy is important in the postoperative period.

Recurrent mandibular dislocation

Acute mandibular dislocation occurs occassionally with minor trauma and in patients with conjenital joint laxity.

Diagnosis

1. The clinical features of chronic or recurrent dislocation of the temporomandibular joint include hypermobility, subluxation and reducible or irreducible dislocation.

2. Aetiology. Often unclear but may include psychogenic or occlusal factors. In the elderly drug induced dystonias may be implicated. Most cases are idiopathic.

Non-surgical treatment

1. Reduction of acute dislocations is performed under liberal local anaesthetic and if necessary, using intravenous sedation. There are several techniques described for manipulation. One technique involves the surgeon positioned behind the patient and applying firm downward traction of the palpable dislocated condylar heads.

2. Chronic and recurrent dislocations may occur and reduce spontaneously. In some patients, remedial exercises encourage reduction of frequent dislocations.

3. Other measures. Physiotherapy and revision of drug treatment may be of benefit. Chemical capsullorraphy and arthroscopic sclerotherapy have been used with reports of success.

Surgical treatment
1. Soft tissue surgery. Interposition of muscle or fascia around the anterior face of the condylar neck or surgical construction of muscle slings using temporalis fibres is described.

2. Eminectomy. Exposure and reduction of the bony eminentia articularis is performed with a view to removal of the anterior limit of the glenoid fossa. Although foward positioning of the condylar head is possible there is no block to its posterior movement during mouth closing. Dislocation is therefore no longer possible.

3. Dautrey procedure. Downward fracture of a segment of the zygomatic arch augments the bulk and steepness of the slope of the articular eminence. Dislocation is prevented.

4. Bone grafts. Augmentation of the articular eminence may be achieved using bone grafting techniques.

Related topics of interest

Bone grafts (p. 25)
Mandibular surgery (p. 238)
TMJ dysfunctional disorders (p. 403)

Revision points

Physiology of mouth opening and closing
Principles of joint disease
TMJ anatomy

TRACHEOSTOMY

A tracheostomy is a surgically created portal into the anterior wall of the subcricoid trachea. There are several different types of openings into the trachea. Tracheotomy by distinction is a simple incision through the subcricoid trachea. Cricothyrotomy and laryngotomy involve incision through or puncture into the cricothyroid membrane. A tracheostome is a permanent stoma fashioned after laryngectomy.

Functions of tracheostomy

To bypass upper airway
Congenital lesions, such as pharyngeal webs, tracheal stenoses, trauma to face, tongue, neck and larynx and foreign bodies may all constitute indications for emergency tracheostomy. Inflammation and infection such as Ludwig's angina, epiglottitis, laryngotracheobronchitis and diphtheria as well as burns and ingestion of corrosives may all constitute a threat to airway patency. Tumours of larynx, pharynx, thyroid and bilateral adductor vocal cord paralysis may all result in a need for planned tracheostomy.

Facilitate assisted ventilation
Tracheostomy will decrease anatomical dead space by up to 50%, reduce airway resistance, protect against aspiration by provision of a cuffed tracheostomy tube, and will permit suction and bronchial toilet. It is a useful technique in pre-term infants, patients with head injuries, burns of the face and neck, overdoses, and patients with severe chest wall injuries.

As part of another surgical procedure
Important in laryngectomy and head and neck tumour surgery.

After an unsuccessful extubation or decannulation
May be necessary, especially in children.

Techniques

Tracheostomy may be peformed under local or general anaesthesia. The patient is positioned with full neck extension. The skin incision is made and deepened through platysma and deep cervical fascia. The pre-tracheal fascia is incised and the thyroid isthmus is either retracted out of the operative field or divided. The incision should be vertical in the emergency situation or when performed by the surgically inexperienced. For surgeons, the horizontal incision is preferred. In children under 10, tracheotomy only, rather than full tracheostomy is performed with a simple incision through the second tracheal ring. In adults a formal fenestration is often required with a ring of tracheal tissue being removed. A Bjork flap is an option in adults with a tracheal fenestration performed but retaining an attached tracheal flap inferiorly. Stay sutures are useful in adults and mandatory in infants. The tracheostomy tube is secured with skin sutures and tapes and dressing are placed as required.

Percutaneous techniques are available and most often performed by anaesthetists. A Seldinger technique is employed with percutaneous puncture of the trachea and dilatation of the track prior to insertion of the tracheostomy tube. In head and neck surgery, formal surgical tracheostomy remains the preferred option in most units.

Postoperative care

Nursing	Most patients are comfortable nursed in the sitting position.
Cuff care and suction	Regular and frequent suction and cuff deflation every 15 minutes are important measures to prevent crusting and tracheal stenosis.
Humidification	Humidified, inspired gases administered via a T-piece or mask are employed to prevent drying, crusting and cilial paralysis. Warm or cold water atomizers may be used.
Tube change	The initial tube change is usually performed within 48 hours (24 hours in some units). However, it is not mandatory and if all is well the first tube may remain for up to 7 days. Thereafter it will need changing regularly.
Feeding	Dysphagia is common after tracheostomy. Formal nasogastric tube feeding may be required initially.
Speech	Tubes which are planned as longer term measures can be replaced with siver or plastic outer tubes which will house an inner tube with a speaking valve. In short term tracheostomies, the patient can be encouraged to speak during periods of cuff deflation by finger occlusion of the tube orifice.
Sutures	Wound sutures should be removed after 5–7 days but the stay sutures should remain, especially in children.

Tracheostomy removal and wound closure

Trials of tube occlusions should be performed and gradually increased in duration. When the patient can tolerate 12 hours with the tube occluded, formal removal can be planned. Even in those with tracheostomies the track will close rapidly in a matter of days with an airtight dressing.

Complications

- Haemorrhage
- Infection
- Tube displacement
- Surgical emphysema
- Pneumothorax or pneumomediastinum
- Tracheal stenosis
- Dysphagia

Tracheostome

There are a number of important distinctions to be made between those with a tracheostomy and those with a post-laryngectomy stoma. Post-laryngectomy patients have no communication from their pharynx to their lower airway and they usually need no indwelling tube. Loss of the larynx requires extensive rehabilitation to achieve acceptable speech. There are several devices available including hand held amplification devices, implantable valves and tracheostome washers.

Related topic of interest

Neurology of the head and neck (p. 275)

TUMOURS OF THE PHARYNX

Anatomically the pharynx is divided into three sub-sections; naso-pharynx, oro-pharynx, and hypo-pharynx. The subdivisions are useful because both pathologically and surgically the three sites are very different in the tumours which may present and in the treatment options used. In excess of 90% of pharyngeal tumours are squamous carcinomas. Non-Hodgkin's lymphomas account for 7 or 8% and minor salivary gland lesions for the remainder.

Oro-pharynx

Anatomy

The oro-pharynx extends craniocaudally from the hard palate at the upper limit to the level of the hyoid bone inferiorly. Its anterior limits are the faucial pillars and the retromolar trigone. For purposes of pathological description it has an anterior wall comprising the base of the tongue, the lateral wall comprising the anterior pillar of the fauces or palatal glossal fold, the posterior palatopharyngeal fold and the tonsil. The roof is formed by the soft palate and its musculature and the posteror wall extends down the posterior pharyngeal wall from the level of hard palate to the hyoid bone.

Tumours of the oro-pharynx Squamous carcinoma of the pharynx in the UK occurs at a rate of about 8 new cases per million per annum. The most significant aetiological factor is tobacco but ethanol is synergistic. Betel or araca nut chewing is a significant factor in the aetiology of carcinomas of the floor of the mouth but less so in the causation of oro-pharyngeal tumours. Distant metastases occur in approximate proportion to the depth of tumour invasion and lymphoid spread occurs in step-wise fashion from upper to lower cervical lymph nodes. Distinct from other head and neck tumours, 10% of patients have distant metastases at presentation; a higher rate than expected with other squamous carcinomas of the head and neck. Posterior triangle lymphadnopathy is related to a poorer prognosis and bilateral lymphatic drainage does occur with soft palate and base of tongue tumours.

Patterns of tumour spread Lateral wall tumours are most common and spread directly to the contiguous tissues of the retro-molar region and buccal mucosae. Lesions of the inferior pole of the tonsil are difficult to diagnose and 50% of patients have metastatic nodes at initial presentation. Base of tongue tumours frequently present late as they are asymptomatic until quite large. They spread anteriorly to the genioglossus region and quickly involve the entire tongue. Displacement and swelling of the tongue is often the presenting feature at this stage. Twenty per cent of patients may present with isolated cervical lymphadenopathy without an obvious primary lesion.

Soft palate tumours

Carcinoma of the soft palate occurs typically on the anterior surface. It may be heralded by many years of leucoplakia or lichen planus and is most common in heavy smokers. Half of the patients have cervical lymph nodes at presentation and 15% have bilateral nodes.

Minor salivary gland tumours

Soft palate tumours may be of salivary gland origin. Most are benign and typically pleomorphic in histology, however adenoid cystic carcinomas invading perineural lymphatics are well described and the rich innervation of this region provides a good route for tumour spread along the palatine and the dental nerves.

Clinical presentation. Chronic pharyngitis, referred otalgia or dysphagia are common complaints. Some present with leucoplakia, lichen planus or an ulcer. Other patients notice a mass in the neck.

Base of tongue tumours

These tumours often present very late with referred otalgia or deep pharyngitis. Forward displacement of the tongue by an infiltrating carcinoma occurs and approximately 70% of patients have metastatic nodal disease on initial presentation. Of those with nodal disease, 25% have bilateral neck nodes and 20% of patients with nodal disease with an occult primary tumour will subsequently be discovered to have tongue base lesions.

Lateral wall tumours

This region is the most common site for pharyngeal lesions. These tumours spread to the retromolar region, tongue and buccal tissues. Tumour spread to the pterygoid region and inferior alveolar nerve involvement produces pain, sensory disturbance and trismus. Over 50% of patients have positive neck lymph nodes at diagnosis and tonsillar lesions may remain occult with nodal disease until quite advanced.

Posterior wall tumours Uncommon lesions. They may be diagnosed as extensions from naso or hypopharyngeal disease. Bilateral neck nodes may be present.

Lymphomas These are typically non-Hodgkin's in pattern but unilateral enlargements in tonsils in young people may the herald the onset of Hodgkin's disease.

Investigation

Radiology *Plain radiographs.*

- *OPG.* To assess inferior alveolar nerve and mandibular bone involvement.
- *Chest X-ray.* Permits diagnosis of metastases, second primaries and as staging procedure in lymphoma.
- *CT scan.* Is a good method of determining the extent of disease.
- *MRI scan.* Assessment of degree of soft tissue invasion and presence and extent of neck nodal disease.

Endoscopy Panendoscopy including fibre-optic nasendoscopy and EUA with rigid pharyngolaryngoscopy and oesophagoscopy is useful. Endoscopic biopsy is possible.

Tissue diagnosis Incisional biopsy of the primary tumour, micro-biopsy at endoscopy or fine needle aspiration of cervical lymph nodes may all be required.

Base line laboratory investigations Routinely required preoperatively and as part of lymphoma assessment.

Principles of treatment

Treatment options for squamous carcinomas are determined by the patient's clinical state, age, concomitant medical condition, histological diagnosis of the tumour and its clinical stage.

Primary surgery	This modality yields an acceptable cure rate but high morbidity because the necessary excision of tongue and pharyngeal musculature during excision of the tumour commonly results in impairement of speech, swallowing and in overspill of salivary secretions into the chest. The 'commando' operation was first described as an operation for lateral wall tumours of pharynx.
Primary radiotherapy	This method results in an overall cure rate of 70% at 5 years but because many of these tumours present late as T3 or T4 lesions the results are often disappointing.
Base of tongue tumours	Extensive resection is often required due to the late presentation of the tumour. Curative surgery may require complete or subtotal glossectomy with extension of the excision margin inferiorly so close to the larynx that postoperative overspill of saliva is almost inevitable and laryngectomy has therefore to be considered as part of the excision. Radical neck dissection is frequently required. Reconstruction with pectoralis major or a free flap is possible.
Posterior wall tumours	In common with hypopharyngeal tumours, these lesions require pharyngolaryngectomy. These excisions are extensive operations and usually require reconstruction with gastric or colonic 'pull up' procedures. Free jejunal flaps are an option. If bulk is required, pectoralis major flaps are possible but subsequent surgical debulking may be required.
Soft palate tumours	The first line treatment is usually primary radiotherapy. Palate excision is possible but swallowing and speech is severely impaired postoperatively. Reconstruction with galeal pericranial flap is possible and temporary obturation is usually required.
Inoperable tumours	Tumour extension high into the nasopharynx, poor underlying medical condition, advanced metastatic disease or refusal for treatment suggest that the lesion should be considered inoperable.

Operations

'Commando' operation

1. *Acronym.* Combined mandible and oral cavity resection.

2. *Indications.* Squamous carcinoma of lateral wall with nodal disease, recurrent lateral wall or tonsil lesion after radiotherapy or minor salivary gland disease of pharynx.

3. *Preparations.* Perioperative hyperbaric oxygen if previous radiotherapy has been used. Tracheostomy and PEG.

4. *Incision.* Schöbinger or extended 'T' incision.

5. *Excision.* Hemimandible, attached muscles, tumour with adequate margin.

6. *Neck dissection.* Usually a radical dissection is required.

7. *Reconstruction.* Pectoralis major, deltopectoral, latissimus dorsi or contralateral tongue flap.

Complete glossolaryngectomy

1. *Preparations.* Tracheostomy and PEG.

2. *Incisions.* As for bilateral neck dissections.

3. *Approach.* Midline mandibulotomy, lateral commando pattern or trans-cervical approach.

4. *Excisions.* Standard laryngectomy in continuity with tongue and oral floor. A more limited glossectomy excising the tongue base to the pre-epiglottic space is possible. This preserves the larynx but the risk of aspiration remains.

Related topics of interest

Carcinoma of the oral floor and lower alveolus (p. 52)
Neck dissection (p. 267)
Reconstruction – principles (p. 323)

Revision point

Anatomy of the pharynx and larynx

VASCULAR LESIONS OF THE HEAD AND NECK

Atheroma

1. Carotid atheromatous plaques are very common in Western populations. These lesions occur in patients with an associated increase in risk for coronary, cerebrovascular and distal arterial disease.

2. Diabetes, smoking, hypertension and hyperlipidaemia all predispose. There is an associated risk of embolization of platelet and lipid rich tissue to the cerebral circulation. Transient ischaemic attacks (TIAs) and strokes may occur. Low dose aspirin, dipyridamole and warfarin are preventative.

3. The benefits of carotid endarterectomy in stroke prevention is disputed as the risk of stroke in the postoperative period is approximately equal to that of a patient who has already suffered an episode of TIA.

4. In maxillofacial surgery, the problems associated with extensive atheromatous vessels in a patient planned for tumour ablation and free flap reconstruction are considerable. The risks of myocardial infarction perioperatively are much increased in comparison with the non-affected population. The affected vessels, if required as recipients during free tissue transfer may mitigate against successful microvascular anastomosis.

Haemangiomata

1. Cavernous haemangiomata occur typically in young patients. They enlarge slowly throughout childhood and adolescence and can become very large. Extensive lesions may involve facial skin, oral and pharyngeal mucosa, larynx and bone. The lesions are liable to rupture and massive spontaneous haemorrhage is a risk. If GA or endotracheal intubation is required in patients with extensive oropharyngeal lesions, performing the intubation may itself provoke haemorrhage. Surgery may prove difficult and hazardous where complex vascular anatomy is present.

2. *Investigation*. CT or MRI scanning with enhancement will demonstrate the extent of the lesion. Angiography in conjunction with embolization is available in some centres.

3. *Embolization* requires radiological catheter insertion, angiography with non-oily contrast medium to demonstrate the details of vascular anatomy serving the lesion and injection of foam, polymeric material, wire mesh or coils. These materials occlude the feeding vessels and formation of a blood clot will complete this process of occlusion and result in shrinkage and involution of the haemangioma. Post-embolization excision and reconstruction of the defect may require use of local flaps or free tissue transfer.

4. *Capilliary haemangiomata*. These lesions may occur as isolated congenital lesions or as part of the Sturge–Weber anomaly. They may be extensive and disfiguring if the face is affected. Excision usually leaves unacceptable scarring although laser ablation is advocated by some.

Arteriovenous fistulae

There are several types including congenital, post-traumatic, iatrogenic or Pagetoid. These lesions may be high or low throughput. Cardiac failure may occur in Pagetoid type if the malformation is sufficiently extensive and of the high throughput type. Excision is possible with separation of the arterial and venous circulations. Interpositional fascia, fat or muscle may be required to prevent reformation. False aneurysm formation is associated with the post-traumatic type.

Glomus tumours

These are rare lesions. The tumour contains tissue of mixed cellular origin. Angiomatous and smooth muscle elements are present and the lesion may be tender due to abundant non-medullated neurones which are intermingled with the tumour cells.

Chemodectomas. Anatomically associated with the carotid and aortic bodies there is a variant involving the jugular and vagal bulbs. Lesions are usually non-chromaffin paraganglionomas and considered to be derived from the embryonic neural crest. They are related to the adrenal medullary lesions which secrete a variety of hormone-like agents. These latter lesions include neuroblastoma, ganglioneuroma and phaeochromocytoma. The non-chromaffin paraganglionomas present as pulsatile and expansile masses in the upper neck or as middle ear polyps. Intra-cranial presentation is described. Malignant variants are very rare. Excision may be required but these lesions are very vascular and biopsy should be avoided preoperatively. Excision may require intra-operative shunting.

Varicosities

Sublingual varicosities are common with increasing age, after excisional surgery and in alcoholics. They are of no significance and require no treatment.

Vascular neoplasms

Haemangiopericytoma, haemangiosarcoma and Kaposi's sarcoma may all occur in the head and neck. In patients with squamous cell malignancies, vascular invasion may occur and be diagnosed in the postoperative histology of the resected specimen. The prognosis is poor where this occurs. Some tumours exhibit a degree of angioblastosis and marked neovascularization is commonly apparent at excision or neck dissection. Obstruction of the superior vena cava or jugular venous system may occur if tumour extension is advanced. Facial oedema may be marked if this occurs. Involvement of the carotid arterial tree by adjacent malignancy may result in rupture or carotid 'blow out'. This is commonly a terminal event and appropriate analgesia and sedation may be required. Techniques for ligation under local anaesthesia are described and may be considered if the vascular event is due to radiation damage rather than involvement by tumour.

Vascular inflammation

Arteritides. Temporal arteritis, Wegener's granulomatosis and the collagen vascular disorders may all typically present with lesions in the head and neck. Post-radiotherapy radiation endarteritis is well described.

Investigations

- Doppler flow studies
- Duplex ultasound scans

- Digital subtraction angiography
- Gadolinium enhanced MRI scans

Operative techniques
- Vascular reconstruction
- Intra-operative hypothermia
- Intra-operative shunting

Related topics of interest

Imaging (p. 206)
Microvascular surgery (p. 256)

Revision points

Development of the vascular tree in the head and neck
Pathology of atheroma and arteritis

VELOPHARYNGEAL INCOMPETENCE

Intelligible speech requires an anatomically and functionally intact velopharyngeal sphincter. Normal separation of oral and nasal cavities is essential. The anatomical elements of the sphincter mechanism include soft palate, posterior and lateral pharyngeal wall musculature and Passavant's ridge. Soft palate elevation, reduction in pharyngeal lumen dimensions by lateral and posterior wall muscles and generation of intra-luminal negative pressure all improve the efficiency of vocal cord action and are all essential functional components for normal speech.

Velopharyngeal incompetence (VPI) is a clinical problem which arises due to a combination of anatomical, neuromuscular and psychological events.

Causes of VPI

1. Idiopathic muscle insufficiency. On endoscopy where posterior wall insufficiency occurs a slit-like orifice remains. With lateral muscle insufficiency, lateral port-like defects occur. Hypernasality of speech is common.

2. Congenital palatal length deficiency. It remains unclear whether the palate length or the overall pharyngeal volume is the problem. Neuromuscular function is usually normal in these patients.

3. Submucous clefts. This condition occurs where mucosal union of the palatal shelves has occurred but the muscle insertions are typical of a true cleft. The direction of muscle action during palatal shelf elevation produces a V-shaped midline cleft and the pharynx may fail to close effectively. A bifid uvula is common. Hypernasal speech and nasal air escape are usual. Occult submucosal clefts are diagnosed with difficulty by oral examination. They are best visualized from the nasal aspect of the palate by nasendoscopy.

4. After cleft palate repair. A short, tight velum may occur after surgery and failure to close the pharyngeal port then occurs. Scarring and associated functional deficits contribute to poor speech postoperatively.

5. After pharyngoplasty. Too narrow a flap design may leave residual failure of lateral port closure and residual nasal air escape.

6. After UVPPP. Uvulopalatopharyngoplasty is an operation designed for reduction of snoring and as part of the treatment of obstructive sleep apnoea. Excision of the posterior soft palate margin in continuity with the tonsils may produce postoperative sphincter dysfunction. This complication may be permanent in some patients. In addition to the marked speech defect, passage of air, liquids and even solid food down the nasal passages is troublesome.

7. After midface advancement. In patients with previous cleft palate repairs high level midface osteotomies are associated with a risk of postoperative VPI.

8. Neurogenic. In children with marked hypernasality in speech but normal swallow there is a poorly defined syndrome of neuromuscular incoordination. Surgery is ineffective in these patients. Intensive speech therapy may improve speech.

9. Hysterical. A rare manifestation of a psychiatric or personality disorder. Hypernasal speech with normal clinical and endoscopic examination is expected in these patients.

Management

Assessment of the underlying defect, the functionality available in the veolpharyngeal musculature, the presence of sucking or swallowing habits and the psychiatric condition of the patient are all noted.

Early initiation of speech therapy is helpful for all patients. This step helps to identify those whose speech pattern will resolve without surgery, those whose compliance with postoperative speech therapy is likely to be poor and those whose problem is other than purely anatomical.

Assessment
- Speech assessment
- Swallowing assessment
- Fibre-optic nasendoscopy
- Nasal airflow measurement
- Hearing and audiometry
- Videofluoroscopy
- CT or MRI scans

Surgical approaches

1. Palate lengthening procedures. The classical palatal push back operations of Passavant or Gillies and Fry are all well described. Use of an obturator to close the anterior defect created may also be required. Later described operations, the best documented of which is the Veau–Wardill–Killner operation require no obturation but used intervening muscle flaps and levator palati transplantation. There are may variations on this type of operation.

2. Pharyngeal flaps. The use of posterior ridge adhesion has been superseded by use of posterior pharyngeal flaps. The principle of raising a cranially based mucosal flap from the prevertebral fascia is widely used.

3. Pharyngoplasty. The most frequently cited pattern include Hynes and the oroticochea crossed posterior wall flaps. Some operations use a split velar design and introduce posterior pharyngeal wall tissue. Others create a pocket in the velum between oral and nasal mucosa into which posterior pharyngeal wall flap tissue is secured. The importance of preserving the lateral pharyngeal ports should be considered during surgery.

4. Posterior wall augmentation. Use of silicone or injectable PTFE into Passavant's ridge has replaced the use of earlier materials.

5. Sphincter reconstruction. Suture encirclage is described. Use of muscle bearing flaps developed from medial pterygoid or salpingopharyngeus are effective when used to construct lateral slings.

6. Obturators. Prosthetic obturators may be used particularly in acquired palatal defects but in cleft related VPI this is a less attractive option.

Surgery

1. Diagnosis. All surgery should be tailored to clinical, radiological and endoscopic findings.

2. Nasendoscopy. Sphincter defect patterns observed on nasendoscopy include central or circular, slit like, asymmetric, and combined patterns.

VELOPHARYNGEAL INCOMPETENCE **429**

- *Central pattern defects* are amenable to posterior wall augmentation or palatal repair or revision of earlier surgery.
- *Slit-like* palatal elevation failure or inadequacy is likely to respond to use of a central, superior based pharyngeal flap.
- *Asymmetric defects* are uncommon and often associated with craniofacial asymmetry. Laterlized posterior pharyngeal flaps may be appropriate.
- *Gross functional defects* respond poorly to surgery and are often best managed with enthusiastic speech therapy.

Adjuncts
- Insertion of grommets
- Lip, nose corrections
- Scar revisions
- Midface or mandibular osteotomies
- Alveolar bone grafts

Related topics of interest

Cleft palate surgery (p. 78)
Obstructive sleep apnoea (p. 279)
Speech and speech disorders (p. 351)

Revision points

Speech physiology
Swallowing physiology
Velar anatomy

XEROSTOMIA

The sensation of dry mouth is a common complaint but in relatively few patients there is a significant, objective reduction in saliva production demonstrable. The precise reason for the sensation of mucosal dryness in patients with normal saliva flow is not clear; it may represent one form of oral dysaesthesia and in some patients, xerostomia may co-present with oral causalgia.

Causes

1. Developmental defects. Congenital absence, aplasia or hypoplasia of the salivary glands results in marked reduction in saliva production. Complete absence of functioning salivary tissue is very rare and xerostomia is not a common complaint after surgical resection of a single major salivary gland.

2. Cystic fibrosis. A congenital disease affecting the mucus glands of the bronchial and gastro-intestinal tracts. The acinar glands are inflamed and fibrotic and produce inspissated mucus which obstructs lumens and accelerates glandular atrophy. The pancreas is typically affected but the salivary glands may be equally involved.

3. Infections. Glandular destruction by infection is described. Viral causes include paramyxovirus infections which in adult mumps may be severe enough to result in loss of parotid gland cells. In males a painful orchitis may be associated. Ascending peri-ductal bacterial infections are quite common and intra-parotid abscesses may result. Submandibular glands may also be the focus of pyogenic bacterial infections. Tuberculosis sialadenitis may occur.

4. Postsurgical. Postoperative dehydration and inadequate postoperative fluid management may be associated with mucosal dryness, xerostomia and parotitis.

5. Inflammatory gland disease. Sjögren's syndrome, a triad of xerostomia, keratoconjunctivitis sicca and a collagen vascular disease typically affects females in their fourth to sixth decades. Sjögren's syndrome in males is uncommon, the female:male incidence ratio is about 9:1. The connective tissue disorder is a rheumatoid like arthropathy in about 50% of patients although associations with systemic lupus erythematosus (SLE), scleroderma and polymyositis are described. CREST syndrome may be implicated. Miculicz syndrome is a limited form of Sjögrens with keratoconjunctivitis and xerostomia without evidence of connective tissue disorder. Other associations include lymphoma, Waldenstrom's macroglobulinaemia, chronic active hepatits and primary biliary cirrhosis. It is suggested that there is a common pattern of autoantibody production which mediates the hepatic, biliary and salivary gland damage in this group of patients.

6. Heerfordt's syndrome. Sarcoid infiltration of the major salivary glands may result in xerostomia. Uveitis and systemic sarcoidosis with fever are characteristic of the full syndrome.

7. Tumours and radiotherapy. Malignant destruction or infiltration of salivary glands may occur. Primary salivary gland lesions may be very advanced before significant loss of salivary function is noted by the patient. Secondary deposits in the major salivary glands or their associated lymph nodes may occur in primary lesions of breast, kidney and lung. The major cause of complaints of dry mouth in oncology are from patients who have undergone radiotherapy for a head and neck malignancy. This mode of treatment may result in severe oral mucositis and salivary gland destruction with disabling irreversible symptoms of dry mouth.

8. Duct obstruction. Transient duct occlusion due to calculus impaction occurs and is associated with painful gland swelling followed by relief of pain once the obstruction is passed. Chronic obstruction or long-term flow reduction due to scarring or duct stricture may be associated with gland atrophy and xerostomia.

9. Neuropsychiatric. Sympathetic nervous system activity in relation to fear, anxiety or panic is associated with the sensation of dry mouth in many people.

10. Organic neurology. Multiple sclerosis may exhibit xerostomia as part of the symptom complex.

11. Drugs. Many psychotropic drugs exhibit antimuscarinic side effects including the phenothiazines, tricyclic antidepressants and the anticholinergic antiparkinsonian agents such as benztropine. Antisialogogues used in anaesthetic practice may be given as part of preoperative premedication or during sedation for minor procedures around the upper airway. Drugs include atropine, scopolamine and glycopyrrolate. Some indirect sympathomimetics cause dry mouth as a side effect.

12. Other causes. Vitamin deficiencies, systemic toxaemia, diabetes mellitus, hypothyroidism, some anaemias may each result in a degree of xerostomia.

Investigations

1. Oral dryness. Mucosal dryness and lichenification may be demonstrable.

2. Saliva flow. Expressed saliva flow from major duct orifices may be examined.

3. Saliva sampling for culture and cytology is sometimes useful.

4. Tissue examination. FNAC of salivary gland masses or chronically inflamed major salivary glands may be diagnostic.

5. Imaging. Ultrasound and sialography if gland is not infected.

6. Serology. Extractable nuclear antigens, serum immunoglobulin estimation and angiotensin converting enzyme (ACE) assay are useful in xerostomic patients with Sjögren's syndrome, connective tissue disorders and sarcoidosis respectively.

7. Other tests. Conjunctival lachrimal flow by Schirmer's test may demonstrate keratoconjunctivitis sicca, and may be positive in Sjögren's syndrome. Labial gland biopsy for minor salivary gland tissue is a useful investigation in diagnosis of sarcoidosis.

Treatment

1.   Anticipation and prevention. Anticipate and explain before commencing radiotherapy.

2.   Underlying conditions. Treatment of rheumatoid or connective tissue disorders is important. Steroids relieve dry mouth effectively in such patients but have significant side effects particularly in elderly females in whom osteoporosis is a potential serious problem.

3.   Saliva substitute. There are a many available preparations given either as a mouth rinse or spray.

4.   Drugs. Stop the offending medication if possible.

5.   Dental treatment. Chronic dry mouth predisposes to accelerated dental caries and poor denture retention.

6.   Surgery. Excision of a painful gland may occasionally be appropriate.

Related topics of interest

Salivary gland disease (p. 336)
Salivary gland surgery (p. 340)

Revision points

Immunology of connective tissue disorders
Pharmacology of parasympathomimetic drugs

INDEX